COMPUTED TOMOGRAPHY OF THE BODY

With Magnetic Resonance Imaging

Second Edition

Albert A. Moss, M.D.

Professor and Chairman, Department of Radiology
University of Washington School of Medicine
Seattle, Washington

Gordon Gamsu, M.D.

Professor of Radiology and Medicine
University of California, San Francisco, School of Medicine
San Francisco, California

Harry K. Genant, M.D.

Professor of Radiology, Medicine, and Orthopaedic Surgery; Chief of the
Musculoskeletal Section; Director of the Osteoporosis Research Group
University of California, San Francisco, School of Medicine
San Francisco, California

Volume Two
Bone and Joint

W.B. SAUNDERS COMPANY

A Division of Harcourt Brace & Company

Philadelphia   London   Toronto   Montreal   Sydney   Tokyo

W.B. SAUNDERS COMPANY
A Division of
Harcourt Brace & Company

The Curtis Center
Independence Square West
Philadelphia, Pennsylvania 19106

Library of Congress Cataloging-in-Publication Data

Moss, Albert A.

Computed tomography of the body with magnetic resonance
imaging / Albert A. Moss, Gordon Gamsu, Harry K. Genant.
— 2nd ed.

     p.   cm.

Rev. ed. of: Computed tomography of the body / Albert A.
Moss, Gordon Gamsu, Harry K. Genant.

Includes bibliographical references and index.

ISBN 0–7216–2415–4 (set)

1. Tomography.   2. Magnetic resonance imaging.
I. Gamsu, Gordon.   II. Genant, Harry K.
III. Moss, Albert A.   Computed tomography of the body.
IV. Title.

[DNLM: 1. Anatomy, Regional.   2. Magnetic
Resonance Imaging.   3. Tomography, X-Ray Computed.
WN 160 M913c]

RC78.7.T6M68   1992

DNLM/DLC   91–32837

Editor: Lisette Bralow
Designer: W.B. Saunders Staff
Production Manager: Peter Faber
Manuscript Editors: Lorraine Zawodny and Kendall Sterling
Illustration Coordinator: Walter Verbitski
Indexer: Nancy Newman
Cover Designer: Michelle Maloney

Computed Tomography of the Body With
Magnetic Resonance Imaging, 2/e.

ISBN Volume I 0–7216–4358–2
Volume II 0–7216–4359–0
Volume III 0–7216–4503–8
Three Volume Set 0–7216–2415–4

Printed in the United States of America

Last digit is the print number: 9   8   7   6   5

DEDICATION FOR VOLUME TWO

This volume is dedicated to my wife, Gail,
and to our children, Laura, Justin, and Jonathan

HARRY K. GENANT

CONTRIBUTORS FOR VOLUME TWO

NEIL I. CHAFETZ, M.D.
Associate Clinical Professor, University of California, San Francisco, School of
Medicine, San Francisco, CA
  THE SPINE

KENNETH G. FAULKNER, Ph.D.
Adjunct Assistant Professor, Department of Radiology, University of
California, San Francisco, School of Medicine, San Francisco, CA
  OSTEOPOROSIS

HARRY K. GENANT, M.D.
Professor of Radiology, Medicine, and Orthopaedic Surgery; Chief of the
Musculoskeletal Section; Director of the Osteoporosis Research Group;
University of California, San Francisco, School of Medicine, San Francisco, CA
  THE JOINTS
  THE SPINE
  OSTEOPOROSIS
  MUSCULOSKELETAL TUMORS

CLAUS-C. GLÜER, Ph.D.
Adjunct Assistant Professor, Department of Radiology, University of
California, San Francisco, School of Medicine, San Francisco, CA
  OSTEOPOROSIS

CLYDE A. HELMS, M.D.
Professor of Radiology, University of California, San Francisco, School of
Medicine, San Francisco, CA
  MUSCULOSKELETAL TUMORS

JAY A. KAISER, M.D.
Assistant Clinical Professor of Radiology, University of California,
San Francisco, School of Medicine, San Francisco, CA; Medical Director,
San Francisco Neuroskeletal Imaging Center, Daly City, CA
  THE SPINE

BRUCE A. PORTER, M.D.
Associate Clinical Professor, Diagnostic Radiology, University of Washington
School of Medicine; Medical Director, First Hill Diagnostic Imaging Center;
Seattle, WA
MARROW-INFILTRATING DISORDERS

STEPHEN L. G. ROTHMAN, M.D.
Consultant Radiologist, Spinal Injury Service, Rancho Los Amigos Hospital,
Downey, CA
THE SPINE

PETER STEIGER, Ph.D.
Adjunct Assistant Professor of Radiology, University of California,
San Francisco, School of Medicine, San Francisco, CA
OSTEOPOROSIS

LYNNE S. STEINBACH, M.D.
Assistant Professor of Radiology, University of California, San Francisco,
School of Medicine; San Francisco, CA
MUSCULOSKELETAL TUMORS

DAVID W. STOLLER, M.D.
Assistant Clinical Professor, Radiology, University of California, San
Francisco, School of Medicine; Director, California Advanced Imaging Center,
San Francisco, CA
THE JOINTS

PREFACE

The second edition of *Computed Tomography of the Body* has been extensively updated and is presented as a comprehensive, state-of-the-art text on computed tomography (CT) of the body that now includes an integration of magnetic resonance (MR) imaging in all sections of the book. Since the first edition, there have been great advances in CT and its application to patient care. Although the impact of CT has been enormous, magnetic resonance imaging is undergoing explosive growth and is having an ever-increasing impact on body imaging.

As in the first edition, this text is organized so that basic anatomy and CT and MR techniques are discussed for each region of the body. The features of disease entities in these two imaging modalities are described and illustrated, and the relationship of CT to MR and other imaging techniques is discussed in depth. Recommendations are offered as to the role of each modality in specific clinical situations. The book presents an integrated approach, reflecting our current standard of practice. Knowledge of CT and MR imaging will continue to expand, and recommendations, techniques, and patterns of use will undoubtedly change in the future.

In writing this book, now expanded to three volumes, there have been many people without whose support, guidance, insight, and help this work could not have been completed. We thank our colleagues who contributed their time and case material, and we acknowledge the illustration departments at the University of California, San Francisco, and the University of Washington, as well as the secretarial and editorial support of Jan Taylor, Isabel Rosenthal, and Denice Nakano.

ALBERT A. MOSS, M.D.
GORDON GAMSU, M.D.
HARRY K. GENANT, M.D.

INTRODUCTION TO VOLUME TWO

Computed tomography (CT) has made an enormous impact on musculoskeletal imaging in general and orthopaedic diagnosis in particular. The technical advances achieved during the 1980s provide the basis for rapid, efficient, and reliable performance, and now CT is used routinely and universally in a broad array of musculoskeletal applications.

Magnetic resonance imaging (MRI), developed in the early 1980s and refined for musculoskeletal application in the late 1980s, is now a primary diagnostic modality in orthopaedic practice and to a lesser extent in rheumatologic practice. The technical developments in MRI have been explosive and continue to drive this modality to ever more diverse and exacting applications. Today, MRI may be viewed as the most important advance of the century in orthopaedic diagnosis.

In Volume Two, the major and important applications of CT and MRI are combined in chapters covering The Joints, The Spine, Osteoporosis, Musculoskeletal Tumors, and Marrow-Infiltrating Disorders. Each topic is handled in depth and illustrated extensively.

I would like to thank my many colleagues and collaborators at the University of California, San Francisco, and at other centers around the country and around the globe who have contributed directly or indirectly to this volume. Without their wisdom, insight, and support, this work would not have been possible.

HARRY K. GENANT, M.D.

CONTENTS

THE JOINTS

DAVID W. STOLLER ▪ HARRY K. GENANT

Computed tomography (CT) and magnetic resonance imaging (MRI) are advanced imaging modalities used in the diagnosis of musculoskeletal disorders. The utilization of CT and MRI has modified and enhanced clinical diagnostic imaging and subsequent patient management. Accurate radiologic assessment relies on an understanding of the use of specific, yet complementary, imaging techniques individualized and tailored to the disease process under consideration.

Although conventional radiography is frequently the most cost-effective initial screening tool in selected cases of trauma, infection, arthritis, and neoplasia, its limitations must also be considered. Conventional radiography is limited in the early detection of infiltrative and destructive processes prior to significant cortical destruction and provides suboptimal visualization of intra- and extraarticular soft tissue structures (tendons, ligaments, and fibrocartilage). The conventional radiograph remains an effective modality for fracture detection and identification of calcification.

Computed tomography has a wide range of applications in the musculoskeletal system and is partic-ularly effective in evaluating trauma, soft tissue and bony lesions, infection, low back pain syndrome, and metabolic bone disorders. For studying the soft tissues and areas of complex bony anatomy such as the spine, shoulder, and pelvis, CT may be superior to conventional radiographic techniques (Fig. 11–1). It provides a cross-sectional view of the anatomy, has excellent density discrimination, and eliminates superimposed structures. CT is especially useful in the evaluation of small joints that require thin-section (1.5 mm) evaluation (e.g., foot and wrist). CT provides high bone detail in cross-sectional display. CT is sensitive to matrix calcification and subtle erosions that may be overlooked on plain film radiography. Bone mineralization may also be determined with quantitative CT techniques. Patients undergoing arthrography may benefit from the addition of CT scanning to increase soft tissue discrimination (e.g., CT shoulder arthrotomography) and spatial resolution (detection of intraarticular loose bodies). Reformatting capabilities and three-dimensional display of CT are functions that facilitate the understanding of complex anatomy and spatial relationships. CT offers an alternative for those patients who do not fulfill

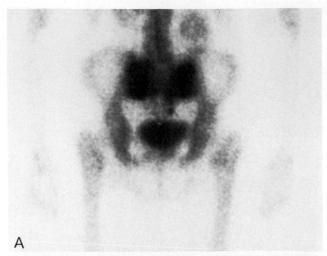

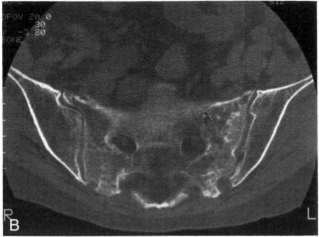

FIGURE 11–1 ■ Bilateral sacral stress fractures in an osteoporotic woman with normal conventional radiographs and identification of bilateral fractures on CT scan *(A)* and with characteristic positive technetium bone scan *(B)*.

MRI screening criteria (e.g., those with claustrophobia or cardiac pacemaker).

The drawbacks to CT scanning include utilization of ionizing radiation, narrow range of soft tissue contrast, and indirect marrow assessment. Nonorthogonal imaging capabilities result in a loss of resolution when reformatting cross-sectional images. Routine use of thin-section CT images to increase the resolution of reformatted images is not practical in studies of larger anatomic boundaries.

MRI allows for direct multiplanar imaging of the appendicular joints in nonorthogonal planes with off-axis fields of view and can differentiate fat, fluid, muscle, cartilage, and cortical bone in both normal and pathologic states. The ability to noninvasively image and characterize early changes in marrow, subchondral bone, and cartilage provides for more precise evaluation in patients presenting with trauma, arthritis, infection, and neoplasia.

MRI can be acquired in a two-dimensional (2D) or three-dimensional (3D) Fourier transform. Three-dimensional volume data can be postprocessed and reformatted into any orthogonal or oblique axis orientation. The introduction of fast scan imaging techniques have complemented conventional spin-echo imaging in providing effective T1- and T2-weighted contrast in reduced acquisition times. Anatomy and pathology specific to tissue T1 and T2 values can be selectively enhanced by the choice of the proper pulse sequence. Contrast resolution of MRI is superior to that of CT, and spatial resolution is equivalent to that obtained with high-resolution CT scanners. The requirement for intraarticular contrast is obviated by the capability to selectively highlight synovial fluid as bright signal intensity on T2-weighted images and articular hyaline cartilage on fast scan sequences. Fat suppression and inversion recovery pulse techniques are utilized in direct marrow imaging. Fast scan imaging techniques have facilitated kinematic studies of the temporomandibular joint (TMJ), patellofemoral joint, and wrist.

MRI is limited in that it has greater sensitivity to motion than CT. The identification of small soft tissue or joint calcification is inferior to that of CT. Cortical edge detail of CT is superior to MR imaging of bony cortex. MRI requires more detailed imaging protocols tailored to both anatomy and pathology; often these must be joint specific.

Technical Considerations

CT

The advantages of CT over conventional radiography are the capabilities for three-dimensional imaging, good contrast resolution, accurate measurement of tissue attenuation coefficient, noninvasive nature, and in many instances, reduced radiation exposure to the patient.[1] All of these factors combine to make CT a powerful tool in the assessment of the musculoskeletal system. CT scanners have the capability for submillimeter resolving power in high-contrast tissue such as bone. This resolution, coupled with the use of thin sections (1 to 3 mm), means that high-quality images of bony structures can be readily obtained. The contrast resolution of CT is recognized as superior to that of conventional films. Motion artifacts are minimized with average scanning time of less than 5 sec. Rapid-sequence scanning in the dynamic mode facilitates the performance of studies requiring 40 to 50 contiguous scans. These scans can be generated in times of 5 to 10 min. With dynamic scanning, back-to-back scans are obtained at a relatively low milliamperage, with 1- to 2-sec interscan delay for table incrementation.[2, 3] Thus for high bone detail, contiguous stacked scans 1 to 3 mm thick provide not only excellent axial images, but also the basis for high-quality sagittal, coronal, or multiplanar reformations,[4] supplanting conventional polytomography for delineating subtle structural changes in anatomically complex regions of the skeleton.

Variable reconstruction algorithms are available that can be used to reconstruct original projection data to optimize high-contrast resolving power, low-contrast detectability, or other parameters. These options are especially useful for imaging cortical structures.[1] The use of extended scales (-1000 to $+3000$ Hounsfield units [H]) permits visualization of the entire range of densities in bone. Computed radiographic localization systems are also widely offered and greatly facilitate studies in musculoskeletal disease. The two-dimensional projection radiograph, indexed to the table location, can be used to specify precise scanning location and gantry angulation. This computed radiograph can additionally be used to select planes for postprocessing reformatting or reconstructions. External localization systems provide an accuracy of 0.5 to 1.0 mm in the table location, so the limiting factor becomes patient motion between the time the computed radiograph is obtained and the time the axial scans are done.

Three-dimensional CT has been utilized in displaying spatial relationships in complex fractures, including hamate fractures in the wrist, tibial plateau depression fractures, and tibiotalar or subtalar joint extension in ankle fractures. Three-dimensional CT may be helpful in defining acetabular and femoral head anatomy in congenital dislocation of the hip (CDH) and trauma. Surface or volume extrapolations, projections, and renderings are obtained at specified rotations. Disarticulation of defined anatomy and depth encoding with varying gray scale intensities permit more accurate 3D viewing. Through the generation of separate composites, multiple structures can be rendered in the final 3D image.[5, 6]

In performing CT examinations, both the normal and abnormal sides can be scanned simultaneously to evaluate for bony and muscular symmetry of the extremities or joints. Large anatomic areas can be scanned with 5- to 10-mm slices, whereas more complex anatomy may require 1.5-cm beam collimation. Separate cortical and soft tissue windows increase contrast in the evaluation of cortical bone and soft tissue (fibrous tissue, muscle, and fat). The bone windows are particularly valuable in the evaluation of intracortical lesions such as osteoid osteoma and sequestra, which can be visualized using high window levels and wide window widths. CT arthrotomography demonstrates the anatomy of the glenohumeral ligament labral complex. Optional scanning with intravenous contrast using drip infusion or rapid bolus injection may be used to assess vascularity.

Thus the combination of projection-computed radiography, high-resolution scanning, dynamic rapid-sequence scanning, thin-section capability, biplanar reformation, and three-dimensional display has created an exciting array of possibilities for CT imaging of the musculoskeletal system.

MRI

The physical and technical principles of magnetic resonance imaging are completely different from those of CT, which depends on ionizing radiation.[7–9] The generation of the imaging signal intensity in MRI is based on events that occur at the molecular level. This has the potential to provide physiologic and biochemical, as well as anatomic, information that may be tissue specific. In contrast to CT, MRI is capable of obtaining direct multiplanar acquisitions with off-axis or oblique imaging using a 2D or 3D volume Fourier transform, with the options of cine, dynamic display, and specialized vascular imaging techniques. Magnetic resonance imaging is free from the restraints of rigid imaging (plane-of-section and reconstruction) without ionizing radiation. It is advantageous to evaluate small and complex musculoskeletal structures with directly acquired multiplanar and oblique imaging at reduced fields of view using high-resolution matrices (192 to 512). Thin-section 2D (3-mm) and 3D (less than 3-mm) sections can provide high spatial resolution with comprehensive joint coverage.

Magnetic resonance imaging requires specialized protocols and specific technical parameters tailored to the individual patient and specific pathologic processes. The selection of appropriate parameters—resolution time (TR) and echo time (TE), field of view, matrix, number of excitations (NEX), slice thickness, and plane and axis designations—is required to optimize imaging for the specific pathologic condition and regional anatomy. Two-dimensional MR techniques utilize separate acquisitions for each plane of section or type of tissue contrast required. A 3D technique acquires data from a volume of tissue and can be subsequently reformatted.

Dedicated extremity coils and surface coils that are positioned near the anatomic region of interest are necessary to optimize signal-to-noise ratios. This is especially important when imaging smaller joints that require higher spatial resolution using small fields of view and thin-section protocols.

A 90° to 180° radio frequency pulse pair is used to generate T1- or T2-weighted images based on the selected TR and TE parameters in conventional spin-echo imaging. Although a T1-weighted image provides superior tissue contrast and anatomic detail, a T2-weighted image is more sensitive to tissues with longer T1 and T2 values. Fluid, edema, and inflamed tissues are characterized by prolonged T2 values and therefore demonstrate increased signal intensity on T2-weighted images. Cortical bone generates a low signal intensity on all pulse sequences because of limited proton motion within its hydrogen lattice. Yellow or fatty marrow, however, generates increased signal intensity on short TR or T1-weighted acquisitions. Signal intensity decreases with progressive T2 weighting. Collagen-containing ligaments and tendons (low spin density) image with low signal intensity, whereas adjacent muscle or hyaline articular cartilage demonstrates an intermediate signal intensity on a T1-weighted sequence. The selection of a long TR sequence produces an increased signal-to-noise ratio, and such sequences require prolonged acquisition times. Decreasing the TR will reduce imaging time, but images will be subjected to greater noise. Gradient-echo and fast scan techniques replace the conventional 90° to 180° pulse pair with a theta flip angle, most commonly less than 90°, to achieve effective T2- or T2*-weighted contrast in a fraction of the time required for traditional spin-echo sequences. Gradient-echo techniques can be used to achieve effective T1- or T2-weighted contrast with reduced imaging time. Three-dimensional volumetric techniques require the application of gradient-echo acquisitions to minimize the TR and thus reduce scan times.[10, 11] Gradient-echo images displayed in page mode can be made to simulate dynamic joint motion. As with CT, magnetic resonance imaging data may be used to produce three-dimensional reconstructed images on a postprocessing work station to enhance spatial relationships and disarticulate regions of anatomy (Fig. 11–2). Chemical shift imaging, a technique that uses a chemical shift between fat and water protons to subtract relative contributions of fat and water, can be useful in distinguishing a variety of pathologic processes.

The presence of orthopedic hardware is not a contraindication for MRI examination. Localized signal intensity loss and artifacts may be produced by both ferromagnetic and nonferromagnetic metals or alloys without compromising adjacent anatomy.[12] Conventional spin-echo techniques are less sensitive to magnetic susceptibility and thus may be more useful than gradient-echo techniques in the postsurgical joint. The artifact generated by metallic hardware is a function of orientation, number, composition, and size of metallic implants.

The Knee

CT

Although not the study of choice, CT may be used to examine ligamentous and meniscal injuries of the knee joint.[8–13] Direct off-axis scans or sagittal reformatted images derived from contiguous axial CT scans can be used to evaluate the cruciate ligaments. Normal anterior and posterior cruciate ligaments should be visualized by reformatting several sagittal slices through the intercondylar notch. A torn cruciate ligament is visible as either an interruption or an absence of the ligament. Cross-sectional scanning with 1.5-mm thin-section air contrast CT has been used to identify meniscal tears and cysts, but without widespread clinical acceptance.

The evaluation of complex patellofemoral compartment disorders by CT has been explored.[13, 14] Chondromalacia patellae may be suggested by irregular imbibition of contrast material, roughening of cartilage surfaces, and generalized articular narrowing. Lateral subluxating and subtle tracking abnormalities may be evaluated by placing the knee in varying degrees of flexion-extension with and without quadriceps relaxation while axial images are taken through the midplane of the patella. This principle has also been applied in kinematic magnetic resonance imaging of the patellofemoral joint.[15] Successful detection and classification of plica syndromes have also been reported using axial CT images.

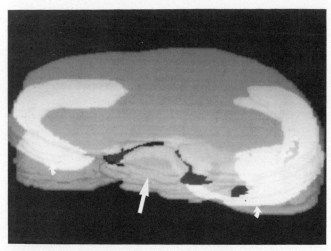

FIGURE 11–2 ■ Three-dimensional MR rendering of the knee joint with a posterior tibial plateau fracture *(large arrow)*. Meniscal cartilages are identified by the small arrows.

Thin-section high-resolution CT has been utilized in the evaluation of tibial plateau fractures. Reformatted coronal and sagittal scans can assess cortical depression as an adjunct to preoperative planning (Fig. 11–3).[16] However, CT is limited in characterizing associated ligamentous, meniscal, and articular cartilage injuries.

CT can be used to determine the location and extent of infection in and about the knee joint. Cortical or periosteal involvement can be differentiated from intramedullary involvement. Bone erosions and soft tissue abscess formation can be demonstrated.

MRI

MRI is replacing arthrography in the evaluation of internal joint derangements of the knee.[17–26] Except in evaluating prosthetic loosening or obtaining synovial fluid samples for culture and Gram's stain, MRI is superior to arthrography in the evaluation of the knee joint. Even plateau fractures are best demonstrated on direct multiplanar MR images, superceding axial CT. The ability to visualize hyaline articular cartilage directly with MRI has been instrumental in characterizing synovial-based and cartilage-based disorders.

IMAGING PROTOCOLS

A routine knee protocol should contain axial, sagittal, and coronal images.[24] The patellofemoral compartment is demonstrated on axial T1- or T2-weighted images. The collateral ligaments are demonstrated on coronal images, and the menisci and cruciate ligaments are defined in the sagittal imaging plane.

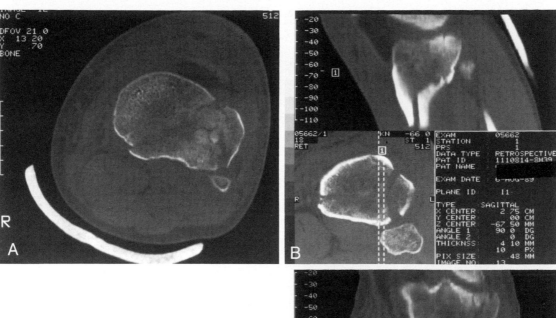

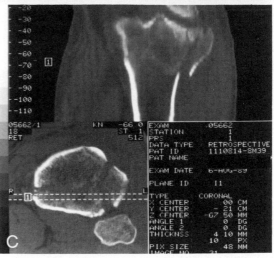

FIGURE 11–3 ■ Medial and lateral tibial plateau fracture demonstrated on direct transaxial CT scan *(A)* and reformatted sagittal *(B)* and coronal *(C)* scans. Cortical depression can be measured on reformatted displays.

Meniscus ■ The normal meniscus is imaged with uniform low signal intensity (Fig. 11–4).[27–29] Meniscal degenerations and tears are imaged with increased signal intensity. An MR grading system rating the morphology of the increased signal intensity relative to an articular surface has been developed and correlated with a pathologic model.[29] Grade I signal intensity represents a focal area of increased signal intensity within the substance of the fibrocartilaginous meniscus. Patients with grade I signal intensity are asymptomatic and have no changes on arthrography or at arthroscopy. The meniscus with grade II signal intensity demonstrates linear signal intensity (usually horizontally oriented) that does not communicate with a meniscal surface. Although a small percentage of patients with grade II signal intensity may be symptomatic, there is no fibrocartilaginous tear (Fig. 11–5). Grade I and II signal intensities thus represent degeneration and should never be termed *tears*. Grade III signal intensity represents signal intensity that communicates with an articular surface of the meniscus and pathologically is a defined tear. Six per cent of patients with grade III signal intensity have closed meniscal tears that may not be identified at arthroscopy without probing. This explains the 6 per cent false-positive result in rating grade III signal intensity. The increased signal intensity observed on T1- and intermediate-weighted images results from increased local proton density and a shortening of T1 relaxation time caused by synovial fluid absorbed into degenerative or torn meniscal surfaces. Thus conventional T2-weighted images may not be as sensitive as T1-weighted images to grade I, II, and III signal intensities. T2* contrast, however, always demonstrates meniscal degenerations and tears as bright signal intensities (Fig. 11–6). With MRI studies, histologic alterations in the fibrocartilaginous meniscus can thus be assessed prior to the appearance of the surface changes seen on arthrographic or arthroscopic examinations. Incorrect interpretation of meniscal tears can be caused by the transverse ligament of the knee (which simulates an oblique tear adjacent to the anterior horn of the lateral meniscus) and the popliteal tendon sheath (Fig. 11–7).

Cruciate Ligaments ■ Knee examinations are usually performed in 15° of external rotation to better align the anterior cruciate ligament (ACL) into the sagittal orthogonal plane.[30] In complete tears of the anterior

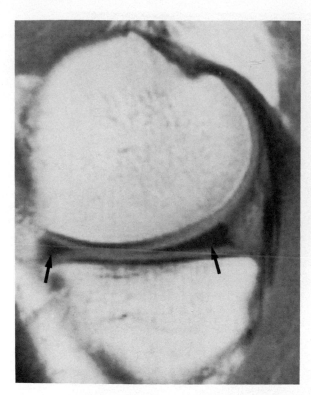

FIGURE 11–4 ■ Intact anterior and posterior horns of the medial meniscus *(arrows)*. The normal low-spin-density fibrocartilage is imaged with uniform low signal intensity.

FIGURE 11–5 ■ Grade III signal intensity in a meniscal tear in the posterior horn of the medial meniscus *(arrow)*.

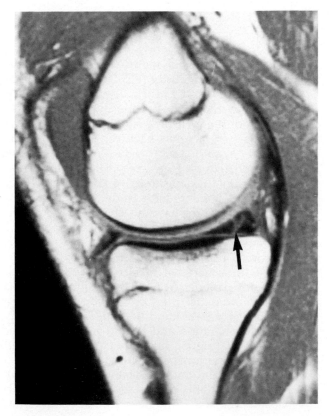

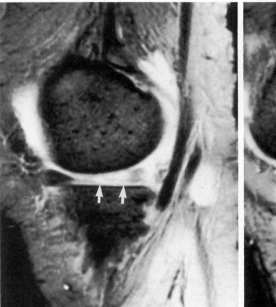
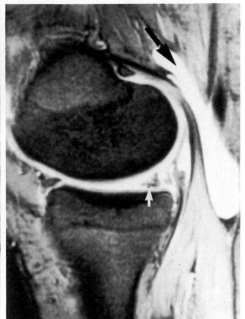

FIGURE 11–6 ■ T2* sagittal gradient-echo images demonstrating body and posterior horn tears of the medial meniscus *(white arrows)* with associated popliteal cyst *(black arrow).*

cruciate ligament, there is discontinuity in the low signal intensity band, with loss of its normally taut parallel margins (Fig. 11–8). Partial or complete ligamentous disruptions may be associated with blurring of the cruciate ligament's fascicles because of edema or hemorrhage. In acute tears or strains, fluid and edema image with high signal intensity on T2- or T2*-weighted images. Posterior bowing of the ACL or buckling of the posterior cruciate ligament (PCL) may be associated with increased laxity or with a chronic tear of the anterior cruciate ligament.

The anatomy of the PCL is not as sensitive to positioning as is that of the ACL (Fig. 11–9). Within this normally low-signal-intensity ligament, any increase in signal intensity on either T1- or T2-weighted images should be interpreted as abnormal (Fig. 11–10).

Collateral Ligaments ■ Partial tears or sprains of the medial collateral ligament (MCL) are seen as increased distance between the subcutaneous tissue and cortical bone.[24] T2-weighted images demonstrate high-signal-intensity edema or hemorrhage around

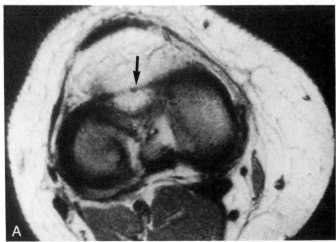
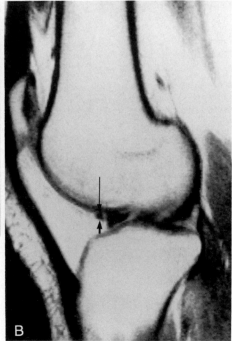
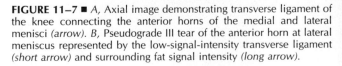

FIGURE 11–7 ■ *A,* Axial image demonstrating transverse ligament of the knee connecting the anterior horns of the medial and lateral menisci *(arrow). B,* Pseudograde III tear of the anterior horn at lateral meniscus represented by the low-signal-intensity transverse ligament *(short arrow)* and surrounding fat signal intensity *(long arrow).*

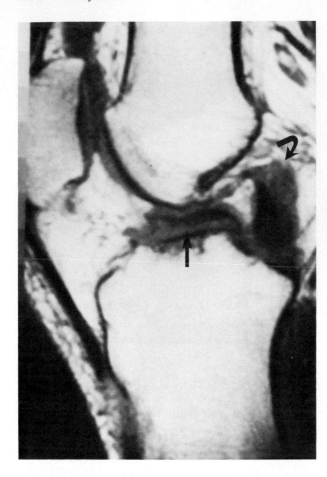

FIGURE 11–8 ■ Disrupted anterior cruciate ligament *(straight arrow)* and high-arched posterior cruciate ligament *(curved arrow)* on T1-weighted sagittal image.

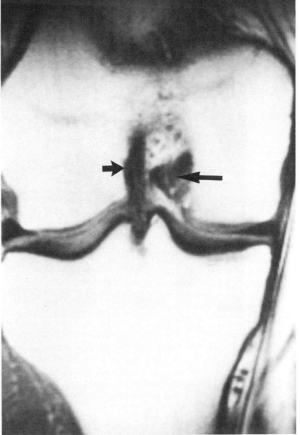

FIGURE 11–9 ■ Intact anterior *(short arrow)* and posterior *(long arrow)* cruciate ligaments on T1-weighted coronal image.

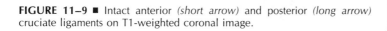

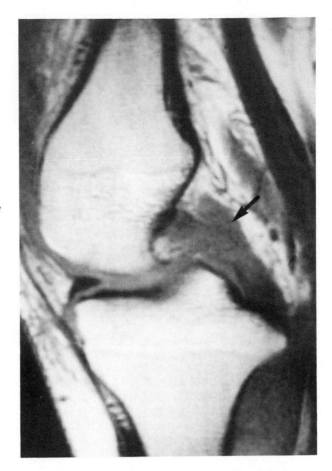

FIGURE 11–10 ■ Increased signal intensity in disrupted posterior cruciate ligament *(arrow).*

low-signal-intensity ligamentous fibers (Fig. 11–11). Tears are identified by a loss of continuity of ligament fibers.

The lateral collateral ligament (LCL) is best seen on posterior coronal images and is visualized as a band of low signal intensity. In complete disruptions, the LCL may be imaged with a wavy contour and loss of ligamentous continuity.

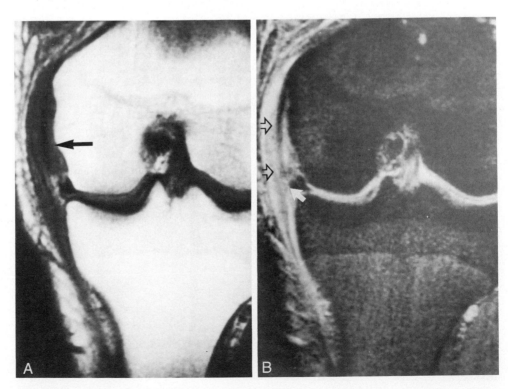

FIGURE 11–11 ■ Medial collateral ligament tear. *A,* Torn medial collateral ligament *(arrow)* shown as a thickened band of low signal intensity with increased separation between the subcutaneous tissue and cortical bone on T1-weighted coronal image. *B,* Corresponding T2* gradient-echo coronal image delineates disrupted medial collateral ligament and meniscocapsular separation *(solid arrow).* Surrounding edema shown with high signal intensity *(open arrows).*

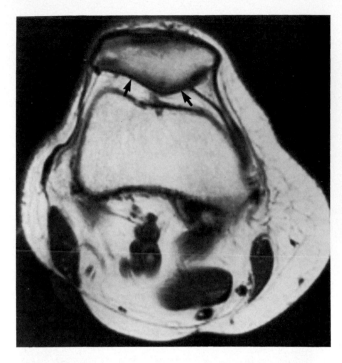

FIGURE 11–12 ■ Chondromalacia patellae with attenuated hyaline articular cartilage *(arrows)* of the patellar facets on T1-weighted axial image.

Chondromalacia Patellae ■ On axial MR images, early articular cartilage attenuation or erosions can be appreciated in either the medial or lateral facets (Fig. 11–12).[31] Sagittal images, which are less sensitive to cartilage erosions, may show a straightening or loss of the normal convex curve seen in patellar hyaline cartilage when viewed in profile.

Cartilage ■ On conventional T2-weighted images, hyaline cartilage maintains an intermediate signal intensity. With gradient-echo, chemical shift and fast, low-angle shot (FLASH) techniques, however, hyaline cartilage images with high signal intensity. With these techniques it is possible to detect early stages of hyaline cartilage degeneration (Fig. 11–13).[30]

The Infrapatellar Fat Pad Sign ■ Synovial reaction and proliferation are imaged as changes in the contour of synovial reflections.[24] Irregularity, with loss of the smooth posterior concave-free border of the infrapatellar fat pad, can be observed with a variety of synovial reactions and is referred to as the *irregular*

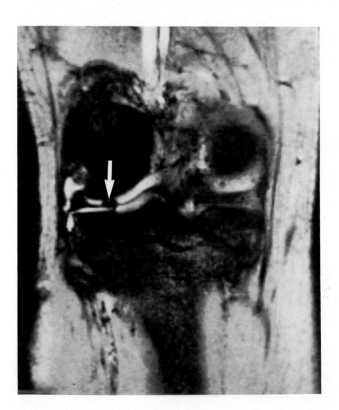

FIGURE 11–13 ■ T2* gradient-echo coronal image identifying femoral articular cartilage defect *(arrow).*

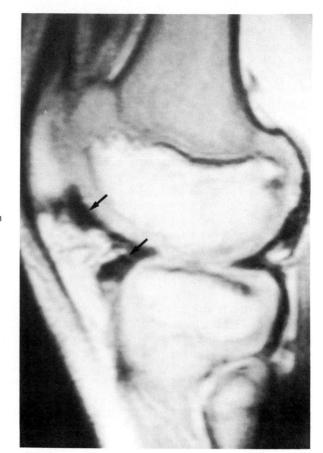

FIGURE 11–14 ■ Hemophilia with dark hemosiderin deposits seen along an irregular infrapatellar fat pad *(arrows)*.

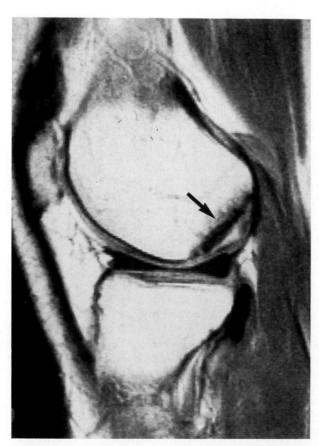

FIGURE 11–15 ■ Osteochondritis dissecans of the knee visualized as a low signal intensity involving the non–weight bearing portion of the medial femoral condyle *(arrow)*.

infrapatellar fat pad sign (Fig. 11–14). The irregular fat pad sign has been seen in patients with hemophilia, rheumatoid arthritis, pigmented villonodular synovitis (PVNS), Lyme arthritis, inflammatory osteoarthritis, and hemorrhagic effusions (from arthritis or trauma), all caused by reactive synovium.[24]

Osteonecrosis, Bone Infarction, and Fractures ■ Spontaneous osteonecrosis of the knee typically affects older patients, predominantly females, and presents with acute medial joint pain. Most commonly, spontaneous osteonecrosis involves the weight-bearing surface of the medial femoral condyle. Osteochondritis dissecans differs from spontaneous osteonecrosis of the knee in that it primarily affects young male patients and involves the non–weight bearing surface of the medial femoral condyle (Fig. 11–15). On MRI scans the focus of osteochondritis images with low signal intensity on T1- and T2-weighted images before it is detectable on conventional radiographs.[24]

Bone infarcts are usually metaphyseal in location but have also been imaged in more epiphyseal and diaphyseal locations. The MRI appearance of a bone infarct is characteristic, with a serpiginous, low-signal-intensity border of reactive bone and a central compartment of high signal that is isointense to surrounding yellow marrow (Fig. 11–16).

MRI easily detects a spectrum of trabecular bone contusions, stress fractures, and plateau fractures, even when conventional radiographs are negative (Fig. 11–17).[33] Bone changes on MRI are classified as type I (diffuse marrow involvement), type II (involving cortical fracture), and type III (focal area of low signal intensity, as seen with osteonecrosis).

Infection ■ Capsular distention and joint effusions are identified on MRI scans as signs of joint infection but are nonspecific.[34, 35] Septic joints may be further

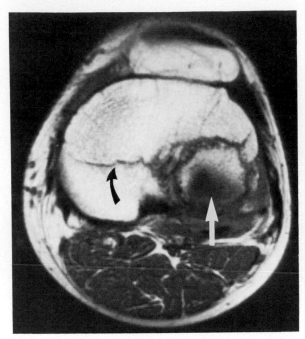

FIGURE 11–17 ■ T1-weighted axial image identifying tibia fracture site *(white arrow)* and radiating fracture segments *(black arrow)*.

characterized by intraarticular debris and synovitis from hematogenous seeding.

The Hip

CT

TRAUMA

Computed tomography has an important role in the evaluation of pelvic and hip trauma (Figs. 11–18 through 11–20).[36, 37] Surgical management of fracture-dislocations of the hip is based on the stability of the joint space, presence or absence of intraarticular fragments, congruity of fracture fragments, and the general condition of the patient.[38–42] In patients with hip trauma, the condition of the femoral head and acetabulum is frequently difficult to evaluate by means of conventional radiography or polytomography. Often, anteroposterior views are obtained using a portable apparatus, resulting in suboptimal image quality. Special views described by Judet and coworkers,[43] including anterior and posterior oblique projections, provide additional important information but cannot always be obtained. Furthermore, they do not adequately define the joint space or the integrity of the medial acetabulum.

Mack and colleagues[39] analyzed the capability of CT for assessing acetabular fractures and showed that the traditional classification[44] of hip fractures into anterior column, posterior column, and complex two-column fractures was greatly facilitated by this modality. The prognosis of acetabular fractures was shown to depend on the type of fracture, the condition of the weight-bearing part of the joint, the persistence of displaced or intraarticular fragments,

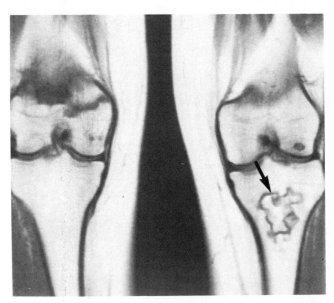

FIGURE 11–16 ■ Metaphyseal-based bone infarct demonstrating peripheral rim of low-signal-intensity sclerosis on T1-weighted coronal image *(arrow)*.

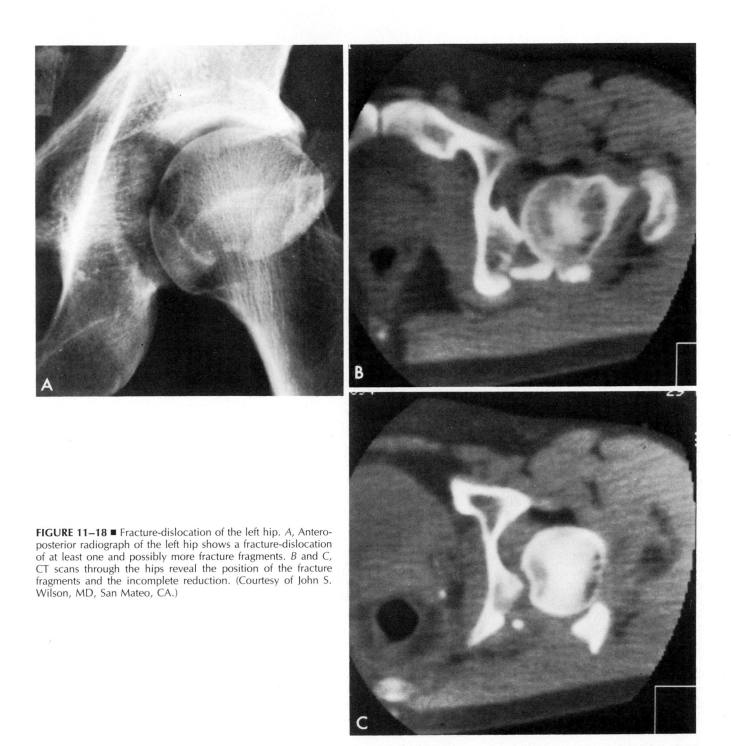

FIGURE 11–18 ■ Fracture-dislocation of the left hip. *A,* Antero-posterior radiograph of the left hip shows a fracture-dislocation of at least one and possibly more fracture fragments. *B* and *C,* CT scans through the hips reveal the position of the fracture fragments and the incomplete reduction. (Courtesy of John S. Wilson, MD, San Mateo, CA.)

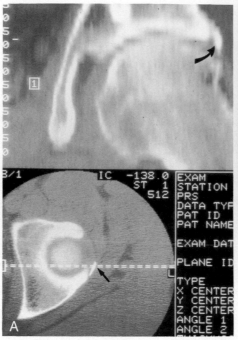

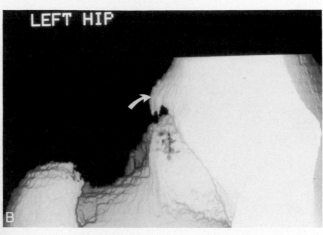

FIGURE 11–19 ■ *A,* Posterior acetabular rim fracture displayed on transaxial CT *(straight arrow)* and reformatted coronal CT scan *(curved arrow).* *B,* Three-dimensional CT reconstructed posterior coronal image demonstrates posterior acetabular fragment *(arrow).*

and the presence of additional fractures that further destabilize the pelvis. For each of these factors, CT provides essential and often unique information so that appropriate surgical intervention can be undertaken and long-term patient prognosis can be improved. In two-column fractures, CT provides useful information concerning the configuration of the fracture, integrity of the acetabular dome and quadrilateral surface, and position of the stable fragment. CT has been shown to be comparable to conventional radiography in the detection of fractures of the iliac wing, anterior pelvic column, posterior pelvic column, and pubic rami.[38] However, CT shows greater sensitivity than plain radiography in detecting fractures involving the sacrum, quadrilateral surface of the acetabulum, the acetabular roof, and the posterior acetabular lip.

In the evaluation of complex pelvic fractures, the capability of CT to demonstrate, in cross-sectional array and with good contrast resolution, the surrounding muscle and soft tissue planes greatly facilitates the detection and evaluation of posttraumatic hematomas, which at times may be massive and life threatening.[43]

The ability of CT to show subtle differences in tissue density generally allows differentiation of fat, muscle, blood, serous and purulent fluids, and faint calcification not possible on plain radiographs (Fig. 11–21). Subtle circumferential ossification in the early stages of myositis ossificans can be diagnostic and thus obviate additional workup. This ossification may or may not be visible on plain radiographs, and even if visualized, its circumferential nature can be difficult to ascertain (Fig. 11–22). Soft tissue swelling caused by a hematoma can occasionally be related to an adjacent vascular structure, which may be the source of the mass. Intravenous injection of contrast material

enhances vascular areas and allows easy differentiation of some vascular masses, such as a pseudoaneurysm (Fig. 11–23).

JOINT ASSESSMENT INCLUDING THE FEMORAL HEAD AND OSTEONECROSIS

The assessment of femoral anteversion or torsion by CT has been reported, with studies showing highly accurate, reproducible, and technically straightforward methodology for measuring the angle between the head, neck, and shaft of the femur.[45–47] Using scout localization, single axial images through the femoral neck and femoral condyles are sufficient to determine the degree of femoral anteversion.

The status of the capsular and periarticular structures of the hip in degenerative and inflammatory disorders by CT evaluation has been described.[48] Capsular thickening, edema, or effusion can be assessed.

Conventional tomography has traditionally been used in children to determine the position of the femoral head after placement in an abduction cast for congenital dislocation of the hip. However, this technique involves considerable radiation to the gonads and often does not show whether the femoral head is covered by the acetabulum. Computed tomography (Fig. 11–24) and, more recently, magnetic resonance imaging have been used to locate the femoral head through the plaster cast.[49–51] MRI is more accurate in demonstrating the morphology of the incompletely ossified femoral epiphysis. CT may be useful in preoperatively assessing the quantity of cortical and trabecular bone in adult patients with congenital hip dysplasia (Fig. 11–25).

Thin-section high-resolution CT has been applied to the evaluation and staging of femoral head osteo-

Text continued on page 453

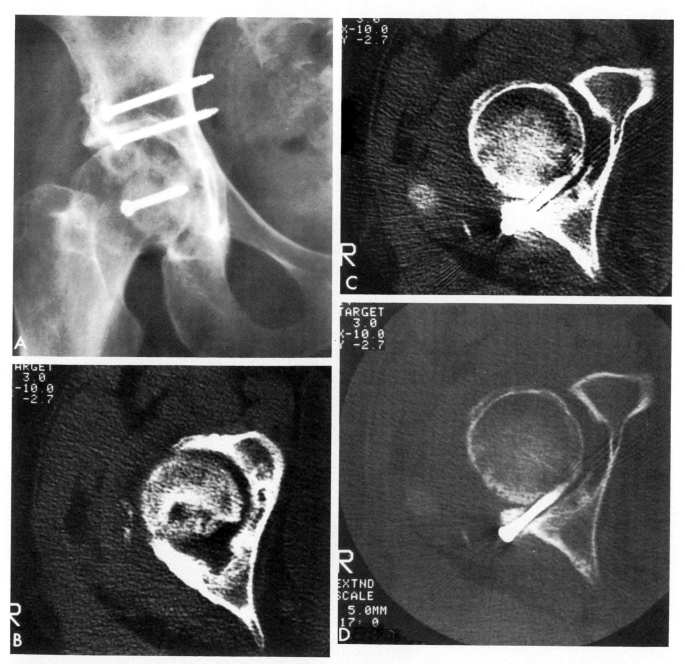

FIGURE 11–20 ■ *A,* Conventional radiograph demonstrates abnormal right hip 3 months after open reduction and internal fixation of an acetabular fracture. *B* and *C,* CT images demonstrate osseous and articular destruction resulting from screw extending into hip joint. *D,* CT image using extended gray scale better displays relationship of the screw to the hip joint.

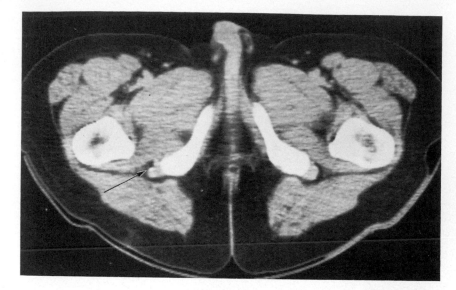

FIGURE 11–21 ■ CT scan through the ischial tuberosity. The patient had pain, muscle atrophy, and reflex loss in the distribution of the right sciatic nerve. Scan shows faint calcifications (arrow) around the ischial tuberosity. The sciatic nerve running adjacent to the ischial tuberosity on the right was found in surgery to be entrapped by a calcific inflammatory process of the ischial bursa caused by trauma from a paddleball racquet.

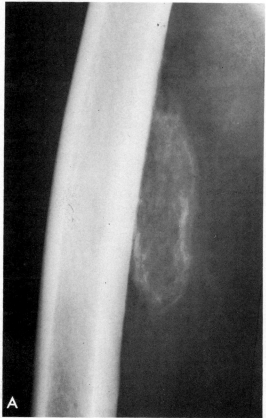

FIGURE 11–22 ■ Myositis ossificans. A, Radiograph of the femur in a patient with a slightly painful, enlarging mass in the thigh shows an ossified soft tissue mass without definite bone destruction. A diagnosis of myositis ossificans was made, even though the history of trauma was equivocal. B, CT scan through the mass shows peripheral ossification and ill-defined centrum, the classic features of myositis ossificans. The CT findings made biopsy unnecessary.

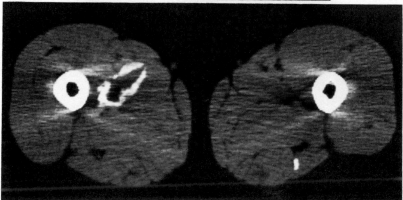

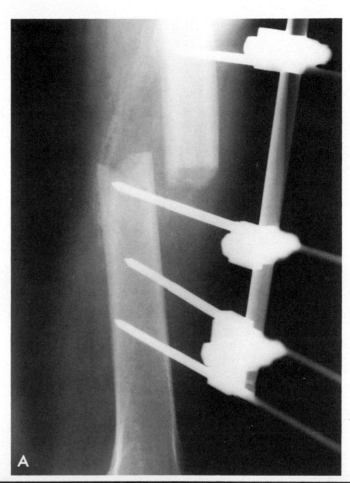

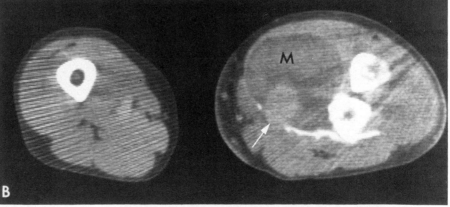

FIGURE 11–23 ■ Posttraumatic pseudoaneurysm. *A,* Radiograph of the femur taken 2 weeks after fracture shows internal traction pins and exuberant callus formation. This patient developed fever, pain, and swelling in his thigh over a 24-hour period and was considered to have an abscess. *B,* Before the surgical drainage, a CT scan through the mass showed a large, low-density soft tissue mass (M) surrounding a contrast-enhanced dilated artery *(arrow).* The diagnosis of pseudoaneurysm of the femoral artery with rupture and bleeding in the soft tissue was confirmed at surgery.

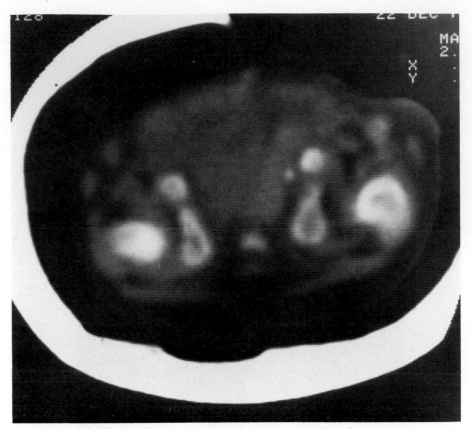

FIGURE 11–24 ■ Computed tomography may be used to demonstrate the adequacy of reduction of congenital hip dislocations following placement in a spica cast. In this case, CT demonstrates lateral subluxation of the left proximal femur, indicating inadequate reduction.

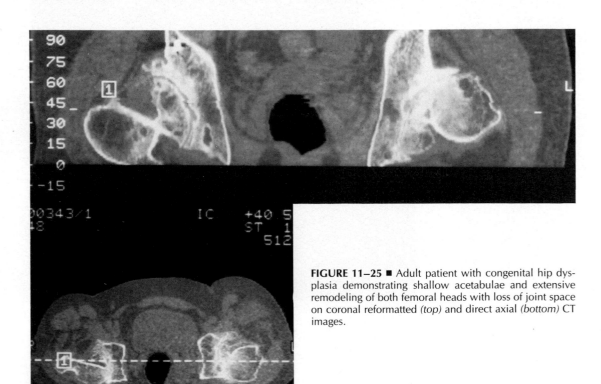

FIGURE 11–25 ■ Adult patient with congenital hip dysplasia demonstrating shallow acetabulae and extensive remodeling of both femoral heads with loss of joint space on coronal reformatted *(top)* and direct axial *(bottom)* CT images.

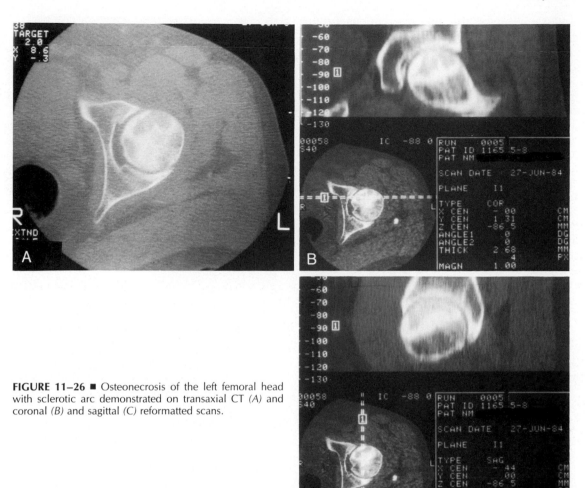

FIGURE 11–26 ■ Osteonecrosis of the left femoral head with sclerotic arc demonstrated on transaxial CT (A) and coronal (B) and sagittal (C) reformatted scans.

necrosis (Fig. 11–26).[51] CT, although less sensitive than MRI, has the potential to identify the focus of sclerosis within the femoral head. Changes in the femoral head and the weight-bearing acetabular dome congruity can be displayed.

PROSTHESES AND INFECTION

The evaluation of metallic prostheses by CT is significantly restricted by image artifacts that result from the presence of the radiographically opaque object in the field. Artifacts can be a deterrent, particularly for imaging structures in the immediate vicinity of the prosthesis. Nevertheless, advanced software methods for reducing scan artifacts in the prosthetic hip have been explored.[52–54] The hope is that the axial representation of the cement-bone and cement-prosthesis interfaces may provide information of importance in biomechanical research, if not in the clinical practice of orthopedics.

In the study of infection CT has value in (1) examining the articular surface of bone and the periarticular soft tissues; (2) delineating the extent of medullary and soft tissue involvement; (3) demonstrating cavities, serpiginous tracks, and sequestra or cloacae in osteomyelitis; and (4) sometimes demonstrating soft tissue edema or bone destruction not seen on conventional radiographs.[55]

MRI

Magnetic resonance imaging has been successfully used to examine several pathologic processes in the hip. Its excellent spatial and contrast resolution facilitates early detection and evaluation of femoral head osteonecrosis, definition of hyaline articular cartilage in arthritis, identification of joint effusions, and characterization of osseous and soft tissue lesions about the hip. In addition, the cartilaginous epiphysis in an infant or child, which is not visible on routine radiographs, can be demonstrated on MR images.

IMAGING PROTOCOLS

The body coil is used in most MRI examinations of the hip, allowing comparison of both hips when large fields of view are used. T1-weighted images can be acquired in the axial, sagittal, or coronal planes. T2-weighted images are particularly useful in evaluating arthritis, infection, and neoplasia. Smaller fields of view should be used to obtain high spatial resolution when imaging the hip in the sagittal plane.

Surface coil imaging of the hip may be useful to delineate high-resolution structures such as the acetabular labrum.

Osteonecrosis ■ Evaluation of patients with osteonecrosis can be accomplished with a T1-weighted axial localizer and either a T1- or T2-weighted spin-echo coronal sequence.[55-57] Imaging in the sagittal plane is optional. Short T1 inversion recovery (STIR) pulse sequences, which negate yellow marrow fat signal, provide excellent contrast to detect marrow replacement, fluid, and necrotic tissue (Fig. 11–27). Fatty marrow alterations associated with osteonecrosis can be detected using chemical shift imaging techniques. On fat-selective and water-selective images, fatty and hematopoietic marrow and the distribution of water within the ischemic focus can be differentiated.

Mitchell and co-workers have described a MR classification system for avascular necrosis (AVN) based on alterations in the central region of MR

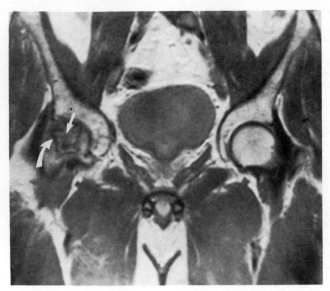

FIGURE 11–28 ■ Right femoral head osteonecrosis *(straight arrow)* is visualized with intermediate-to-high signal intensity. The lesion is demarcated by a peripheral rim of low signal intensity *(curved arrow)*.

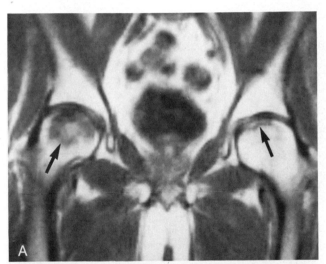

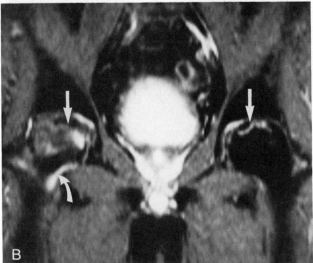

FIGURE 11–27 ■ Avascular necrosis. *A,* Bilateral osteonecrosis of the hip images with low signal intensity *(arrows)* on T1-weighted image. *B,* On fat suppression image, avascular necrosis *(straight arrows)* and associated joint effusion *(curved arrow)* are visualized with a bright signal intensity.

signal intensity in the osteonecrotic focus (Fig. 11–28).[58-61] In MR class A, the osteonecrotic lesion demonstrates signal intensity analogous to fat (a central region of high signal intensity on short TR/TE settings [T1-weighted] and intermediate signal intensity on long TR/TE settings [T2-weighted]). Class B indicates a signal intensity characteristic of blood or hemorrhage (high signal intensity on both short and long TR/TE images). Hips identified as class C demonstrate fluid signal intensity properties (low signal intensity on short TR/TE images and high signal intensity on long TR/TE images). Class D indicates a signal characteristic of fibrous tissue (low signal intensity on short and long TR/TE sequences). A peripheral band of low signal intensity demarcates the central focus of avascular necrosis in all classes. This border is most visible on T1-weighted images of class A and B hips, where the central focus is of high signal intensity, and on T2-weighted images of class C hips. Therefore MR signal intensity can be seen to follow a chronologic progression from acute (class A) to chronic (class D) osteonecrosis. A characteristic double line sign can be observed in up to 80% of lesions and is not attributed to a chemical shift artifact on T2-weighted images.

MR findings can also be correlated with histologic changes. The central region of high signal intensity corresponds to necrosis of bone and marrow prior to development of capillary and mesenchymal ingrowth. The low-signal-intensity peripheral band corresponds to a sclerotic margin of reactive tissue at the interface between necrotic and viable bone. Low signal intensity on T1-weighted images and intermediate-to-high signal intensity on T2-weighted images can be attributed to high water content of mesenchymal tissue and thickened trabecular bone.

Fractures ■ Fractures about the hip and pelvis may be associated with significant morbidity, especially

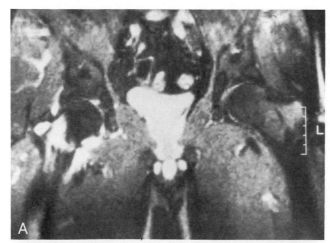

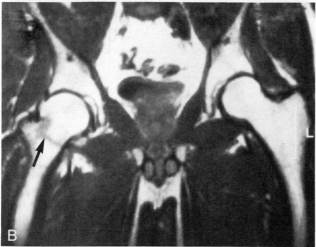

FIGURE 11–29 ■ Normal conventional radiographs of femoral neck fracture. Detection and delineation of fracture morphology are possible on T1 (A) and T2* (B) coronal images (arrow).

the medial and lateral joint capsule is distended and is imaged with convex margins. Joint effusions are also easily identified on axial and sagittal images.

Muscle Trauma ■ Muscle tears and avulsions image with high signal intensity on T2-weighted images in areas of edema or hemorrhage (Fig. 11–30).[64–66] MR axial imaging is useful for the demonstration of associated muscle retraction and atrophy. Coronal or sagittal images provide a longitudinal display of the entire muscle on a single image.

Osteoarthritis ■ Articular cartilage attenuation is best demonstrated on either sagittal or coronal images, but separation of acetabular and femoral head articular cartilage is better displayed in the sagittal plane. Trabeculae thickened by stress can be seen with low signal intensity on T1- and T2-weighted images before there is evidence of subchondral sclerosis on conventional radiographs. Small subchondral cystic lesions can be identified on MR scans before there is superior joint space narrowing, lateral acetabular and femoral head osteophytes, and medial femoral buttressing.

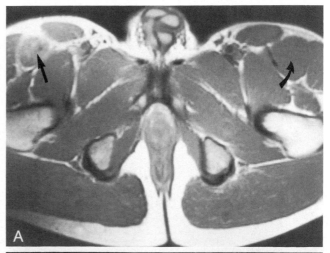

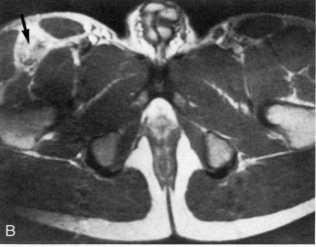

FIGURE 11–30 ■ Torn right rectus femoris muscle with atrophy and edema (straight arrows) on intermediate-weighted (A) and T2-weighted (B) axial images. Edematous muscle fibers display increased signal intensity on T2-weighted image. Normal-size left rectus femoris shown for comparison (curved arrow).

when diagnosis and treatment are delayed. Femoral fractures are classified as either intra- or extracapsular. Intracapsular femoral neck fractures are subcapital, transcervical, or basicervical in location. The incidence of posttraumatic osteonecrosis increases as the fracture site nears the femoral head, culminating in a 30% incidence for fractures in closest proximity to the femoral head. MR imaging has been particularly useful in identifying nondisplaced proximal femoral fractures that require surgical treatment but are not detectable on routine radiographs (Fig. 11–29).[62]

Acetabular Labrum ■ High spatial resolution with anatomic detail of the acetabular labrum is made possible with surface coil imaging. The normal labrum, triangular on cross section, is visualized on coronal planar images as a low-signal-intensity triangle located between the lateral acetabulum and femoral head. Labral tears present with symptoms of pain, decreased range of motion, and clicking.

Joint Effusions ■ On coronal MR images, joint fluid first accumulates in the recess bordered superiorly by the labrum of the acetabulum and inferomedially by the transverse ligament.[63] With larger effusions

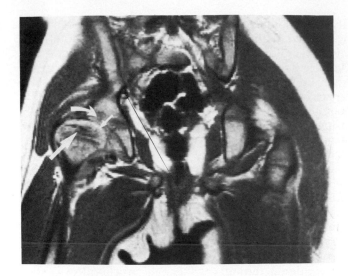

FIGURE 11–31 ■ Congenital dislocation of the hip with superolateral subluxation of the right femoral head and interposed soft tissue *(curved arrow)* within the acetabulum. Osteonecrosis *(large straight arrow)* and flattening of the cartilaginous epiphysis *(small straight arrow)* are visualized.

Congenital Dislocation of the Hip ■ MRI has been used in the evaluation of congenital dislocation of the hip (CDH).[67] T1-weighted coronal and axial images display the exact position of the intermediate-signal-intensity cartilaginous femoral head (Fig. 11–31). This is important when the position of the femoral head is uncertain on plain radiographs and when serial follow-up examinations, in or out of plaster casts, are required. It further obviates the need to expose the child to ionizing radiation. T2-weighted images are helpful when evaluating complications associated with CDH, such as ischemic

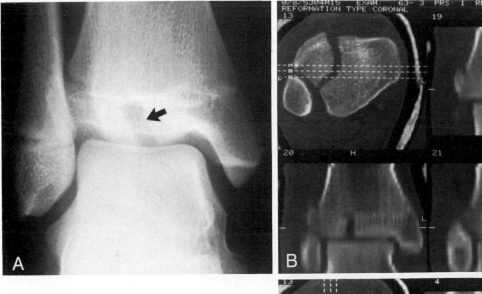

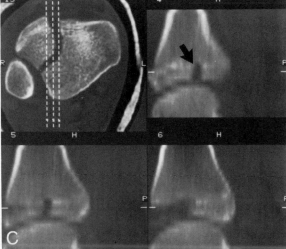

FIGURE 11–32 ■ Tibial plafond fracture with lateral displacement shown on AP radiograph *(A)* and coronal *(B)* and sagittal reformatted *(C)* CT scans *(arrow)*. Displacement and fracture obliquity are best defined on CT.

necrosis and associated effusions. With MR imaging, the origin of CDH and the failure to achieve adequate reduction can be determined without the use of invasive arthrography.

The Ankle

CT

The complex anatomic relationships of the ankle, which includes the talocalcaneal, transverse tarsal, and tibiotalar joints, are best examined on 1.5-mm high-resolution CT scans.[68, 69] Multiplanar reconstruction in the coronal and sagittal planes is superior to conventional tomographic evaluation. Three-dimensional image reconstruction facilitates visualization of complex spatial relationships in fractures and coalitions.

TRAUMA

CT is effective in assessing calcaneal fractures, including trabecular stress fractures and complicated fracture-dislocations.[70–73] Subtalar fracture extension can be evaluated on reformatted sagittal images. Sustentacular anatomy is isolated on coronal reformatted scans, whereas sagittal reformations display the anterior, middle, and posterior facets. The integrity of the tibial plafond and ankle mortise is best demonstrated in the coronal plane (Fig. 11–32). Fracture diastasis and articular surface depression can be directly measured. Fracture-dislocation of the tarsometatarsal joints (Lisfranc's joint) and trauma to the metatarsophalangeal joints are best studied in axial and coronal (reformatted) scans. CT aids in the assessment of fracture complications, including displacement of fragments, in which it can specify position and number and identify loose bodies, degenerative arthrosis, and avascular necrosis (Fig. 11–33). Complex articular injuries may require bilateral scanning for comparison with the normal anatomy of the contralateral ankle. CT identifies osteochondral fragments associated with transchondral fractures of the talar dome; the morphology of the talar lesion and extent of reactive subchondral sclerosis can be characterized.

TARSAL COALITIONS

CT is effective in classifying tarsal coalitions that may be fibrous or osseous (Figs. 11–34, 11–35).[74–78] Calcaneonavicular coalitions may be associated with hypoplasia of the talar head. Talocalcaneal coalition most frequently involves fusion at the level of the sustentaculum tali that is appreciated on coronal reformations free of superimposed bony structures. Cortical irregularity, subchondral sclerosis, and close apposition of the middle facet surfaces may be seen in association with fibrous unions not identified on conventional radiographs. Talar beaking is demonstrated on sagittal reformation.

ARTHRITIS AND INFECTION

Joint space narrowing, eburnation, osteophytosis, subchondral degenerative cysts, and loose bodies can be shown by CT in degenerative arthrosis (Fig. 11–36). Osteoporosis, erosions, and subluxations may characterize rheumatoid disease.

The spectrum of CT findings of infection includes lytic erosions, soft tissue swelling, periosteal reac-

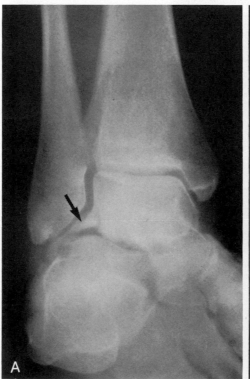
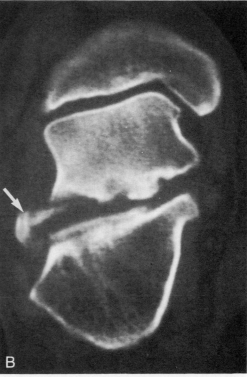

FIGURE 11–33 ■ Inferolateral talar fracture (arrow) with subtalar extension identified on conventional radiograph (A) and transaxial CT scan (B).

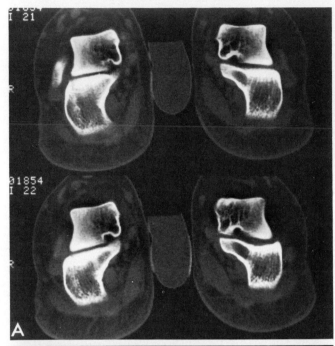

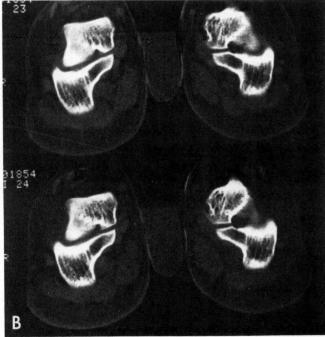

FIGURE 11–34 ■ *A, B,* CT scans through the hind foot demonstrate the posterior and medial facets of the subtalar joint without evidence of tarsal coalition.

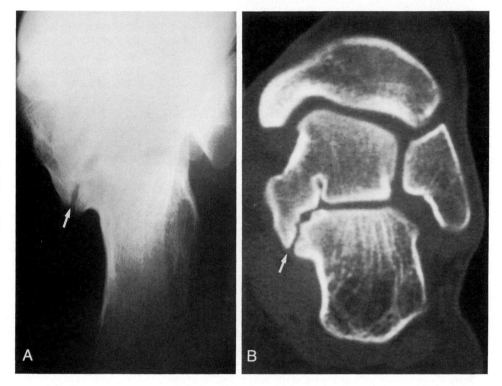

FIGURE 11–35 ■ Talocalcaneal coalition (fibrous) with irregular morphology and cortical surface irregularity of the sustentaculum tali *(arrow)* in the middle facet. This form of coalition is shown on an angled view of the calcaneus using conventional radiography *(A)*. *B,* A better view, obtained with transaxial CT, shows bone detail.

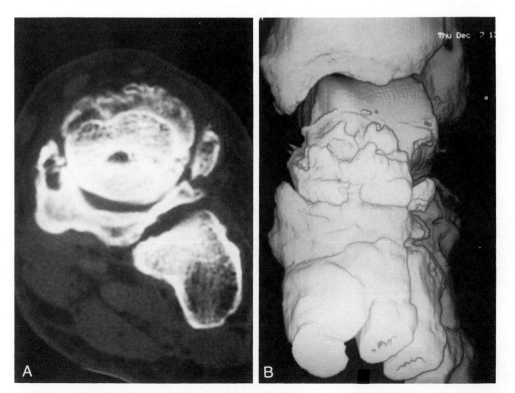

FIGURE 11–36 ■ Posttraumatic talonavicular degenerative arthrosis with osteophytosis and subchondral cysts shown on direct axial CT *(A)* and three-dimensional CT *(B)* scans.

tion, and sequestra. Bone involvement may be demonstrated adjacent to an overlying diabetic ulcer. Soft tissue findings in infection include obliteration of fat planes, diffuse soft tissue swelling, and presentation of a discrete soft tissue mass.

MRI

The use of a circumferential extremity coil for magnetic resonance imaging of the ankle provides high tissue contrast and excellent spatial resolution, affording superior depiction of complex soft tissue anatomy, including muscles, ligaments, and tendons (Fig. 11–37).[79, 80] In addition, marrow and cortical bone definition permits detection of fractures, cysts, and infections (Fig. 11–38). The unique ability to image hyaline articular cartilage directly with MR has made MR valuable in assessing arthritis and transchondral fractures and in identifying intraarticular loose bodies. By placing both legs within the circular extremity coil, comparison with the contralateral ankle and foot can be achieved. Alternatively, when smaller fields of view are needed, the extremities may be imaged one at a time by repositioning the surface coil. The foot is usually placed in neutral position, or a partial plantarflexion may be used when comparing MR images with a CT ankle examination performed with 45° tibiotalar orientation.

TRANSCHONDRAL FRACTURES

Transchondral fracture is the accepted term for several osteochondral lesions, including osteochondral fracture, osteochondritis dissecans, and talar dome fracture.[81] Transchondral fractures of the medial or lateral talar dome involve the articular cartilage and subchondral bone and have a high association with antecedent trauma. Conventional radiographs and CT scans cannot assess the integrity of hyaline articular cartilage surfaces in osteocartilaginous defects. Detachment with a loose osteochondral fragment characterizes an advanced stage in the Berndt and Harty classification (Fig. 11–39).[81]

With MR imaging tibiotalar anatomy can be displayed in the coronal, axial, or sagittal plane to identify the talar defect and the presence of an avulsed bony fragment.[82] The hyaline articular cartilage surface of the talar dome images with intermediate signal intensity on T1- and T2-weighted images, but a detached cortical fragment will remain low in signal intensity. Peripheral areas of low signal intensity within the subchondral bone on T1- and T2-weighted images have been correlated with reactive bone sclerosis on plain radiographs. The accumulation of high-signal-intensity joint fluid within or undermining the articular cartilage surface indicates small fissures or breaks in the articular cartilage (Fig. 11–40). Abnormalities of the articular cartilage surface include regions of cartilage thinning, bowing, nodularity, or disruption. The presence of an intact articular cartilage surface could obviate the need for surgical excision and curettage and permit more conservative treatment (e.g., drilling).

TENDINOUS AND LIGAMENTOUS STRUCTURES

Preliminary investigations have shown potential applications of MR imaging in the evaluation of tendinous and ligamentous structures about the ankle.[83] Intact tendons and ligaments image with low signal intensity on all pulsing sequences. The Achilles tendon is the largest tendon in the body and is formed from the confluence of the gastrocnemius and soleus muscle complexes. The Achilles tendon

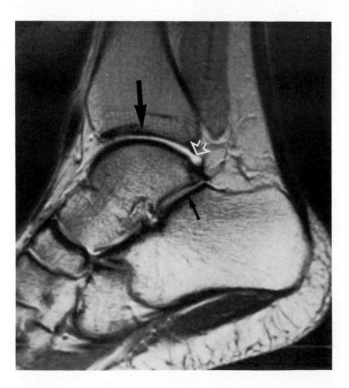

FIGURE 11–37 ■ T2-weighted sagittal image demonstrates the anatomy of the tibiotalar joint *(large solid arrow)* and subtalar joint *(small solid arrow)*. Bright-signal-intensity fluid is visualized within the tibiotalar articulation *(open arrow)*.

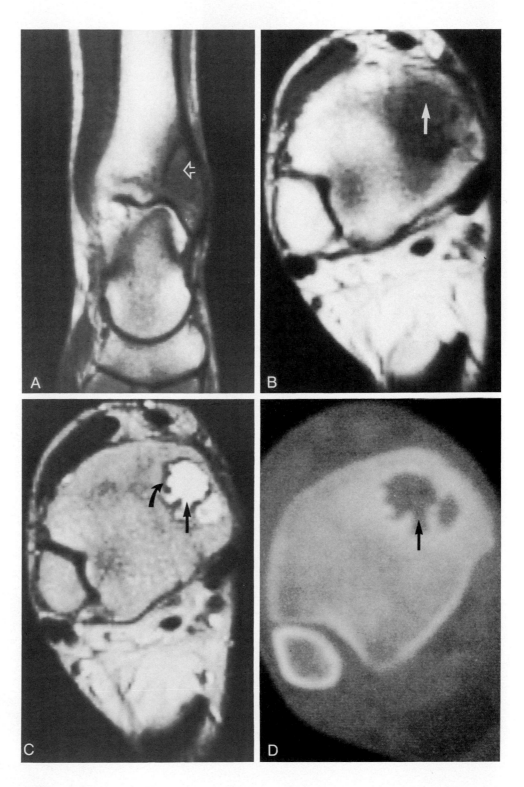

FIGURE 11–38 ■ *A,* Low-signal-intensity subchondral cyst *(open arrow)* visualized on T1-weighted coronal image. Synovial fluid contents demonstrate low signal intensity and bright signal intensity on T1- *(B)* and T2-weighted *(C)* axial images, respectively. Synovial fluid content *(straight arrow)* is surrounded by peripheral low signal intensity sclerosis *(curved arrow). D,* Corresponding axial CT scan defines sclerotic edge of the tibial cyst *(arrow).*

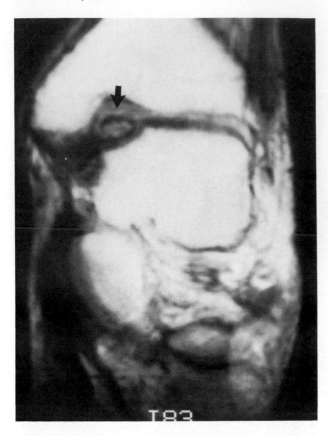

FIGURE 11–39 ■ Transchondral fracture *(arrow)* with upward bowing of medial talar hyaline articular cartilage surface. (Courtesy of Robert Princenthal.)

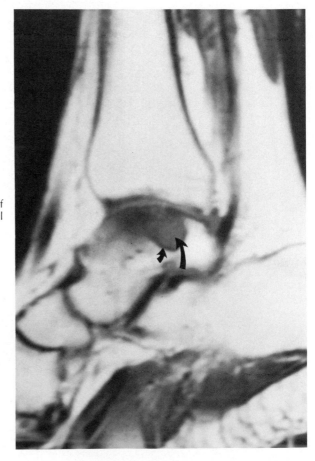

FIGURE 11–40 ■ Osteochondral defect with low-signal-intensity periphery of reactive bone *(small arrow)* and intermediate-signal-intensity viscous synovial fluid contents *(large arrow).*

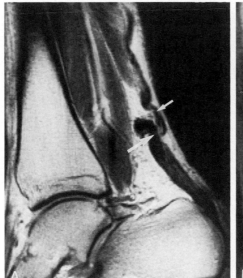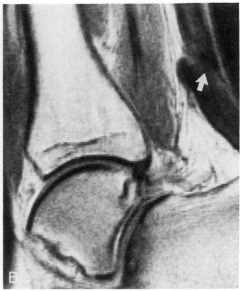

FIGURE 11–41 ■ *A*, Complete rupture of the Achilles tendon with proximal *(small arrow)* and distal *(large arrow)* tendinous fibers identified in close proximation. *B*, Complete fibrous healing with apposition of torn tendon after 4 months of cast treatment *(arrow)*.

is most susceptible to rupture 2 to 6 cm superior to the os calcis, with acute rupture associated with forced dorsiflexion of the foot against a contracting force generated by the triceps surae group. The Achilles tendon is clearly demonstrated on sagittal and axial MR images.[84, 85] The normal Achilles tendon images with uniform low signal intensity. Axial images show the tendon in cross section with a mildly flattened anterior surface and convex posterior surface. In ruptures of the Achilles tendon, the relationship of the proximal and distal portions of the torn tendon can be seen in either pre- or postplaster casting MR studies (Fig. 11–41). More patients with tendon tears are being conservatively managed with serial casting, and thus MRI has become invaluable in documenting the degree of apposition in the disrupted proximal and distal tendon fragments.

INFECTION

Acute and chronic osteomyelitis of the calcaneus, cuboid, metatarsals, and distal tibia and fibula has been studied with MRI.[86] On T2-weighted sequences in the acute or subacute phase, a diffuse or patchy increase in the medullary bone indicates marrow involvement. A peripheral rim of low signal intensity, representing reactive bone, may demarcate the focus over time. Alterations in signal intensity may also be seen at sites of cortical transgression, periosteal reaction, soft tissue mass, and sequestra.

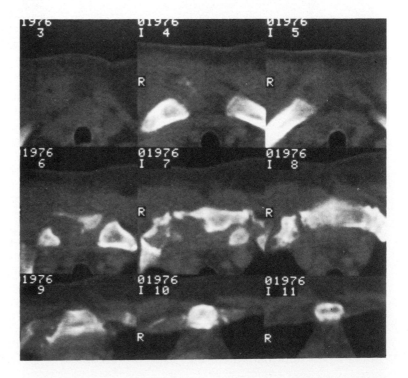

FIGURE 11–42 ■ Manubriosternoclavicular abscess. CT scan demonstrates destruction of the right manubriosternoclavicular articulation and a large associated soft tissue mass with fluid density, indicating abscess formation.

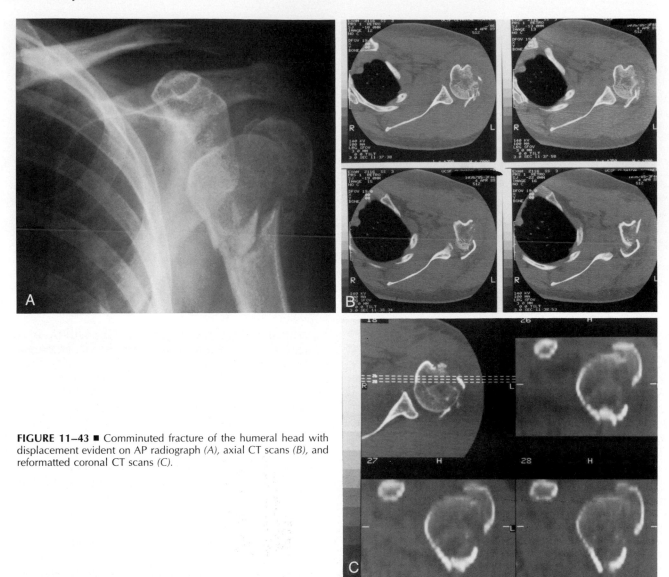

FIGURE 11–43 ■ Comminuted fracture of the humeral head with displacement evident on AP radiograph *(A)*, axial CT scans *(B)*, and reformatted coronal CT scans *(C)*.

The Shoulder

CT

The shoulder girdle represents a complex articulation including the glenohumeral joint (shoulder joint proper), the acromioclavicular joint, the sternoclavicular joint, and scapulothoracic mechanics.[87, 88] CT can be performed without intraarticular contrast in the evaluation of soft tissue masses (these may require intravenous contrast), cystic lesions, infection (Fig. 11–42), and fractures (Fig. 11–43).

The rotator cuff muscles, the supraspinatus, infraspinatus, teres minor, and subscapularis provide important structural support to the glenohumeral joint. CT, although not the study of choice to identify rotator cuff lesions (demonstrated satisfactorily by conventional arthrography), will show the communication of contrast with the subacromial-subdeltoid bursa when reformatted coronal scans are used.

CT in combination with arthrography (computed arthrotomography) has proven useful in the evaluation of the glenohumeral joint, specifically the glenoid labrum.[89] Computed arthrotomography requires minor modification of the double-contrast technique, with the injection of 1.0 to 1.5 mL of contrast and approximately 10 mL of air. After double-contrast injection, 3-mm to 4-mm contiguous scans are obtained from the midacromioclavicular joint to the inferior glenoid. By positioning the contralateral shoulder more superiorly (i.e., with the arm extended), streak artifacts may be minimalized. The integrity of the rotator cuff is assessed on postarthrographic films, and subsequent CT scanning is used to evaluate the glenoid labrum, glenohumeral ligaments, bursae, and joint capsule.

The normal glenoid labrum, part of the glenohumeral ligament labral complex, is a fibrous structure displaying anterior labral (triangular-shaped) and posterior labral (more rounded outline) morphology

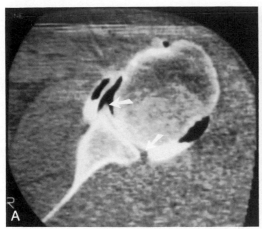
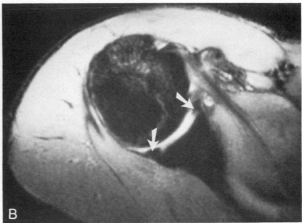

FIGURE 11–44 ■ Normal anterior and posterior glenoid labrum *(arrows)* on axial air contrast CT scan *(A)* and T2*-weighted axial MR image *(B).*

(Fig. 11–44). The anterior labrum may be torn in patients who present with anterior and multidirectional instability patterns. CT is accurate in demonstrating detachment of the capsule and labral tears or fraying at sites of imbibed iodinated contrast (Fig. 11–45A).[90–93] The use of intraarticular contrast facilitates the assessment of articular cartilage and its attenuation in degenerative disease.

CT is an excellent modality to display associated Hill-Sachs compression fractures involving the posterolateral humeral head. This lesion may occur after a single or repeated episodes of anterior glenohumeral dislocation and is best shown at the level of the coracoid, with loss of normal posterolateral humeral head convexity. A posterior glenohumeral joint dislocation may result in a medial humeral head impaction. The Bankart lesion, either cartilaginous or osteocartilaginous, is characterized by disruption of the anteroinferior glenoid rim during anterior glenohumeral dislocations, which are frequently seen in association with Hill-Sachs fractures. CT is superior to conventional radiography in cartilaginous assessment.

The long head of the biceps tendon is outlined by air and contrast in the bicipital groove. The absence of the biceps tendon in its sheath on cross-sectional scans is diagnostic of a tear. Loose bodies may be identified as filling defects on computed arthrotomography.[94] Small cartilaginous fragments, however, may be obscured if surrounded by excessive pooled contrast.

MRI

Magnetic resonance imaging of the shoulder offers the advantages of noninvasive direct imaging of the rotator cuff muscles and tendons of the glenohumeral joint in axial, oblique coronal, and oblique sagittal planes (Fig. 11–46).[95–99] With its excellent soft tissue and bony discrimination, MRI has shown potential in characterizing the spectrum of changes seen in the shoulder impingement syndrome.

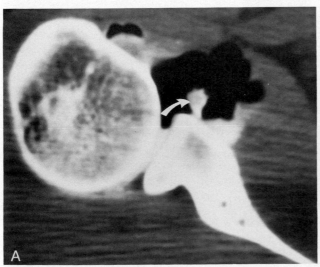
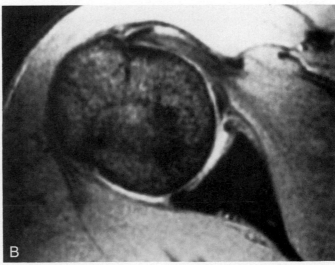

FIGURE 11–45 ■ *A,* Anterior glenoid labral tear on axial air contrast CT scan *(arrow).* This was not identified on corresponding T2* axial MR image *(B).*

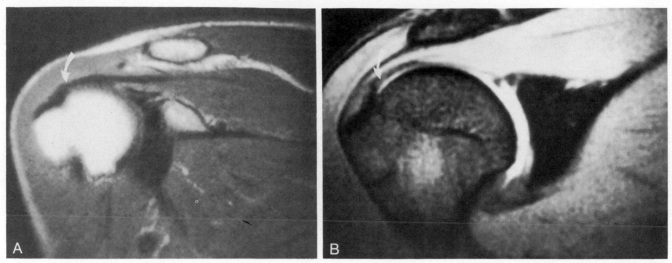

FIGURE 11–46 ■ Normal supraspinatus tendon in two different patients on T1-weighted *(A)* and T2*-weighted *(B)* coronal oblique images. The low-spin-density tendon is low in signal intensity on both pulse sequences *(arrows)*.

High-resolution shoulder imaging is achieved with the use of a dedicated surface coil. T2 weighting in the form of conventional spin-echo imaging or effective T2 weighting using a gradient-echo technique is required in the evaluation of rotator cuff lesions and glenohumeral ligament labral abnormalities. Sagittal images are particularly helpful in evaluating the coracoacromial arch, assessing acromial morphology, and identifying the extent of supraspinatus tears. The supraspinatus tendon is best displayed on oblique coronal images parallel to the supraspinatus muscle.

IMPINGEMENT SYNDROME AND ROTATOR CUFF TEARS

The pathogenesis of cuff tears is thought to involve the shoulder impingement syndrome.[100, 101] Neer has developed a three-tier clinical staging system for shoulder impingement syndrome that helps to establish indications for surgical treatment of rotator cuff lesions.[100] In this system, the pretear impingement lesion represents one end of the spectrum that can culminate in development of a complete rotator cuff tear. In stage I lesions edema and hemorrhage are present within the rotator cuff, and the shoulder responds to conservative management. Stage II is characterized by fibrous and tendinous thickening of the subacromial soft tissue; partial tears may be seen in this stage. In stage III there is a complete rupture or tear of the rotator cuff. Impingement is also classified into three types based on coronal MR images (Fig. 11–47).[100] Type I is characterized by the presence of subacromial bursitis, which is imaged as thickening of the normally high-signal-intensity sub-acromial-subdeltoid bursal line. Signal intensity in the supraspinatus muscle and tendon remains unchanged (intermediate and low, respectively). In type II impingement, signal intensity of the supraspinatus tendon is high on T1-weighted images (Fig. 11–48). Increased or bright signal intensity of the tendon on T2-weighted images represents a type IIb change.

Type III impingement is characterized by the addition of supraspinatus retraction with complete disruption of the rotator cuff. Partial tears have been reported to occur in both type II and III impingement. Secondary signs in rotator cuff tears include supraspinatus muscle atrophy and retraction of the musculotendinous junction medial to the glenoid on coronal oblique images.

Rotator cuff tears are classified as partial or complete. Only complete or full-thickness tears allow direct communication between the glenohumeral joint and the subacromial bursa, which will then contain fluid.[102] The coronal plane is the most sensi-

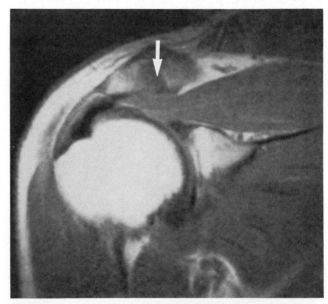

FIGURE 11–47 ■ Impingement syndrome with mild impingement of the supraspinatus muscle/tendon secondary to hypertrophic changes of the acromioclavicular joint *(arrow)*. A mild increase in signal intensity is identified in the involved portion of the supraspinatus muscle.

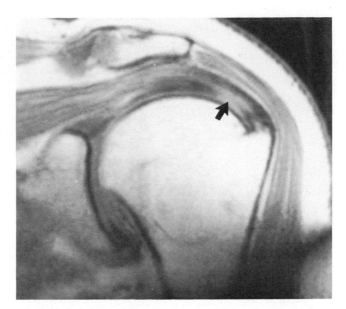

FIGURE 11–48 ■ Focus of tendinitis and partial tear of the supraspinatus with intermediate-signal-intensity edema identified on T1-weighted coronal oblique image *(arrow)*. Subdeltoid peribursal fat is intact.

tive for identifying rotator cuff lesions (Fig. 11–49). On T2-weighted images most tears demonstrate increased signal intensity, and partial tears usually exhibit signal characteristics similar to those described for full-thickness or complete tears.[103] Complete absence of the rotator cuff also indicates massive tears with retraction (Fig. 11–50).

GLENOHUMERAL JOINT

The stability of the glenohumeral joint depends on support by the rotator cuff, the glenohumeral ligaments, and the fibrous glenoid labrum. Glenohumeral joint subluxations and dislocations may be associated with Hill-Sachs compression fractures and tears or detachments of the capsular mechanism in the labrum. Computed tomography air contrast arthrography and MRI have been used to identify labral, capsular, and glenohumeral ligament tears in patients with anterior, posterior, or multidirectional instabilities (Fig. 11–51).[104, 105] Thin-section T2-

weighted axial images demonstrate the low signal intensity (low spin density) of the fibrous anterior and posterior labrum in contrast to the bright signal intensity of the synovial fluid. In the absence of fluid, labral tears may be undetected by MRI (see Fig. 11–45*B*). T1-weighted axial images offer superior contrast resolution in demonstrating bony Bankart lesions.

BICEPS TENDON

The biceps tendon is optimally visualized on images through the glenohumeral joint in the axial plane. Increased fluid in the biceps sheath, nonspecific for inflammation, images with low signal intensity on T1-weighted images and with high signal intensity on T2-weighted images. Bicipital tenosynovitis or inflammation of the biceps tendon synovial sheath can be the result of trauma, calcific deposition, or infection.

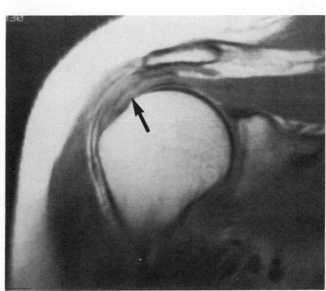

FIGURE 11–49 ■ Complete rotator cuff tear with proximal retraction of the supraspinatus tendon *(arrow)*. Increased fluid signal intensity is identified in the critical zone of the supraspinatus tendon on T1-weighted coronal image.

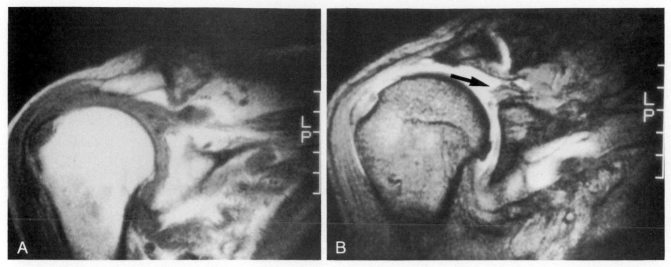

FIGURE 11–50 ■ Complete supraspinatus tendon tear with proximal retraction to glenoid rim shown on T1- (A) and T2*-weighted (B) coronal images (arrow). Advanced arthropathy is present.

The Wrist

CT

CT is especially useful in the evaluation of bone detail in the small, complex wrist joint.[106, 107] Evaluation of carpal bone trauma, including fractures of the hamate, is performed with 1.5-mm thin axial sections from the level of the distal radioulnar joint to the proximal metacarpals. Sagittal and coronal reformations are useful in displaying the articular relationship of the radiocarpal and midcarpal compartments (Figs. 11–52 and 11–53). With proper positioning, direct coronal CT is possible with the wrist supported in dorsiflexion.[106] Three-dimensional images are beneficial in showing complex spatial relationships in different planes and rotations (Fig. 11–54).[108, 109] Articular congruity is shown in coronal or sagittal reformations through intraarticular distal radial fractures. CT demonstrates trabecular and cortical detail and cystic erosions, sometimes before identification on conventional radiography (see Fig. 11–53). The distal radioulnar joint is characterized on cross-sectional scans and can demonstrate ulnar subluxations or dislocations.[110–112] The bony and soft tissue anatomy is defined in sections through the carpal tunnel and Guyon's canal.[113, 114]

MRI

With the selection of a proper surface coil to optimize the signal-to-noise ratio, magnetic resonance imaging can provide the high spatial and contrast resolution of both soft tissue and osseous components that is needed for the evaluation of the small and complex anatomy in the articulations of the wrist.[115–117] MRI can provide high-resolution images of muscles, ligaments, tendons, tendon sheaths, vessels, nerves, marrow, and cortical bone at small

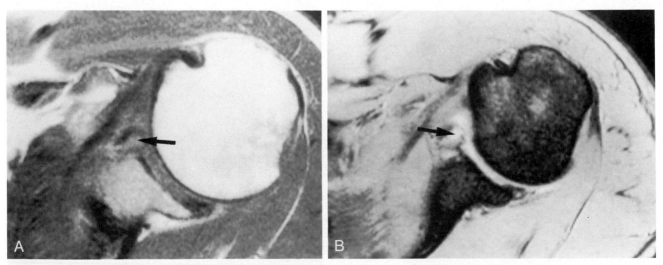

FIGURE 11–51 ■ Tear of the anterior glenoid labrum displayed on T1- (A) and T2*-weighted (B) axial images at the level of the subscapularis tendon (arrow).

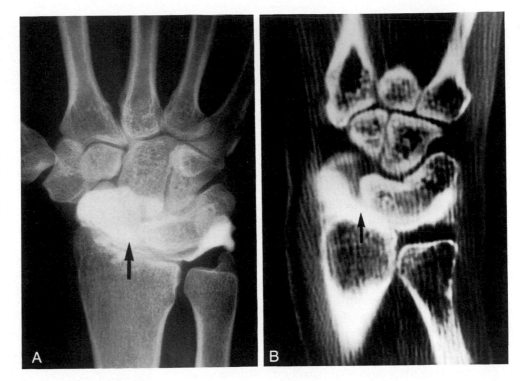

FIGURE 11–52 ■ Wrist arthrogram. AP radiograph *(A)* and coronal reformatted CT scan *(B)* demonstrate the accumulation of contrast within the radiocarpal compartment *(arrows)*. There is no extension of contrast into the inferior radioulnar joint.

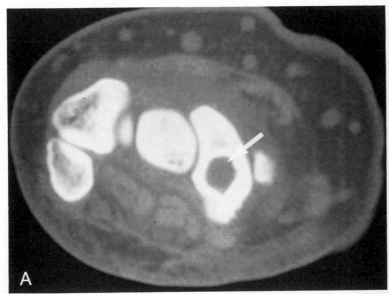

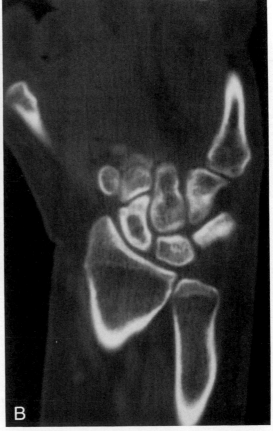

FIGURE 11–53 ■ Scaphoid intraosseous cyst identified on direct axial *(A)* and coronal *(B)* 1.5-mm CT images *(arrow)*.

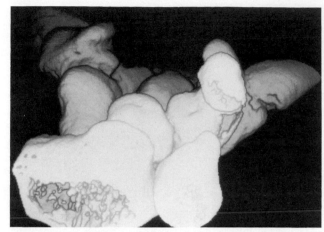

FIGURE 11–54 ■ Normal three-dimensional CT image displaying carpal tunnel osseous anatomy. The three-dimensional image was reconstructed from 1.5-mm thin transaxial scans.

fields of view with uniform depth penetration (Fig. 11–55). In the wrist and hand, MRI has shown application in the study of avascular necrosis; trauma; carpal tunnel syndrome; ligament, tendon, and cartilage abnormalities; arthritis; infection; and neoplasia.

AVASCULAR NECROSIS

AVN in the wrist primarily affects the scaphoid bone (Fig. 11–56) in posttrauma patients and the lunate bone in those with Kienbock's disease (lunatomalacia) (Fig. 11–57). Most scaphoid fractures of the proximal one third and up to 33 per cent of

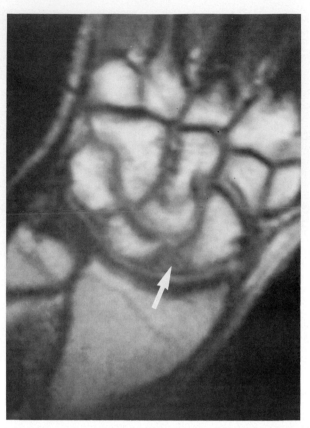

FIGURE 11–56 ■ Scaphoid fracture with avascular necrosis of the proximal pole (arrow). Necrotic segment demonstrates low signal intensity on T1-weighted coronal image.

fractures of the middle one third (waist fractures) are associated with AVN. Nondisplaced fractures may be missed on conventional radiographs, and detection of sclerosis at the fracture site may not be apparent on plain films for as long as 2 weeks after the initial insult. Kienbock's disease of the lunate, especially in the early stages of vascular compromise, may be also particularly difficult to detect by standard radiographic methods.

Abnormal areas of decreased marrow signal intensity can be associated with AVN.[118] MRI has been reported to be as sensitive as bone scintigraphy in the detection of AVN and to possess even greater specificity in diagnosis. The most common imaging pattern in AVN of the scaphoid is low signal intensity in the proximal pole on both T1- and T2-weighted images. It is possible that early marrow edema may be confused with AVN in a patient who has sustained traumatic fracture. With marrow edema, however, a diffuse increase in signal intensity should be evident on T2-weighted sequences.

CARPAL TUNNEL SYNDROME

Impairment of motor or sensory function of the median nerve as it passes through the carpal tunnel (carpal tunnel syndrome) may be caused by fractures and dislocations about the wrist, intraneural hemorrhage, infection, infiltrative disease, and various soft tissue injuries. Up to two thirds of patients with

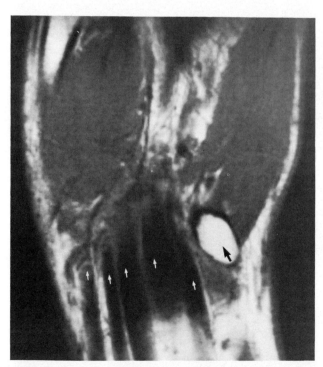

FIGURE 11–55 ■ Normal anatomy of low-signal-intensity flexor tendons (white arrows) seen in carpal tunnel. Pisiform (black arrow) is indicated.

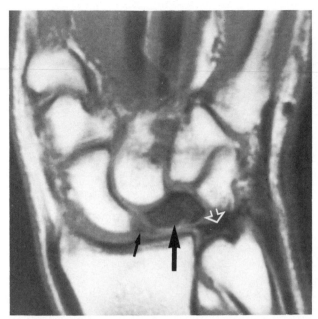

FIGURE 11–57 ■ Kienbock's disease on T1-weighted image with low-signal-intensity necrotic lunate *(large black arrow)* and disrupted scapholunate ligament *(small black arrow)*. Triangular fibrocartilage is identified by the open arrow.

carpal tunnel syndrome have bilateral involvement, rendering comparison with the contralateral wrist for normal anatomy misleading. Edematous changes, which image with high signal intensity on T2-weighted images, have been documented in the median nerve of patients with carpal tunnel syndrome.[119] Attempts have been made to use MRI in the measurement of the diameter and area of affected portions of the median nerve, although clinical application needs further documentation.

TRIANGULAR FIBROCARTILAGE AND INTEROSSEOUS LIGAMENT ABNORMALITIES

Coronal MRI of the wrist with T1- and T2-weighted sequences has identified the triangular fibrocartilage ligament complex and interosseous ligaments of the wrist, including the scapholunate and lunatotriquetral ligaments (Fig. 11–58).[120, 121] MR imaging of the triangular fibrocartilage complex and interosseous ligaments may replace triple-compartment arthrography. The sagittal imaging plane is important in demonstrating dorsal intercollated segmental instability (DISI) and volar intercollated segmental instability (VISI) patterns.

The Temporomandibular Joint

CT

CT of the TMJ offers a noninvasive alternative to arthrography and its associated morbidity.[122–124] Thin-section transaxial CT scans through the TMJ are reformatted into the sagittal plane displaying the mandibular condyle and articular eminence. Through electronic enhancement of surrounding tissue atten-

uation values (the blink mode), soft tissue structures (including the pterygoid muscles, which have lower attenuation values than the TMJ disk) are eliminated to allow indirect assessment of disk position relative to the condylar head. Sharper anatomic detail is possible with direct sagittal CT, but this technique requires more difficult patient positioning.[124] CT assessment of disk abnormalities is thus limited to operator adjustments of attenuation values of surrounding structures. An accurate visualization of true disk morphology and internal structure is not obtained. However, CT does evaluate osseous anatomy, including sclerosis, erosions, osteophytes, and fractures.

MRI

Magnetic resonance imaging is rapidly replacing arthrography and CT as the examination of choice in evaluating the TMJ.[125–127] CT requires the use of ionizing radiation, allows visualization of the TMJ disk only through the use of reformatted sagittal images obtained from a series of transaxial joint scans, and provides no dynamic information. MRI is noninvasive and provides direct sagittal images that not only display the TMJ meniscus, but also differentiate cortex, marrow, hyaline cartilage, muscle, fluid, fibrous tissue, and adhesions. The development of faster imaging techniques has facilitated routine bilateral examinations with functional or dynamic positioning of the joint. Direct sagittal images through the TMJ are acquired with the use of a small-diameter (3-in) surface coil placed over the region of interest.

Bony support of the TMJ, the articular eminence

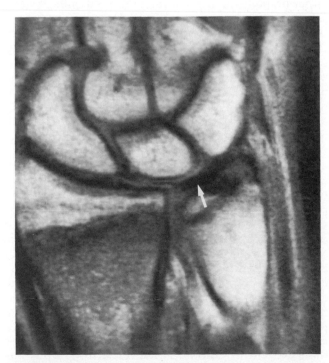

FIGURE 11–58 ■ High-resolution coronal image of the wrist demonstrating intact low-signal-intensity triangular fibrocartilage *(arrow)*.

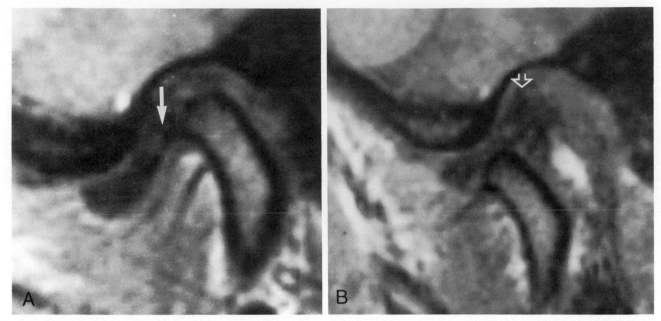

FIGURE 11–59 ■ T1-weighted sagittal image of the TMJ in closed- *(A)* and open-mouth *(B)* positions. In the closed-mouth position the posterior band is anterior to the condylar head *(solid arrow)*, and in the open-mouth position with reduction, the posterior band is identified superior to the condylar head *(open arrow)*.

of the temporal bone, and the condyle of the mandible image with high signal intensity of marrow fat. The fibrous TMJ meniscus is composed of three parts: an anterior band, a thin intermediate zone, and a thicker posterior band. All three parts visualize with low signal intensity (a central portion of intermediate signal intensity may be identified within the posterior band as a normal finding). The anterior band, positioned in front of the condyle, is anchored to the superior belly of the lateral pterygoid muscle. The thick posterior band is attached to a vascularized bilaminar zone in the retrodiscal tissue complex anchored to the temporal bone. In the open-mouth position the posterior band occupies a 12 o'clock position in relationship to the condylar head of the mandible.

Internal derangements of the TMJ usually involve an anteromedial displacement of the meniscus in relationship to the condyle and temporal fossa (Fig. 11–59). Trauma, degeneration, ligamentous laxity, and retrodiscal rents can be contributing factors. Such an anteriorly positioned disk blocks normal forward translation of the condyle, and the patient may present clinically with limited jaw opening and deviation of the mandible toward the affected side. An opening click is usually associated with relocation of the thick posterior band as it moves posteriorly in the open-mouth position and is recaptured by the condylar head. A patient with the jaw locked in the closed-mouth position (closed lock) has a displaced meniscus in both closed- and open-mouth positions, preventing anterior condylar motion. Disk perforations may be more difficult to identify on MR images than with arthrography. However, arthrography has a reported high false-positive rate in the detection of disk perforations.

Osteoarthritis may occur as a sequela to TMJ trauma and internal disk derangements. In osteoarthritis, cortical and articular thinning with flattening and deformity of the condylar head is visualized on MR images. Osteophytes (usually anterior), joint space narrowing, and erosions at both the temporal eminence and the condyle are frequently seen in degenerative joint disease.

Summary

Clinical advances in the fields of orthopedics and rheumatology have necessitated more precise noninvasive radiologic assessment. Magnetic resonance imaging has provided detailed high-contrast and high-resolution images of articular joints, supporting muscles, ligaments, cartilage, and synovium. With the development of advanced systems, hardware, surface coil technology, and flexible software programs (including innovative fast scan pulse sequences and three-dimensional Fourier transform acquisition), MRI has replaced computed tomography in many applications for the evaluation of disorders affecting the appendicular joints. However, CT continues to offer valuable information regarding cortical and cancellous bone, calcification, and mineral quantification.

References

1. Genant HK, Cann CE, Chafetz NI, Helms CA: Advances in computed tomography of the musculoskeletal system. Radiol Clin North Am 19:645, 1981.
2. Brown BM, Brant-Zawadzki M, Cann CE: Dynamic CT scanning of spinal column trauma. AJNR 3:561, 1982.

3. Reese DF, McCullough EC, Balcer HL Jr: Dynamic sequential scanning with table incrementation. Radiology 140:719, 1981.

4. Glenn WV, Rhodes ML, Altschuler EM, Wiltse LL, Lostanek C, Kuo YM: Multiplanar display computerized body tomography applications in the lumbar spine. Spine 4:282, 1979.

5. Woolson S, Dev P, Fellingham L, Vassilindis A: Three-dimensional imaging of bone from computerized tomography. Clin Orthop 202:231, 1986.

6. Totty WF, Vannier MW: Complex musculoskeletal anatomy, analysis using three dimensional surface reconstructions. Radiology 150:173, 1984.

7. Fullerton GD: Basic concepts for nuclear magnetic resonance imaging. Magn Reson Imaging 1:39, 1982.

8. Wehli FW: Principles of magnetic resonance. In Stark DD, Bradley WG (eds): Magnetic Resonance Imaging. St Louis, CV Mosby, 1987, pp 3–23.

9. Winkler ML, Ortendahl DA, Mills TC, Crooks LE, Sheldon PE, et al: Characteristics of partial flip angle and gradient reversal MR imaging. Radiology 166:17, 1988.

10. Solomon SL, Totty WG, Lee JK: MR imaging of the knee: comparison of three-dimensional FISP and two-dimensional spin-echo pulse sequences. Radiology 173:739–742, 1989.

11. Harms SE, Flamig DP, Fisher CF, Fulmer JM: New method for fast MR imaging of the knee. Radiology 173:743–750, 1989.

12. Shellock FG: MR imaging of metallic implants and materials: a complication of the literature. AJR 151:811–814, 1988.

13. Ihara H: Double-contrast CT arthrography of the cartilage of the patellofemoral joint. Clin Orthop 188:50–55, 1985.

14. Martimez S, Korubkin M, Fondren FB, Hediund LW, Foldner JL: Diagnosis of patellofemoral malalignment by computed tomography. J Comput Assist Tomogr 7:1050–1053, 1983.

15. Shellock FG, Mink JH, Deutsch AL, Fox JM: Patellar tracking abnormalities: clinical experience with kinematic MR imaging in 130 patients. Radiology 172:799–804, 1989.

16. Rafii M, Firooznia H, Golimbu C, Bonamo J: Computed tomography of tibial plateau fractures. AJR 142:1181–1186, 1984.

17. Reicher MA, Bassett LW, Gold RM: High-resolution magnetic resonance imaging of the knee joint: pathologic correlations. AJR 145:903–909, 1985.

18. Reicher MA, Hartzman S, Bassett LW, Mandelbaum B, Duckwiler G, Gold RH: MR imaging of the knee. Part I. Traumatic disorders. Radiology 162:547–551, 1986.

19. Gallimore GW Jr, Harms SE: Knee injuries: high-resolution MR imaging. Radiology 160:457–461, 1986.

20. Kean DM, Worthington BS, Preston BJ, et al: Nuclear magnetic resonance imaging of the knee: examples of normal anatomy and pathology. Br J Radiol 56:355–364, 1983.

21. Burk DL Jr, Kanal E, Brunberg JA, Johnstone GF, Swensen HE, Wolf GL: 1.5-T surface-coil MRI of the knee. AJR 17:293–300, 1986.

22. Li DKB, Adams ME, McConkey JP: Magnetic resonance imaging of the ligaments and menisci of the knee. Radiol Clin North Am 24:209–227, 1986.

23. Li KC, Henkelman RM, Poon PY, Rubenstein J: MR imaging of the normal knee. J Comput Assist Tomogr 8:1147–1154, 1984.

24. Stoller DW: Magnetic resonance imaging of the knee. Perspect Radiol 1:21–60, 1988.

25. Mink JH, Levy T, Crues JV: Tears of the anterior cruciate ligament and menisci of the knee: MR imaging evaluation. Radiology 167:769–774, 1988.

26. Tyrrell RL, Gluckert K, Pathria M, Modic MT: Fast three-dimensional MR imaging of the knee: comparison with arthroscopy. Radiology 166:865–872, 1988.

27. Manco LG, Losman J, Coleman ND, Kavanaugh JH, Bilfield BS, Dougherty J: Noninvasive evaluation of knee meniscal tears: preliminary comparison of MR imaging and CT. Radiology 163:727–730, 1978.

28. Beltran J, Noto AM, Mosure JC, Bools JC, Zuelzer W, Christoforidis AJ: Meniscal tears: MR demonstration of experimentally produced injuries. Radiology 158:691–693, 1986.

29. Stoller DW, Martin C, Crues JV III, Kaplan L, Mink JH: Meniscal tears: pathologic correlation with MR imaging. Radiology 163:731–735, 1987.

30. Turner DA, Prodromos CC, Petasnick JP, Clark JW: Acute injury of the ligaments of the knee: magnetic resonance evaluation. Radiology 154:717–722, 1985.

31. Yulish BS, Montanez J, Goodfellow DB, et al: Chondromalacia patellae: assessment with MR imaging. Radiology 164:763–766, 1987.

32. Gylys-Morin VM, Hajek PC, Sartoris DJ, Resnick D: Articular cartilage defects: detectability in cadaver knees with MR. AJR 148:1153–1157, 1987.

33. Yao L, Lee JK: Occult intraosseous fracture: detection with MR imaging. Radiology 167:749–752, 1988.

34. Beltran J, Noto AM, Herman LJ, Mosure JC, Burk JM, Christoforidis AJ: Joint effusions: MR imaging. Radiology 158:133–137, 1986.

35. Berquist TH, Brown ML, Fitzgerald RH, May GR: Magnetic resonance imaging: application in musculoskeletal infection. Magn Reson Imaging 3:219–230, 1985.

36. Fishman EK, Magid D, Mandelbaum BR, et al: Multiplanar (MPR) imaging of the hip. Radiographics 6:7–54, 1986.

37. Magid D, Fishman EK, Brooker AF, Mandelbaum BR, Siegelman SS: Multiplanar computed tomography of acetabular fractures. J Comput Assist Tomogr 10:778–783, 1968.

38. Harley JD, Mack La, Winquist RA: CT of acetabular fractures: comparison with conventional radiography. AJR 138:413, 1982.

39. Mack L, Harley JD, Winquist RA: CT of acetabular fractures: analysis of fracture patterns. AJR 138:407, 1982.

40. Shirkhoda A, Brashear HR, Staab EV: Computed tomography of acetabular fractures. Radiology 134:683, 1980.

41. Lange TA, Alter AJ Jr: Evaluation of complex acetabular fractures by CT. J Comput Assist Tomogr 4:849, 1980.

42. Lasda NA, Levinsohn EM, Yuan HA, Bunnell WP: CT in disorders of the hip. J Bone Joint Surg 60A:1099, 1978.

43. Judet R, Judet J, Letournel E: Fractures of the acetabulum: classification and surgical approaches for open reduction. J Bone Joint Surg 46:1615, 1964.

44. Pennal GF, Davidson J, Garside H, Plewes J: Results of treatment of acetabular fractures. Clin Orthop 151:115, 1980.

45. Bjersand AJ, Eastgate RJ: The accuracy of CT-determined femoral neck anteversion. Eur J Radiol 2:1, 1982.

46. Grote R, Elgeti H, Saure D: Bestimmung des antertorsionswinkels am Femur mit der axialen Computertomographie. Roentgenblaetter 33:31, 1980.

47. Hernandez RJ, Tachdjian MO, Poznanski AK, Diaz LS: CT detection of femoral torsion. AJR 137:97, 1981.

48. Dihlmann W, Nevel G: CT for evaluation of the hip capsule. J Comput Assist Tomogr 7:278, 1983.

49. Padovani J, Faure F, Devred P, Jacquemier M, Sarrat P: Use and advantages of tomodensitometry in testing congenital luxations of the hip. Ann Radiol 22:188, 1979.

50. Padovani FF, Devred MJ, Sarrat P: Interet et indications de la tomodenstometrie dans le bilan des luxations congenitales de la hanche. Ann Radiol 22:188, 1979.

51. Magid D, Fishman EK, Scott WW Jr, et al: Femoral head avascular necrosis: CT assessment with multiplanar reconstruction. Radiology 157:751–756, 1985.

52. Faul DD, Cough JL, Cann CE, Hoaglund FT, Genant HK: An ART approach to reconstructing CT slices through metallic prostheses. Presented at the Radiological Society of North America 67th Annual Meeting, Chicago, IL, November 15–19, 1981.

53. Hinderling TH, Ruegsegger P, Anliker M, Dietschi C: Computed tomography reconstruction from hollow projections: an application in vivo evaluation of artificial hip joints. J Comput Assist Tomogr 3:52, 1979.

54. Seitz P, Ruegsegger P: Bone densitometry in the vicinity of metallic implants. Abstract. J Computed Assoc Tomogr 6:200, 1982.

55. Bassett LW, Gold RH, Reicher M, Bennett LR, Tooke SM: Magnetic resonance imaging in the early diagnosis of ischemic necrosis of the femoral head: preliminary results. Clin Orthop 214:237–248, 1987.

56. Gillespy T III, Genant HK, Helms CA: Magnetic resonance imaging of osteonecrosis. Radiol Clin North Am 24:193–208, 1986.
57. Totty WG, Murphy WA, Ganz WI, Kumar B, Daum WJ, Siegel BA: Magnetic resonance imaging of the normal and ischemic femoral head. AJR 143:1273–1280, 1984.
58. Mitchell MD, Kundel HL, Steinberg ME, Kressel HY, Alavi A, Axel L: Avascular necrosis of the hip: comparison of MR, CT, and scintigraphy. AJR 147:67–71, 1986.
59. Mitchell DG, Kressel HY, Arger PH, Dalinka M, Spritzer CE, Steinberg ME: Avascular necrosis of the femoral head: morphologic assessment by MR imaging with CT correlation. Radiology 161:739–742, 1986.
60. Mitchell DG, Rao VM, Dalinka MK, Spritzer CE, Alavi A, et al: Femoral head vascular necrosis: correlation of MR imaging, radiographic staging, radionuclide imaging, and clinical findings. Radiology 162:709–715, 1987.
61. Lang P, Jergesen HE, Moseley ME, Block JE, Chafetz NI, Genant HK: Avascular necrosis of the femoral head: high-field-strength MR imaging with histologic correlation. Radiology 169:517–524, 1988.
62. Berger PE, Ofstein RA, Jackson DW, Mornison DS, Silvino N, Amadon R: MRI demonstration of radiographically occult fractures. What have we been missing? Radiographics 9:407, 1989.
63. Mitchell DG, et al: MRI of joint fluid in the normal and ischemic hip. AJR 146:1215, 1986.
64. Ehman RL, Berquist TH: Magnetic resonance imaging of musculoskeletal trauma. Radiol Clin North Am 24:291, 1986.
65. Fisher MR, et al: Magnetic resonance imaging of the normal and pathologic musculoskeletal system. Magn Reson Imaging 4:491, 1986.
66. Dooms GC, et al: MR imaging of intramuscular hemorrhage. J Comput Tomogr 9:908, 1985.
67. Lang P, et al: Three-dimensional CT and MR imaging in congenital dislocation of the hip: technical considerations. Radiology 165(P):279, 1978.
68. Lindsjo U, Hemminsgsson A, Sahlstedt B, Danckwardt-Lilliestrom G: Computed tomography of the ankle. Acta Orthop Scand 50:797–801, 1979.
69. Solomon MA, Gilula L, Oloff LM, Oloff J, Compton T: CT scanning of the foot and ankle: 1. Normal anatomy. AJR 146:1192–1203, 1986.
70. Guyer BH, Levinsohn EM, Fredrickson BE, Bailey GL, Formikell M: Computed tomography of calcaneal fractures: anatomy, pathology, dosimetry, and clinical relevance. AJR 145:911–919, 1985.
71. Rosenberg ZS, Feldman F, Singson RD: Intra-articular calcaneal fractures: computed tomographic analysis. Skeletal Radiol 16:105–113, 1987.
72. Heger L, Wulff K: Computed tomography of the calcaneus: normal anatomy. AJR 145:123–129, 1985.
73. Heger L, Wulff K, Sediqi MSA: Computed tomography of calcaneal fractures. AJR 145:131–137, 1985.
74. Deutsch AL, Resnick D, Campbell G: Computed tomography and bone scintigraphy in the evaluation of tarsal coalition. Radiology 144:137, 1982.
75. Deutsch AL, Resnick D, Campbell G: Computed tomography and bone scintigraphy in the evaluation of tarsal coalition. Radiology 144:137–140, 1982.
76. Sarno RC, Carter BL, Bankoff MS, Semine MC: Computed tomography in tarsal coalition. J Comput Assist Tomogr 8:1155–1160, 1984.
77. Pineda C, Resnick D, Greenway G: Diagnosis of tarsal coalition with computed tomography. Clin Orthop 208:282–288, 1986.
78. Marchisello PJ: The use of computerized axial tomography for the evaluation of talocalcaneal coalition. A case report. J Bone Joint Surg 69A:609–611, 1987.
79. Beltran J, Noto AM, Mosure JC, Shamam OM, Weiss KL, Zuelzer WA: Ankle: surface coil MR imaging at 1.5T. Radiology 161:203–209, 1986.
80. Hajek PC, Baker LL, Bjorkengren A, Sartoris DJ, Neumann CH, Resnick D: High-resolution magnetic resonance imaging of the ankle: normal anatomy. Skeletal Radiol 15:536–540, 1986.
81. Berndt A, Harty M: Transchondral fractures (osteochondritis dissecans) of the talus. J Bone Joint Surg 41A:988, 1959.
82. Yulish BS, et al: MR imaging of osteochondral lesions of talus. J Comput Assist Tomogr 11:296, 1987.
83. Daffner RH, Reimer BL, Lupetin AR, Dash N: Magnetic resonance imaging in acute tendon ruptures. Skeletal Radiol 15:619–621, 1986.
84. Reinig JW, Dorwart RH, Roden WC: MR imaging of a ruptured Achilles tendon. J Comput Assist Tomogr 9:1131–1134, 1985.
85. Quinn SF, et al: Achilles tendon: MR imaging at 1.5T. Radiology 164:767, 1987.
86. Berquist TH: Musculoskeletal infection. In Berquist TH, et al (eds): Magnetic Resonance of the Musculoskeletal System. New York, Raven Press, 1987, pp 109–125.
87. Destout JM, Gilula L, Murphy WA, Sagal SS: Computed tomography of the sternoclavicular joint and sternum. Radiology 138:123, 1981.
88. Levinsohn EM, Bunnell WP, Yuan HA: Computed tomography in the diagnosis of dislocation of the sternoclavicular joint. Clin Orthop 140:12, 1979.
89. Shuman WP, Kilcoyne RF, Matsen FA, Rogers JV, Mack LA: Double contrast computed tomography of the glenoid labrum. AJR 141:581–584, 1983.
90. Deutsch AL, Resnick D, Mink JH, et al: Computed and conventional arthrotomography of the glenohumeral joint: normal anatomy and clinical experience. Radiology 153:603–609, 1984.
91. Resnick CS, Deutsch AL, Resnick D, et al: Arthrotomography of the shoulder. Radiographics 4:963–976, 1984.
92. Haynor DR, Shuman WP: Double contrast CT arthrography of the glenoid labrum and shoulder girdle. Radiographics 4:411–421, 1984.
93. Rafii M, Firooznia H, Golimbu C, Minkoff J, Bonamo J: CT arthrography of capsular structures of the shoulder. AJR 146:361–367, 1986.
94. Gould R, Rosenfield AT, Friedlander GE: Loose body within the glenohumeral joint in recurrent anterior dislocation: CT demonstration. J Comput Assist Tomogr 9:404–406, 1985.
95. Seeger LL, Ruszkowski JR, Bassett LW, Kay SP, Kahmann RD, Ellman H: MR imaging of the normal shoulder: anatomic correlation. AJR 148:93–91, 1987.
96. Middleton WD, Kneeland JB, Carrera GH, et al: High-resolution MR imaging of the normal rotator cuff. AJR 148:559–564, 1987.
97. Kneeland JB, Carrera GF, Middleton WD, et al: Rotator cuff tears: preliminary application of high-resolution MR imaging with counter rotating current loop-gap resonators. Radiology 160:695–699, 1986.
98. Kieft GH, Bloem JL, Obermann WR, Verbout AJ, Rozing PM, Doornbos J: Normal shoulder: MR imaging. Radiology 159:741–745, 1986.
99. Huber DJ, Sauter R, Mueller E, Requardt H, Weber H: MR imaging of the normal shoulder. Radiology 158:405–408, 1986.
100. Seeger LL, Gold RH, Bassett LW, et al: Shoulder impingement syndrome: MR findings in 53 shoulders. AJR 150:343, 1988.
101. Kieft GH, Bloem JL, Rozing PM, Obermann WR: Rotator cuff impingement syndrome: MR imaging. Radiology 166:211, 1988.
102. Brems J: Rotator cuff tear: evaluation and treatment. Orthopedics 11:69, 1988.
103. Kneeland JB, Middleton WD, Carrera GF, et al: MR imaging of the shoulder: diagnosis of rotator cuff tears. AJR 149:333, 1987.
104. Seeger LL, Gold RH, Bassett LW, et al: MR imaging of shoulder instability. Radiology 165P:148, 1987.
105. Zlatkin MB, et al: Cross-sectional imaging of the capsular mechanism of the glenohumeral joint. AJR 150:151, 1988.
106. Biondetti PR, Vannier MW, Gilula LA, Knapp RD: Wrist: coronal and transaxial CT scanning. Radiology 163:149–151, 1987.

107. Quinn SF, Murray W, Watkins T, Kloss J: CT for determining the results of treatment of fractures of the wrist. AJR 149:109–111, 1987.

108. Vannier MW, Totty WG, Stevens WG, et al: Musculoskeletal applications of three-dimensional surface reconstructions. Orthop Clin North Am 16:543–555, 1985.

109. Weeks PM, Vannier MW, Stevens WG, Gayou D, Gilula LA: Three-dimensional imaging of the wrist. J Hand Surg 10(A):32–39, 1985.

110. Scheffler R, Armstrong D, Hutton L: Computed tomographic diagnosis of distal radio-ulnar joint disruption. J Can Assoc Radiol 35:212–213, 1984.

111. Mino DE, Palmer AK, Levinsohn M: The role of radiography and computerized tomography in the diagnosis of subluxation and dislocation of the distal radioulnar joint. J Hand Surg 8:23–31, 1983.

112. Cone RO, Szabo R, Resnick D, Gelberman R, Taleisnik J, Gilula LA: Computed tomography of the normal radioulnar joints. Invest Radiol 18:541–545, 1983.

113. Cone RO, Szabo R, Resnick D, Gelberman R, Taleisnik J, Bilula LA: Computed tomography of the normal soft tissues of the wrist. Invest Radiol 18:546–551, 1983.

114. Jetzer T, Erickson D, Webb A, Heithoff K: Computed tomography of the carpal tunnel with clinical and surgical correlation. CT Clin Symp 7(4), 1984.

115. Baker LL, Hajek PC, Bjorkengren A, et al: High-resolution magnetic resonance imaging of the wrist: normal anatomy. Skeletal Radiol 16:128–132, 1987.

116. Weiss KL, Beltran J, Shamam OM, Stilla RF, Levey M: High-field MR surface-coil imaging of the hand and wrist. Part I. Normal anatomy. Radiology 160:143–146, 1986.

117. Weiss KL, Beltran J, Lubbers LM: High-field MR surface-coil imaging of the hand and wrist. Part II. Pathologic correlations and clinical relevance. Radiology 160:147–152, 1986.

118. Reinus WR, Conway WF, Totty WG, et al: Carpal avascular necrosis: MR imaging. Radiology 160:689–693, 1986.

119. Middleton WD, Kneeland JB, Kellman GM, et al: MR imaging of the carpal tunnel: normal anatomy and preliminary findings in the carpal tunnel syndrome. AJR 148:307–316, 1987.

120. Zlatkin MB, Chau PC, Osterman L, et al: Chronic wrist pain: evaluation with high-resolution MR imaging. Radiology 173:723–729, 1989.

121. Golimbu CN, Firooznia H, Melone CP, et al: Tears of the triangular fibrocartilage of the wrist: MR imaging. Radiology 173:731–733, 1989.

122. Thompson JR, Christiansen E, Hasso AN, Hinshaw DB Jr: Temporomandibular joints: high-resolution computed tomographic evaluation. Radiology 150:105–110, 1984.

123. Helms CA, Vogler JB III, Morrish RB Jr, Goldman SM, Capra RE, Proctor E: Temporomandibular joint internal derangements: CT diagnosis. Radiology 152:459–462, 1984.

124. Manco LG, Messing SG, Busino LJ, Fasulo CP, Sordill WC: Internal derangements of the temporomandibular joint evaluated with direct sagittal CT: a prospective study. Radiology 157:407–412, 1985.

125. Katzberg RW, Bessette RW, Tallents RH, et al: Normal and abnormal temporomandibular joint: MR imaging with surface coil. Radiology 158:183–189, 1986.

126. Helms CA, Gillespy T III, Sims RE, Richardson ML: Magnetic resonance imaging of internal derangement of the temporomandibular joint. Radiol Clin North Am 24:189–192, 1986.

127. Harms SE, Wilk RM: Magnetic resonance imaging of the temporomandibular joint. Radiographics 7:521–542, 1987.

CHAPTER 12

COMPUTED TOMOGRAPHY AND MAGNETIC RESONANCE IMAGING OF THE SPINE

NEIL CHAFETZ ▪ STEPHEN L. G. ROTHMAN ▪ HARRY K. GENANT ▪ JAY A. KAISER

The evaluation of the patient with signs or symptoms attributable to spinal disorders has changed dramatically. In the 1980s computed tomography (CT) largely replaced myelography as the initial definitive spinal imaging modality. Magnetic resonance imaging (MRI) has since assumed a premier role in the assessment of spinal disorders; computed tomography remains popular, but myelography has become almost a rarity in medically sophisticated circles.

This chapter describes the planning, performance, and interpretation of state-of-the-art spinal CT and MRI examinations. Computed tomography of the spine was well received because it replaced, in most cases, an invasive procedure (myelography) with a noninvasive one. Magnetic resonance imaging, in turn, has been well received, because it replaced a procedure that employs ionizing radiation with one that does not. The routine sagittal MRI images have particularly helped popularize MRI. Although in many cases computed tomography and MRI can each provide comparable information, there are certain circumstances in which one modality is more likely to demonstrate the underlying pathologic disorder than the other. Consequently, special attention to the appropriate use of MRI and CT is given.

Technical Considerations

Computed Tomography

CERVICAL SPINE

In the routine CT examination of the cervical spine, thin contiguous slices are recommended through the major area of interest. Unless clinical information points to another region, attention is focused on the lower cervical spine. A state-of-the-art scanner is employed to obtain contiguous 1.5-mm-thick slices from the C4 to the T1 level. Survey images through the C2-3 and C3-4 disk spaces are also routinely obtained.

THORACIC SPINE

Thoracic CT is not performed nearly as often as thoracic MRI. Although disk herniation in the thoracic spine is encountered less frequently than in the cervical and lumbar regions, the likelihood of calcification of a disk herniation is greater in the thoracic spine. Recognition of a calcified thoracic herniation is easier with CT than with MRI. Additionally, the assessment of spinal fractures is often optimized by the use of CT. In this setting, 5-mm slices obtained every 3 mm or contiguous 3-mm slices are routine and extend from a level above to a level below the region of interest.

LUMBAR SPINE

In the lumbar spine, 5-mm or 3-mm-thick slices at 3-mm intervals are obtained routinely from the L3 to the S1 level. Survey images at the L1-2 and L2-3 levels are often helpful.

THE USE OF CT REFORMATIONS

Software to perform reformations in the sagittal as well as curved coronal planes is readily available. Such software is routine on all state-of-the-art scanners; more sophisticated packages are available that can be placed on the scanner computer or independent console. Additionally, work stations, many of which are manufactured by companies other than the producers of the scanners themselves, have become relatively widespread and are able to receive and reformat data from a large variety of scanners and, in some cases, for both CT and MRI. The usefulness of reformatted images will be highlighted in the discussion that follows. Contiguous sagittal images photographed at both bone and soft tissue window settings should extend from the lateral aspect of the neural foramen on one side to the lateral aspect of the neural foramen on the opposite side. Similarly, contiguous curved coronal images parallel to the curvature of the spine should extend through the entire central canal and posterior elements (Fig. 12–1). In the presence of surgical fusion, the sagittal and coronal reformations should be extended to encompass the entire fusion mass.

Magnetic Resonance Imaging

CERVICAL SPINE

A cervical spine MRI scan should include T1-weighted sagittal and T2-weighted or T2*-weighted sagittal images. Additionally, axial images from C4 through T1, using either a T1- or T2*-weighted technique, are routinely obtained. If a spinal cord pathologic abnormality is suspected, true T2-weighted sagittal images, rather than T2*-weighted images, should be obtained. Optimal visualization of the cervical neural foramina is difficult, but gradient-echo sequences permit the volumetric acquisition of three-dimensional data in a timely fashion. Using this technique, very thin sections can be generated, which should improve the MRI visualization of the neural formina in the cervical spine.

THORACIC SPINE

T1- and T2- or T2*-weighted sagittal images are used through the thoracic spine. Additionally, axial images localized to the particular region of interest, using either a T1- or T2*-weighted technique, are also standard.

LUMBAR SPINE

T1, T2*, or multiecho sagittal images through the lumbar spine are routinely obtained. Additionally, T1 or T2* or multiecho axial images are routinely obtained from L3 through S1 and at L1-2 and L2-3, if an abnormality is noted on the sagittal plane. Gradient echo images are relatively insensitive to bone marrow abnormalities. Therefore, when intramedullary assessment of the bone marrow is of clinical importance, an MR sequence such as inversion recovery that suppresses fat signal intensity is appropriate.

Axial images are also obtained during the cervical, thoracic, and lumbar MRI examinations at any level at which the sagittal images suggest an abnormality and which is not routinely covered by the axial sequence.

Use of Contrast Agents

CT

CT with intrathecal administration of contrast has been performed primarily to detect pathologic abnormalities involving the spinal cord or to detect arachnoiditis. Although intravenous injection of contrast has been performed with CT to differentiate epidural fibrosis from recurrent disk herniation, MRI with intravenous administration of gadopentetate dimeglumine has become the modality of choice for the detection of central nervous system neoplasms and epidural fibrosis. Furthermore, MRI is the preferred modality for the recognition of arachnoiditis and spinal cord abnormality. Consequently, the need for CT with intrathecal or intravenous contrast is rare (Fig. 12–2). In those few instances where the presence of extensive surgical hardware has prevented visualization of the canal, intrathecal contrast may prove helpful.

MRI

The use of gadopentetate dimeglumine has proved to be particularly helpful when searching for spinal neoplastic lesions and when differentiating epidural fibrosis from recurrent disk herniation in

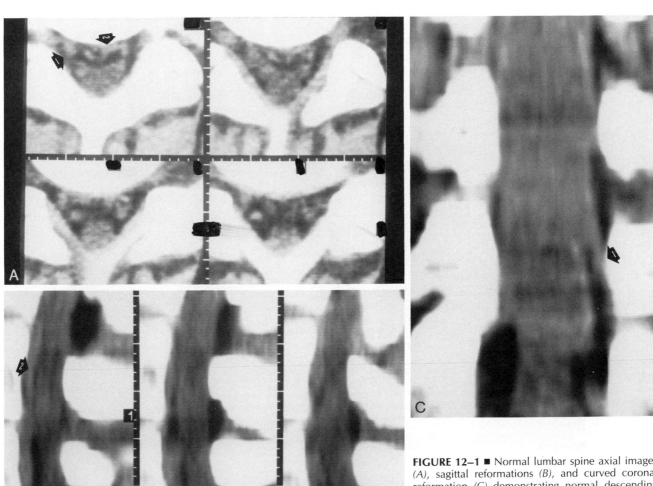

FIGURE 12–1 ■ Normal lumbar spine axial images (A), sagittal reformations (B), and curved coronal reformation (C) demonstrating normal descending nerve roots (1) and prominent epidural veins (2).

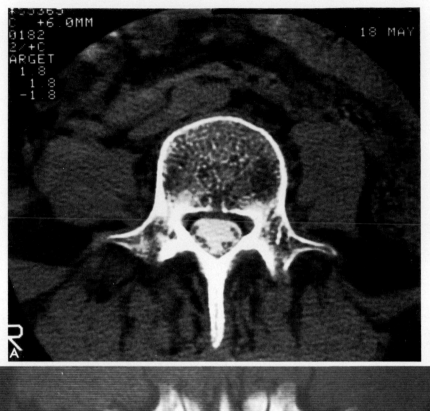

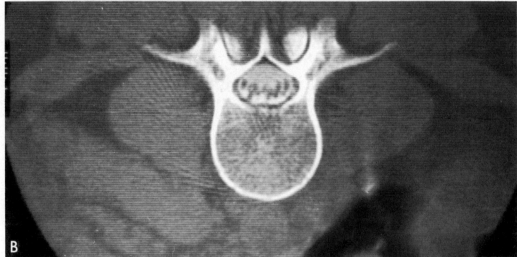

FIGURE 12–2 ■ Normal lumbar CT scans made after intrathecal contrast administration. Scans made in the supine *(A)* and prone *(B)* position demonstrate thin mobile nerve roots.

the postoperative patient (Fig. 12–3).[1, 2] Immediately following the intravenous injection of gadopentetate dimeglumine, T1-weighted sagittal and axial images through the regions of interest permit comparison with the precontrast T1-weighted sagittal and axial images. If scans are delayed, contrast will diffuse into the disk fragment and make differentiation difficult. If the routine examination has already been performed, T1-weighted sagittal and axial images through the region of interest should be generated, both prior and immediately subsequent to the injection of gadopentetate dimeglumine. It is not always necessary to inject gadopentetate dimeglumine to distinguish scar from disk. Often the routine MRI images (especially the T2-weighted axial images) per-

mit differentiation between the two.[3] The decision to use gadopentetate dimeglumine ideally should be left to the radiologist supervising the examination.

Pathology

Fundamentals of Intervertebral Disk Disease

Disk degeneration includes a wide range of pathologic processes that can lead to back and/or leg pain. Torsional injuries are thought to represent the earliest event, leading to small concentric annular tears. Recurrent small torsional injuries, or a significant single one, can lead to coalescence of these concentric tears into a radial annular tear through which nuclear

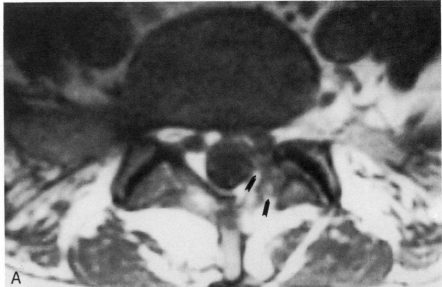

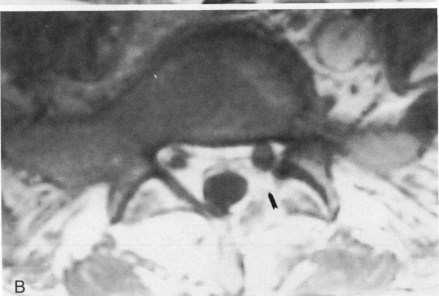

FIGURE 12–3 ■ T1-weighted precontrast L5-S1 axial image *(A)* and a comparable image made after administration of gadopentetate dimeglumine *(B)* demonstrate enhancement of epidural fibrosis immediately posterior to the left S1 nerve root *(arrows).*

material may extend, leading to a herniated disk. The herniated disk is demonstrated on CT or MRI as a focal abnormality in annular contour. Conversely, as a result of breakdown in the annulus over a period of time, the annulus may undergo degeneration with loss of its normal contour and consequent concentric bulging. This can occur as a normal process of aging and rarely causes radiculopathy. The term *bulging disk* should be avoided, as it is possible to differentiate in almost all cases by MRI, and often by CT, between a concentric or diffuse annular bulge and a disk herniation.

It is also possible to differentiate between contained and noncontained disk herniations. Contained herniations, also termed *protrusions*, consist of nuclear material that extends through the inner annular fibers but remains contained by the outer annulus–posterior longitudinal ligament complex. Noncontained herniations consist of nuclear material that has extended through the outer complex into the epidural space. If the herniated nuclear material remains continuous with that within the disk, the term *extrusion* should be used. If the epidural fragment is discontinuous, a "free fragment" or "sequestration" exists. The free fragment often migrates either cranial or caudal to the level of the disk. The location of a herniation may be described as (1) central, (2) posterolateral (meaning lateral to the midline but still within the spinal canal), (3) foraminal, or (4) extraforaminal or "far lateral," indicating a herniation lateral to the foramen.

The CT evaluation of the status of the lumbar disk and its relationship to the thecal sac and exiting nerve roots is made possible by the presence of epidural fat in the spinal canal at the disk levels. The disk is of slightly higher CT density than the thecal sac, enabling the interface between the disk and the thecal sac to be distinguished on a CT scan in most cases. The normal configuration of the posterior aspect of the intervertebral disk from the L1-2

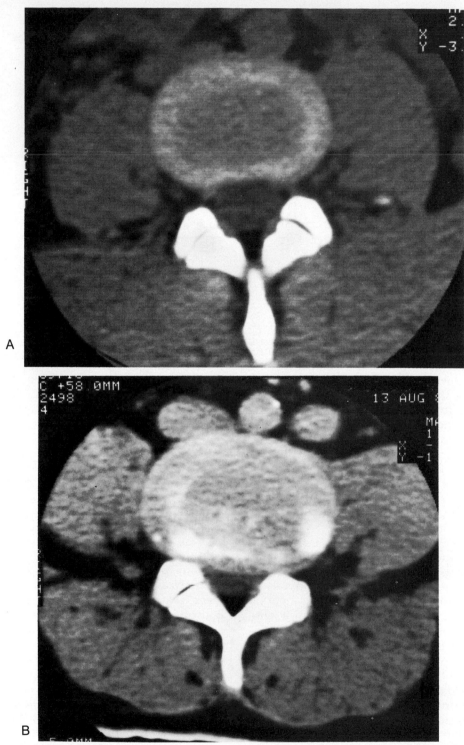

FIGURE 12–4 ■ *A,* Normal L4-5 disk demonstrating posterior disk concavity. *B,* Diffuse annular bulge caused by loss of height from chronic degeneration.

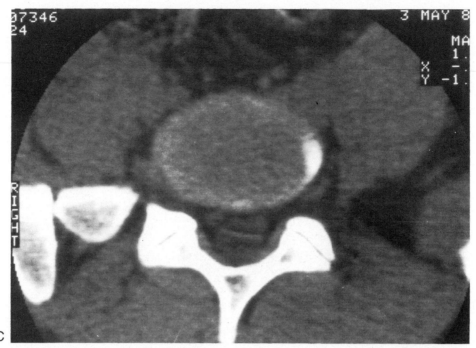

FIGURE 12–4 *Continued* ■ C, Normal L5-S1 disk showing a convex posterior disk border.

through the L4-5 level, as demonstrated on the axial views, is a slight concavity, which becomes flattened with increasing age (Fig. 12–4*A*). It is normal at these levels to visualize virtually no epidural fat separating the disk from the thecal sac. On sagittal views all disks are convex toward the thecal sac. In older patients it is not uncommon to see a mild increase in the degree of convexity, representing minor diffuse annular bulge. We believe, however, that this rarely causes symptoms of neural compression, even when there is slight indentation of the thecal sac (see Fig. 12–4*B*). At the L5-S1 level, the posterior aspect of the normal intervertebral disk has a convex border (see Fig. 12–4*C*). However, abundant epidural fat frequently is present, separating the posterior margin of the disk and the anterior aspect of the thecal sac and S1 roots.[4] Occasionally either the central bony prominence present at the superior S1 segment or merely the lordosis present at the L5-S1 junction presents an image on axial CT images that suggests that the normal disk is protruding centrally. This is a normal variant.

DISK HERNIATION

In contrast to a diffuse annular or concentric protrusion, herniation refers to a disk in which some of the annular fibers are severed, allowing movement of at least some nucleus away from its normal central location (Fig. 12–5).

In a contained intervertebral disk herniation, the displaced nuclear material is confined solely by the outermost fibers of the annulus. The extruded intervertebral disk herniation is one in which the displaced nuclear material has burst through the posterior investing ligament (Fig. 12–6). On axial images the posterior border of the disk has a lumpy or nodular bulge. When large, the extruding disk may touch the thecal sac or the nerve roots. Thecal impingement is clinically irrelevant if there is no associated nerve root compression. In the case of the sequestrated disk, nuclear material may be extruded through the posterior fibers of the annulus and through or around the posterior longitudinal ligament. The fragment lies free in the spinal canal. An extruded disk may therefore be associated with a sequestrated fragment that may remain trapped between a nerve root and the disk or migrate from the site of rupture (Fig. 12–7). The sequestrated fragment may come to lie behind the vertebral body above or below the disk, in the axilla, on the nerve root, in the intervertebral foramen, or in the midline anterior to the dural sac (Fig. 12–8). On occasion, this unattached disk fragment may actually erode or burst through the dura.[4] In L5-S1 lumbar disk rupture, the obliteration of the anterolaterally located epidural fat is the earliest finding on CT. The epidural fat that intervenes between the encroaching disk and neural components must first be displaced before contact between them can occur. The degree of distortion of the normal contour of the thecal sac by the disk, the degree of displacement of the nerve root by the disk, or both, are of high diagnostic importance. Obliteration of epidural fat in the absence of both of these signs suggests abnormality of the disk but does not imply clinical neural compression. Displacement of a nerve root is more commonly appreciated at L5-S1, where the S1 nerve root is usually easily distinguished from the thecal sac. Enlargement of the

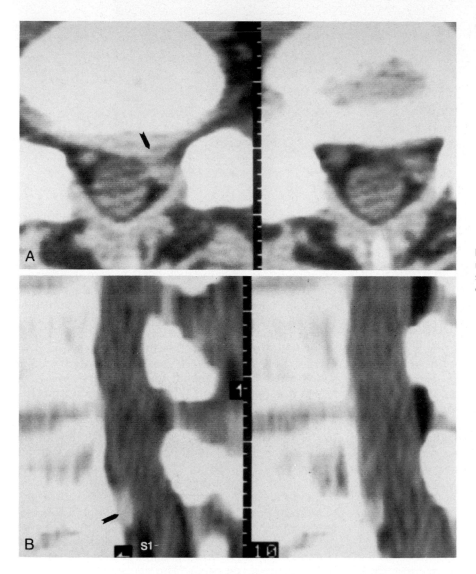

FIGURE 12–5 ■ Axial CT scan *(A)* and lateral reformation *(B)* showing an extruded left-sided L5-S1 disk fragment with displacement of the left S1 nerve root *(arrows)*.

FIGURE 12–6 ■ Axial T1-weighted *(A)*, lateral proton density *(B*, left), and T2-weighted *(B*, right) MRI showing extruded intervertebral disk. Note the torn annular fibers *(arrows)*.

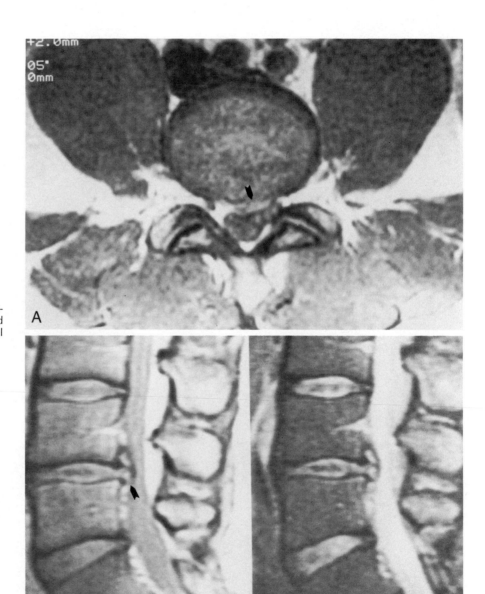

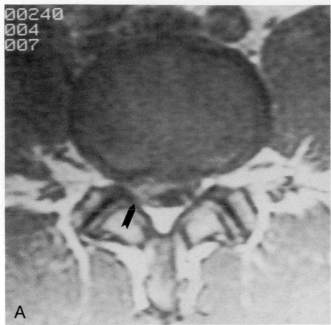

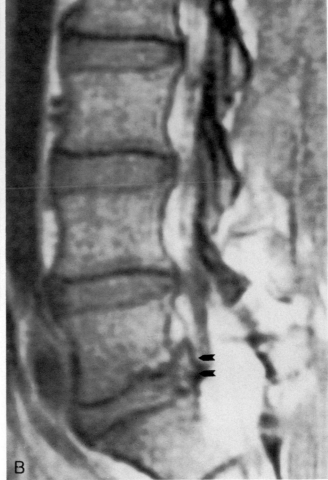

FIGURE 12–7 ■ Axial *(A)* and lateral *(B)* T1-weighted MR scans demonstrating an extruded disk fragment that has partially migrated behind the L5 vertebral body, compressing the right S1 nerve root against the facet *(arrows)*.

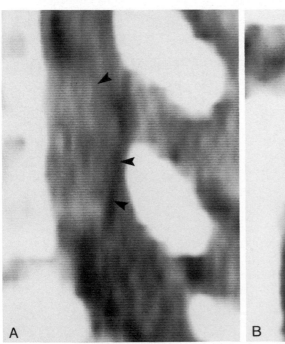

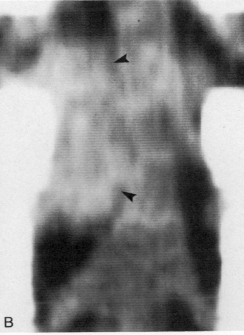

FIGURE 12–8 ■ Lateral *(A)* and curved coronal *(B)* CT reformations demonstrating a huge, totally extruded nuclear fragment that has migrated up behind the L5 vertebral body and displaced the theca to the right *(arrowheads)*.

irritated nerve root may serve as a confirmatory finding. The absolute size of the disk herniation itself has been found to be less meaningful.

It is helpful for the radiologist to correlate clinical information with the findings on the CT or MRI examinations. In order to focus attention on the appropriate anatomical region, familiarity with the relevant spinal anatomy is mandatory. The first seven of the cervical nerve roots exit above the associated vertebral body. The eighth cervical nerve exits below the C7 pedicle. Distal to the T1 vertebra, the nerve roots exit just below the pedicle. In the region of the cauda equina, the nerve roots course obliquely over the intervertebral disk to emerge through the foramina of the vertebra below.

The L4 nerve root exits below the pedicle of L4 and usually escapes compression by the disk that lies between the L4 and L5 vertebrae. It is the L5 nerve root, however, that is most at risk from being compressed by the L4-5 disk. Analogously, therefore, herniation of the L5-S1 disk frequently compresses the first sacral root.

On axial images it is important to trace the extent of an abnormal disk both cephalic and caudal to the disk level itself. Occasionally a laterally herniated nucleus pulposus migrates up into the lateral recess and compresses the nerve root just rostral to the disk space. Similarly, the caudal extent of a disk bulge or herniation may contribute to compromise of the central canal or a lateral recess at the vertebral body level just distal to the disk space.

Nuclear material may herniate anywhere around the circumference of the disk. Disk herniation commonly occurs within or just at the outer margin of the neural foramen, where the disk may compress the sensitive dorsal root ganglion of the exiting nerve.[5] It should be stressed that a foraminal disk fragment compresses the nerve one level higher than usually suspected. For example, a disk fragment within the L3-4 neural foramen causes pain radiating to the thigh above the knee. This is usually associated with an L2-3 central disk herniation.

It is theoretically possible for a far lateral nuclear fragment to compress the root descending from one level higher as it courses past the disk space (Fig. 12-9).

Compression of more than one nerve root may be seen when a large herniation compromises not only the nerve root crossing obliquely behind the disk, but also the nerve exiting through the foramen just cranial to it. Similarly, migration of a sequestered fragment in either a cranial or caudal direction may involve more than one root. A massive central herniation may involve several roots in the cauda equina and result in bowel and bladder paralysis. This type of lesion is more commonly seen at the L4-5 level.[4] On axial CT examination the diagnosis of a massive central herniation may be a difficult one, unless a higher density of the intraspinal canal contents is recognized.

Sometimes bony osteophytes from the vertebral end plates or calcification of the annulus fibrosus is noted (Fig. 12-10). Use of sagittal reformations should readily allow distinction among a calcified annulus fibrosus, a calcified nucleus pulposus, an osteophytic spur, and a posterior limbus vertebra (fracture of the posterior apophyseal ring by a posterior, superior, or inferior herniation of disk) (Fig. 12-11). Less commonly, protrusion of a gas-containing disk into the central canal or neural foramen is seen. On the CT scout view or the conventional radiograph, such a disk may manifest a "vacuum" phenomenon that is difficult to identify on an MR examination.

CT reformations can demonstrate the disk in the sagittal plane so that adjacent levels can be compared with each other. The higher CT density disk is often more apparent on sagittal than on axial views. However, specific information as to the presence of the disk degeneration and the position of the nucleus are not demonstrated on CT.

MRI has added a new dimension to the diagnosis of disk disease. The criteria discussed previously for CT also apply to MRI. However, MRI can readily detect disk degeneration in patients in whom CT has failed to demonstrate it. MRI, both with and without intravenous gadopentetate dimeglumine, has also demonstrated fissures in the architecture of annulus fibrosus—findings not detected by CT.[6, 7] The MRI diagnosis of disk degeneration is made by the presence of lower than normal nucleus pulposus signal intensity on T2-weighted sagittal images (Fig. 12-12).[8] This finding reflects the reduced number of hydrogen atoms present in degenerated disks, which have lower water content than a normal disk. The sagittal plane permits comparison of the degenerated levels with normal levels in one image.

With CT the posterior contour of the disk and the disk space height are the primary determinants of differentiation between degeneration and herniation. With MRI, however, extension of the high-signal-intensity nucleus pulposus through the torn low-signal-intensity annulus fibrosus can frequently be directly visualized. When this finding is present, a herniated nucleus pulposus can be diagnosed with certainty. Thus the differentiation between disk herniation and disk degeneration can usually be made with greater certainty with MRI than with CT. Inflammatory reaction adjacent to a herniated nucleus pulposus may cause the fragment to imbibe water and thereby become relatively well hydrated. The herniated portion of the nucleus pulposus therefore appears high in signal intensity (Fig. 12-13).[9] Long-standing extruded nuclear fragments are degenerated and appear low in signal intensity.

It is important to realize that loss of signal intensity in the nucleus pulposus is extremely common in asymptomatic patients. In fact, in one study degeneration or bulging of at least one lumbar disk level was present in 35 per cent of asymptomatic patients between 20 and 39 years old, in 59 per cent of asymptomatic patients between 40 and 59 years old,

Text continued on page 491

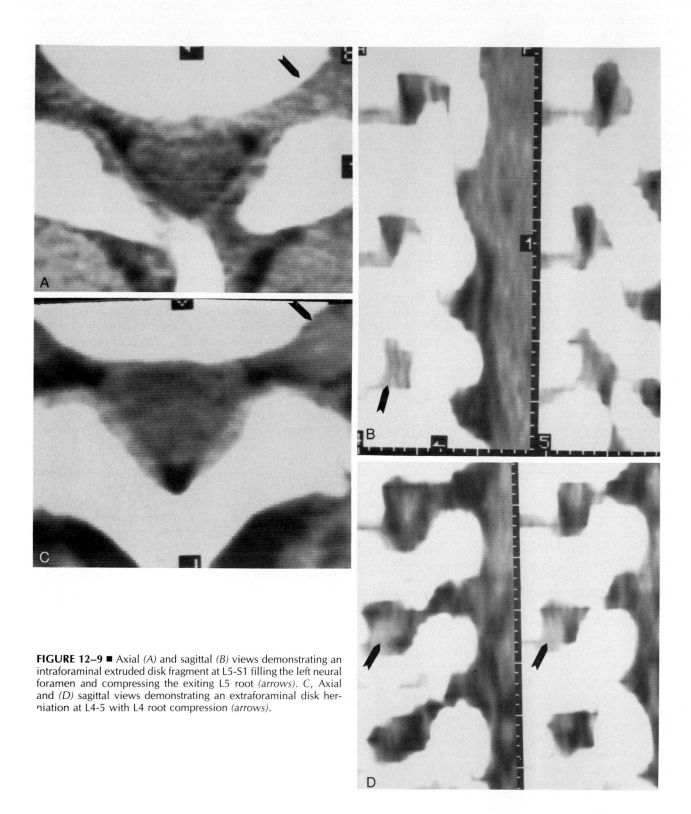

FIGURE 12–9 ■ Axial *(A)* and sagittal *(B)* views demonstrating an intraforaminal extruded disk fragment at L5-S1 filling the left neural foramen and compressing the exiting L5 root *(arrows)*. C, Axial and *(D)* sagittal views demonstrating an extraforaminal disk herniation at L4-5 with L4 root compression *(arrows)*.

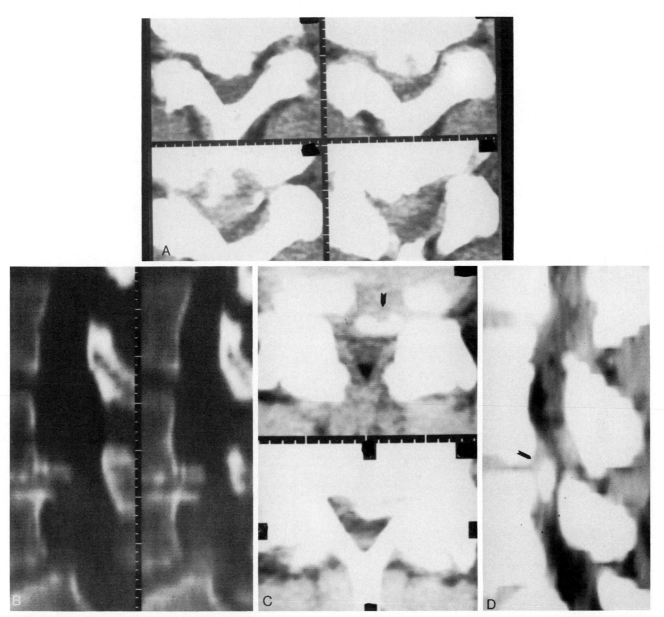

FIGURE 12–10 ■ Axial *(A)* and lateral *(B)* reformations showing a large disk herniation with an apparent calcification on the axial views. The lateral reformatted bone window images demonstrate bony ridges arising from both the superior end plate of L5 and the inferior end plate of L4 in association with this very large disk herniation. This indicates that this is a very long-standing lesion. Axial *(C)* and sagittal *(D)* CT images reveal calcified nuclear herniation. Note that the calcification has no attachment to bone.

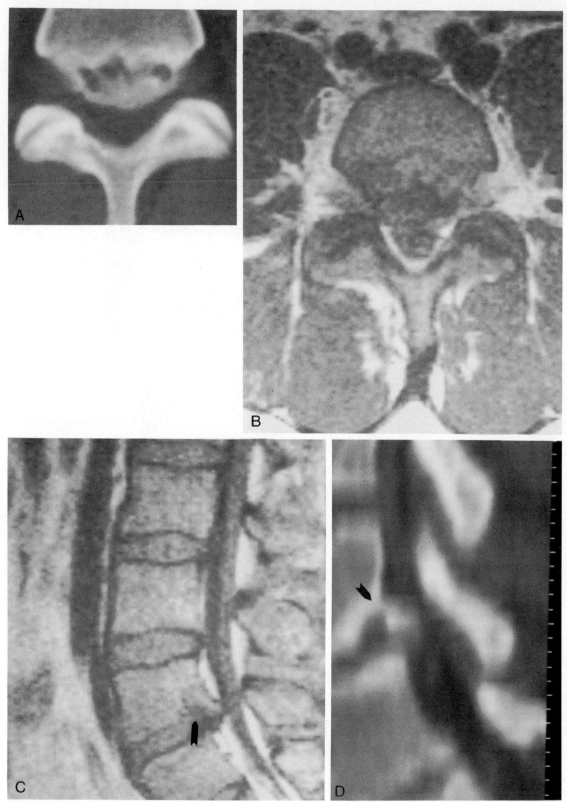

FIGURE 12–11 ■ Axial CT *(A)* and MRI *(B)* scans of a patient with posterior limbus vertebra. On these axial views it is difficult to distinguish a degenerative bony ridge or calcified nuclear herniation from a fracture of the apophyseal ring. Lateral MRI *(C)* and CT *(D)* scan show obvious fracture of the vertebral apophyseal ring, with disk herniation into the vertebra.

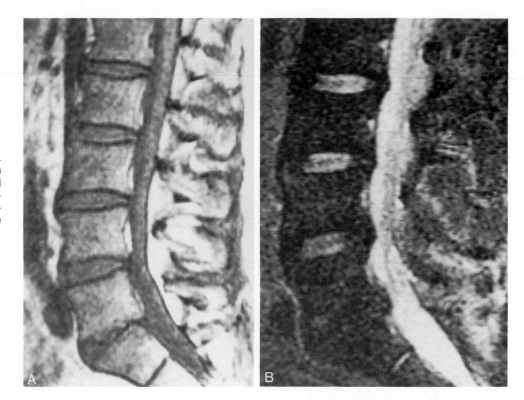

FIGURE 12–12 ■ Lateral T1-weighted *(A)* and T2-weighted *(B)* MRI views reveal narrowing and loss of the normal nucleus pulposus signal intensity within the L5-S1 disk. There is some dehydration of the other disks as well.

and 93 per cent of asymptomatic patients between 60 and 90 years old.[10] Loss of disk signal intensity is therefore a poor indicator of symptoms.

Conjoint nerve roots,[11] although usually only an asymptomatic anomaly, are important to identify for two reasons (Fig. 12–14). Preoperative recognition of the presence of conjoint roots permits the surgeon to avoid injury to one of the roots. As the surgeon moves the more superior of the two conjoint nerves away from the field, inadvertent traction on the attached, more inferior nerve root may damage it. Secondly, a small, strategically located disk bulge of insufficient size to ordinarily cause symptoms may impinge on one or both of the crowded conjoint roots to produce rather significant clinical findings.

Conjoint nerve roots may appear on the axial CT image to represent a normal nerve root and an adjacent disk fragment. However, identification of the "fragment" as having the same CT density as other exiting nerve roots should help avoid this pitfall. Recognition on the axial images of enlargement of the lateral recess adjacent to the conjoint roots should, when present, be confirmatory.

Another potential pitfall to be avoided is mistaking the CT appearance of an epidural hematoma for either a free disk fragment or, less likely, a spinal tumor. The nontraumatic epidural hematoma is thought to occur as a result of tearing of epidural veins resulting from a modest torsion injury which, in turn, results from minor annular disruption or facet disease. Patients with nontraumatic epidural hematoma frequently present with symptoms indistinguishable from those of a herniated disk, symptoms that regress more quickly and without surgery.

Although the CT density of a hematoma is similar to that of nearby neural elements on CT, the bright signal intensity of an acute epidural hematoma on both T1- and T2-weighted MR images is quite characteristic (Figs. 12–15 and 12–16).

Disk Disease of the Cervical Spine

The search for isolated cervical disk herniation should be initially addressed with MRI or noncontrast CT with reformations (Fig. 12–17). Intrathecal contrast-assisted CT is not necessary. CT with adjacent sagittal reformations also demonstrates not only cervical disk ruptures but also degenerative osteophytic ridges. CT may prove to be helpful for those patients (usually older or postoperative) who have a greater likelihood of bony or spinal stenosis or significant facet arthritis. MRI is the study of choice for the patient who is unlikely to demonstrate significant pathologic bony abnormality or for the patient with a possible ruptured disk (Fig. 12–18), but whose symptoms or clinical signs are also compatible with an intrinsic spinal cord abnormality.

It is difficult to recognize abnormal spinal ossification and small but significant cervical osteophytes, especially on the T1-weighted sagittal MRI images. An osteophyte that emanates from the posterior aspect of the vertebral end plate is thought to be secondary to disk degeneration. Sharpey's fibers connect from the outer portion of the annulus to the periosteum of the cortex of the adjacent vertebral body. Because the osteophyte and accompanying disk extend posteriorly, not only the annulus but

Text continued on page 496

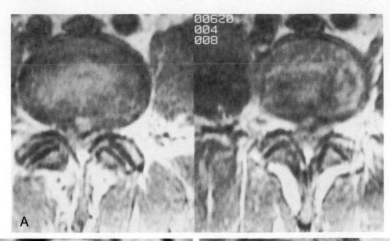

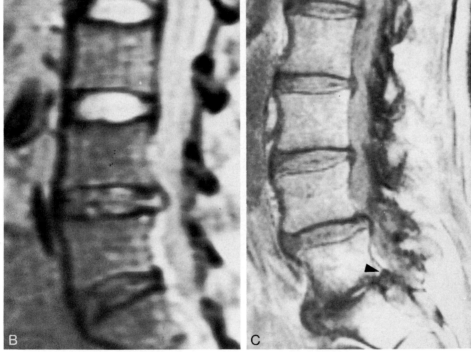

FIGURE 12–13 ■ Axial proton density *(A)* and sagittal T2-weighted *(B)* MR images demonstrate a loss of signal in the L5-S1 intervertebral disk space, indicating dehydration. At L4-5 there is a bright central herniation of disk, indicating an acute, well-hydrated extruded nuclear fragment. *C,* Sagittal image of a different patient with degenerated L4-5 and L5-S1 disks. Note the low signal intensity of the chronically dehydrated L5-S1 nucleus pulposus *(arrowhead).*

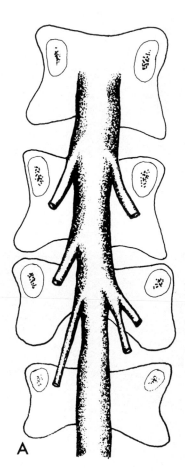

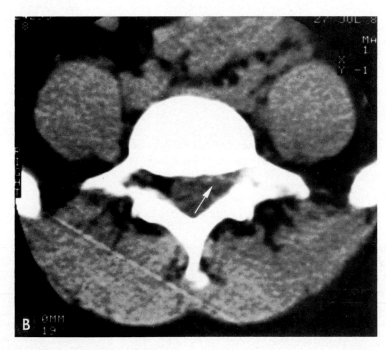

FIGURE 12–14 ■ Conjoined nerve. *A*, Schematically drawn. *B*, Conjoined nerve shown on axial CT image *(arrow)*.

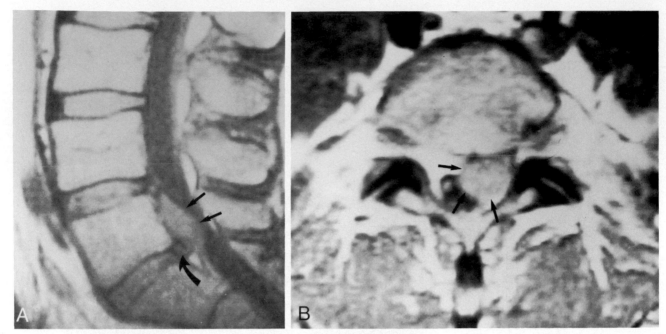

FIGURE 12–15 ■ Epidural hematoma. Sagittal *(A)* and axial *(B)* T1-weighted images demonstrate a large epidural mass *(arrows)* posterior to the L5 vertebral body. The mass is higher in signal intensity than the underlying central disk herniation at L5-S1 *(curved arrow)*. Surgery confirmed the presence of an epidural hematoma.

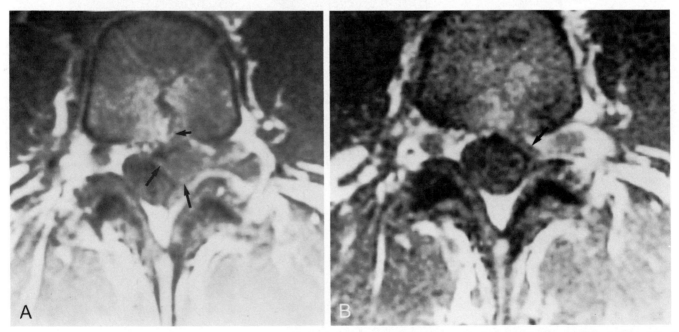

FIGURE 12–16 ■ Epidural hematoma with rapid resolution. The patient presented with sudden onset of severe left radiculopathy. A T1-weighted axial image *(A)* demonstrated a mass of moderate size, intermediate in signal intensity *(arrows)* posterior to the left side of the L4 vertebral body, adjacent to the insertion of the basivertebral vein *(arrowhead)*. The patient's radiculopathy rapidly resolved, and a repeat scan *(B)* 6 weeks later shows almost complete resolution of the mass with only a small residual scar *(arrow)*.

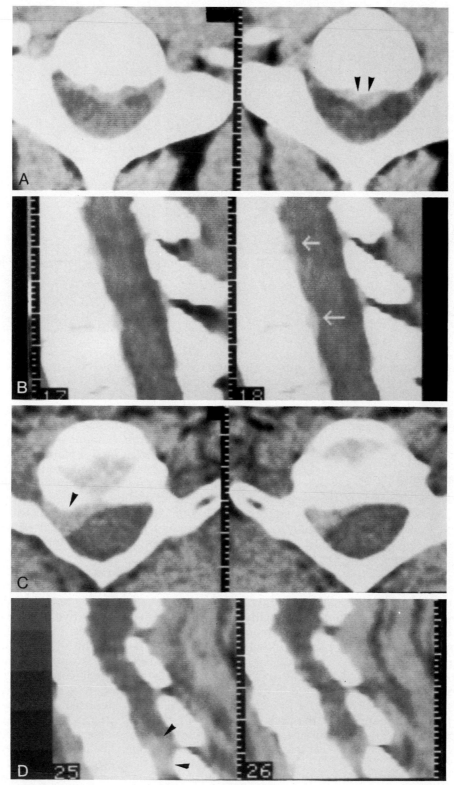

FIGURE 12–17 ■ Central cervical disk protrusion. *A,* Axial CT views demonstrate localized central protrusion of the C5-6 intervertebral disk *(arrowheads). B,* Sagittal reformations demonstrate the local protrusion and allow accurate measurement *(arrows).* Also note the smaller central protrusion at the level above *(arrows). C,* Axial cervical CT scans demonstrate a lateral extruded disk fragment at C5-6 on a different patient *(arrowhead). D,* Lateral reformations demonstrating nuclear fragment out in the lateral gutter *(arrowheads).*

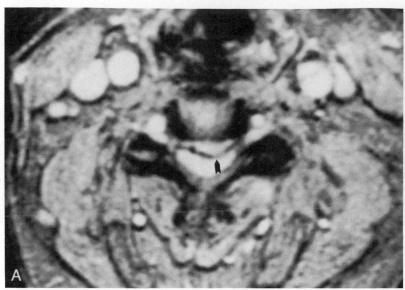

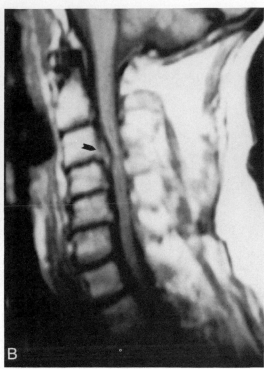

FIGURE 12–18 ■ Axial *(A)* and sagittal *(B)* MR images demonstrating C3-4 disk herniation *(arrow)*.

also the signal from the nucleus pulposus appears to extend posterior to the normal confines. This appearance can easily be misdiagnosed as a disk herniation on MRI (Fig. 12–19). The correct diagnosis is that of a degenerated annular disk bulge and associated osteophyte.

Disk Disease of the Thoracic Spine

MRI is the study of choice for the diagnosis of thoracic disk herniation. A field of view as small as the clinical findings permit should be employed. The trade-off is between seeing a small portion of the thoracic spine in great detail or seeing virtually the entire thoracic spine but in a rather limited fashion. A large-field-of-view sagittal scan that demonstrates a suspicious, but not definite, abnormality should be followed by small-field-of-view axial and sagittal scans through the questionable region. The incidence of thoracic disk rupture is quite low compared with that of the lumbar spine. However, the proportion of abnormal disks that are calcified is higher in the thoracic spine than elsewhere. Therefore if a thoracic disk rupture is identified by MRI and the presence of calcium within the abnormal disk or the presence of a nearby osteophyte is deemed important, then a CT scan localized to the abnormal region may prove helpful.

Spinal Stenosis

A stenotic spinal canal may be defined as one that is abnormally narrowed by a pathologic condition (i.e., disk abnormality, tumor, or bony spurs). Spinal canal stenosis may be congenital or acquired. The term *congenital spinal stenosis* as a clinical entity refers to those patients with a congenitally small canal characterized by short pedicles, trefoil-shaped lateral recesses, and laminae that are more nearly parallel to the posterior element of the vertebral bodies. The congenital form may remain clinically quiescent until superimposed acquired stenosis involving degenerative disease of the motion segment renders the disease clinically symptomatic. Spinal stenosis can also be divided according to the location of spinal narrowing into central canal stenosis, lateral recess stenosis, and foraminal stenosis.

CENTRAL CANAL STENOSIS

The osteophytic changes of degenerative spondylosis, postoperative or posttraumatic osseous overgrowth, and degenerative spondylolisthesis are the most common acquired causes of central canal stenosis (Fig. 12–20). The differentiation of spinal stenosis from congenital and acquired disorders compromising the spinal cord and nerve roots is an important application of computed tomography and MRI. In spinal stenosis, the cross-sectional display of CT permits precise definition of the critically important transverse configuration and size of the canal. Although axial measurements of the anteroposterior, transverse, and cross-sectional area of the lumbar spinal canal have been documented, the application and interpretation of such measurements can be difficult.[12, 13] Wide biologic variation in these measurements makes differentiation between a given patient and a normal population difficult in many cases. In addition, because the window settings of a

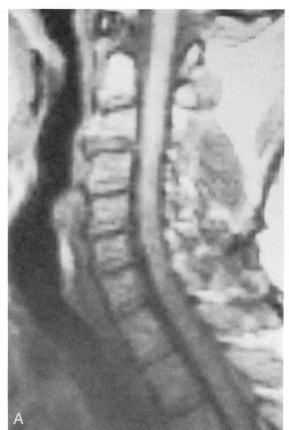

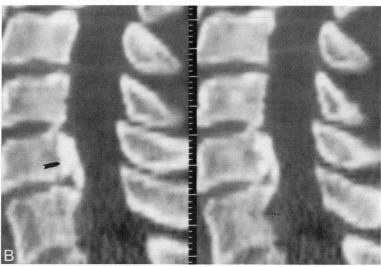

FIGURE 12–19 ■ Sagittal MR scan *(A)* and sagittal CT reformation *(B)* from a patient with severe degenerative disease of the C5-6 disk space with mild disk bulge. MRI fails to demonstrate a very large central ridge of bone. CT does define the lesion as a large area of posterior longitudinal ligament ossification with central canal stenosis *(arrow)*.

FIGURE 12–20 ■ Axial views of central spinal stenosis of the lumbar spine. Note calcification of the ligamentum flavum and bony overgrowth of the articular processes.

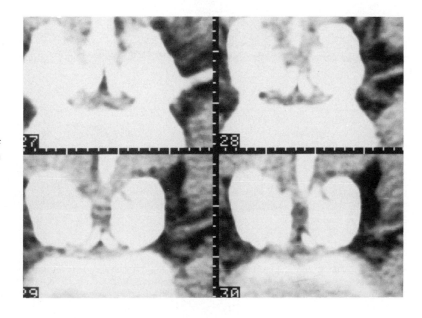

given scanner can affect the linear and area measurements, calibration of the scanner with a phantom of known dimension should be undertaken. In practice, the physician should not rely solely on the measurement of the osseous canal. A qualitative assessment based on how much room the bony canal appears to have to accommodate the neural structures should determine the presence and severity of spinal stenosis. Isolated ligamentum flavum prominence (with normal facet joints) is a rare benign finding that of itself does not cause symptoms.

Paraarticular soft tissue swelling involving the medial aspect of the facet joint and accompanying inflammatory or degenerative arthritis can cause significant central canal compromise. This inflammation of the joint capsule and adjacent ligamentum flavum is often erroneously referred to as *ligamentum flavum hypertrophy* (Fig. 12–21).

LATERAL RECESS STENOSIS

The lateral recess is an area bordered laterally by the pedicle, posteriorly by the superior articular facet, and anteriorly by the posterolateral surface of the vertebral body. The superior aspect of the pedicle marks the level where the lateral recess is most narrow. This is a consequence of the relatively anterior position of the horizontal portion of the supe-

rior articular facet at this point. Therefore it is at the more cephalic aspect of the superior articular facet that hypertrophy is likely to result in nerve root compression (Fig. 12–22). It is here that the anteroposterior dimension of the lateral recess should be measured if measurements are being made.[13, 14]

FORAMINAL STENOSIS

The neural foramina are optimally assessed on sagittal MRI or CT reformations (Fig. 12–23). Both soft tissue and bony encroachment are apparent in this plane. The mere presence of either bone or soft tissue in the neural foramen is not commensurate with symptomatic neural impingement. The sagittal cross-sectional dimensions of the neural foramen are normally approximately six times those of the cross-sectional area of the exiting nerve. Therefore actual contact between the bony spur or disk and the nerve root should be identified before neural impingement is even considered.

The CT evaluation of patency of the neural foramen requires a series of contiguous scans, beginning at the level of the inferior surface of the pedicle and extending through the disk level. Generally the nerve roots appear well outlined by epidural fat immediately adjacent to the inner aspect of the inferior pedicle in the region of the lateral recess. In sections

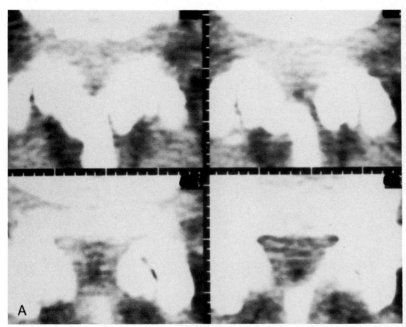

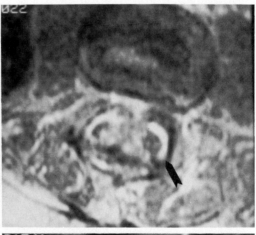

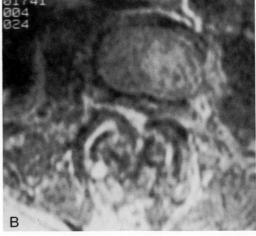

FIGURE 12–21 ■ Joint capsule enlargement. *A*, Axial CT demonstrates the marked paraarticular soft tissue swelling causing severe central canal stenosis. *B*, Axial T2-weighted MR scans demonstrate bilateral facet joint effusion *(arrow)*.

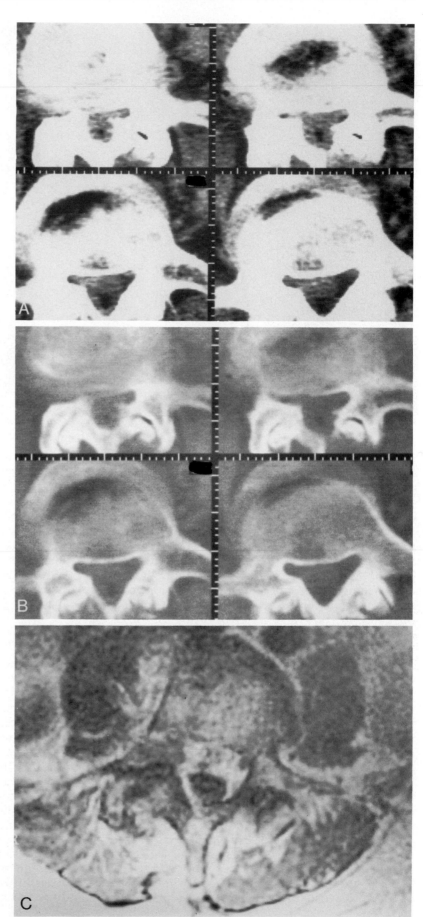

FIGURE 12–22 ■ Soft tissue *(A)* and bone window *(B)* axial CT scans showing severe lumbar spinal stenosis. There is very severe destructive arthropathy of the facets with narrowing of the lateral recesses. Axial MR scan *(C)* of a different patient demonstrates severe facet degeneration.

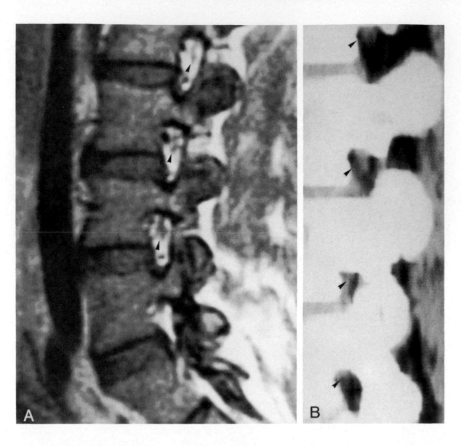

FIGURE 12–23 ■ Sagittal MR *(A)* and CT reformation *(B)* of a normal neural foramen. Note the exiting nerve roots surrounded by fat within the neural foramen *(arrowheads).*

immediately caudal to the lower surface of the pedicle, the neural foramen and the nerve root, which is surrounded by epidural fat, are well seen. As the physician proceeds further caudad, the neural foramina generally become smaller and finally end at the level of the superior surface of the pedicle of the next adjacent vertebra. The finding of a narrow neural foramen at the level of the end plate and the disk does not by itself indicate significant neural foraminal encroachment with nerve root compression, because the nerve generally exits slightly superior to the level of the disk. The entire series of contiguous axial CT or MR images must be evaluated to determine significant foraminal encroachment. Neurologically significant foraminal stenosis may be caused by any soft tissue or bony space–occupying lesion that compresses the nerve root as it exits from the central canal. Neural impingement caused by a bony spur intruding into the neural foramen is usually the result of either an osteophytic spur that has evolved over a considerable period of time or an acute episode (i.e., through some activity the patient has impaled the nerve on the spur, thereby causing acute symptoms). The MRI or CT findings of bone in the neural canal demonstrate the chronic underlying cause that predisposes a particular patient to sciatic symptoms (Fig. 12–24). Bony encroachment may be caused by an osteophyte from the posteroinferior aspect of the vertebral body or the anterosuperior aspect of the superior articular facet. In the overwhelming majority of instances, osteophytic compromise of the neural foramen is caused by a bone spur from the vertebral end plate rather than from the articular process.

Occasionally an important finding of a lateral herniating disk encroaching laterally on the exiting nerve root in the neural foramen may be encountered.[5] The encroachment is readily depicted by CT or MRI. It is very unlikely that diffuse bulging of the disk into the neural foramen will compress the exiting nerve. The only time in which even a moderate likelihood of neural compression occurs is with marked disk space narrowing.

Facet Joint Disease

Radiologic and orthopedic literature has emphasized the role of the lumbar apophyseal joint in causing low back pain and sciatica that is clinically indistinguishable from that caused by a herniated lumbar disk.[15–17] The facets produce symptoms by impingement when hypertrophic bone or an osteophyte encroaches on either a neural foramen or the central canal, compromising either an exiting or descending nerve root, respectively.

The apophyseal joint is surrounded by a synovial capsule that is innervated by branches of the posterior primary ramus from the dorsal root ganglion, with components from the level of the facet joint and the level immediately cranial to it. Inflammation and consequent destruction of the facet joint from osteoarthritis or other arthropathy has been shown to cause pain. These synovial joints may fill with fluid

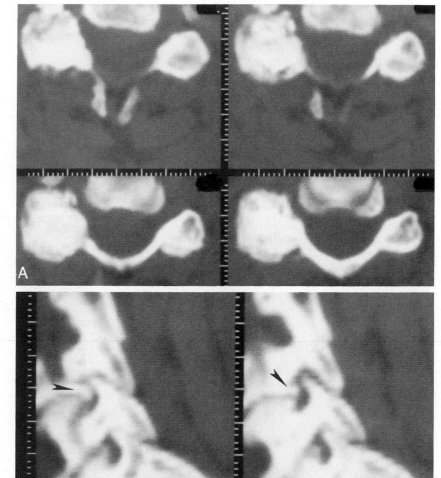

FIGURE 12–24 ■ Destructive facet arthropathy. *A*, Axial cervical CT showing very severe destructive hypertrophic changes of the right facet with foraminal compression. *B*, Cervical CT sagittal reformation demonstrates severe C5 and C6 foraminal stenosis. Note downward-projecting osteophytes *(arrowheads)*.

Illustration continued on following page

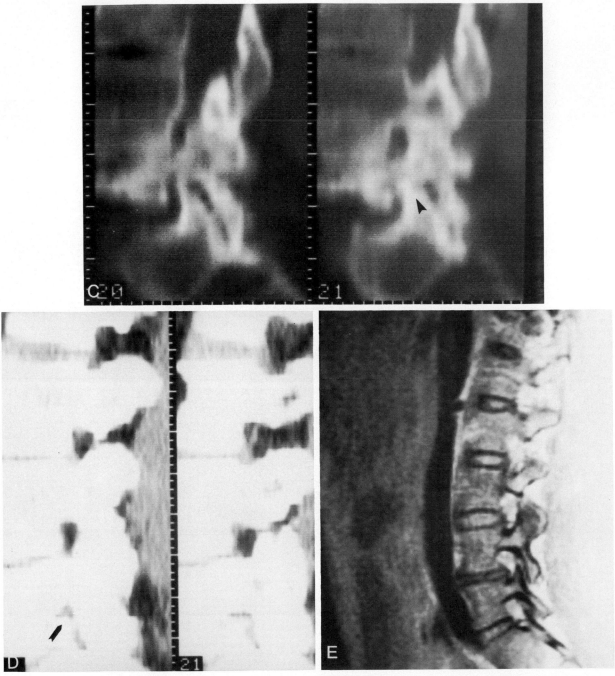

FIGURE 12–24 *Continued* ■ *C*, Sagittal lumbar CT reformation showing upward subluxation of the superior articular process of S1 into the L5 neural foramen *(arrowhead).* The patient complained of L5 radiculopathy. *D*, Lateral CT reformation of a patient with L5 radiculopathy resulting from bony foraminal stenosis. *E*, Sagittal MR scan showing diffuse bulge of the L4-5 disk into the inferior aspect of the neural foramen. Root compression is very unlikely.

and distend, leading to stimulation of the sensitive capsular nerve endings and subsequent pain (Fig. 12–25). Additionally, enlargement of the medial and lateral facet joint recesses during the inflammatory episode may impinge on the lumbar nerve root exiting through the nearby intervertebral foramen and the posterior ramus of the spinal nerve, respectively, thus accounting for the radicular pattern of facet pain and its similarity to pain caused by a herniated disk.

Spondylolysis

The presence of spondylolysis (pars defects), degree of neural foraminal narrowing, and amount of spondylolisthesis are best identified on sagittal CT reformations. They can be recognized on sagittal MR images, but not with the same sensitivity and certainty demonstrated on sagittal CT. Diffuse back pain in the patient with spondylolysis is most likely caused by the abnormal motion segment.

In contrast, radicular symptoms are caused by either neural compression from a bulging disk at the level above the pars fracture or a narrowed neural foramen at the level of the spondylolisthesis (Fig. 12–26). Sagittal images are of particular aid in assessing the presence of the neural foraminal stenosis in the patient with spondylolisthesis. The potential for entrapment of the exiting nerve by downwardly projecting callus from the pars pseudarthrosis is occasionally realized and is most readily seen on sagittal CT reformations.

Spondylolysis may be seen on axial CT scans. Bony defects in the pars interarticularis are more apparent when a spondylolisthesis is present. The bony defect, when accompanied by significant osseous overgrowth, can be mistaken for normal facet joints. However, careful attention to the anatomy of the articular processes as displayed on sequential axial scans should lead to the correct interpretation. The coronal orientation of most, but not all, of the bony

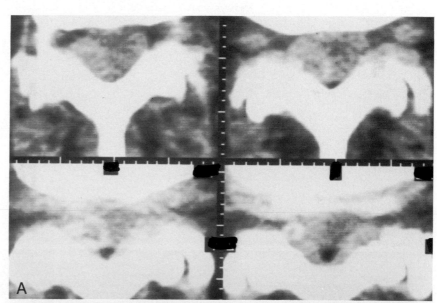

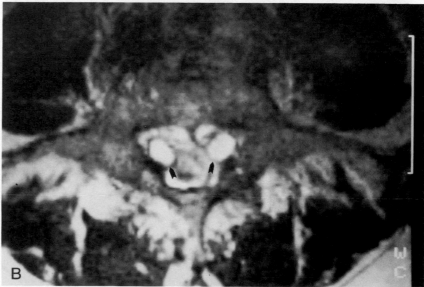

FIGURE 12–25 ■ *A*, Axial CT scan showing partially calcified synovial cyst causing profound spinal stenosis. *B*, Axial MR image of a different patient demonstrates fluid-filled synovial cysts *(arrows)*. (Courtesy of P. Berger, MD; W. Bradley, MD; and J. Amster, MD; Long Beach, CA.)

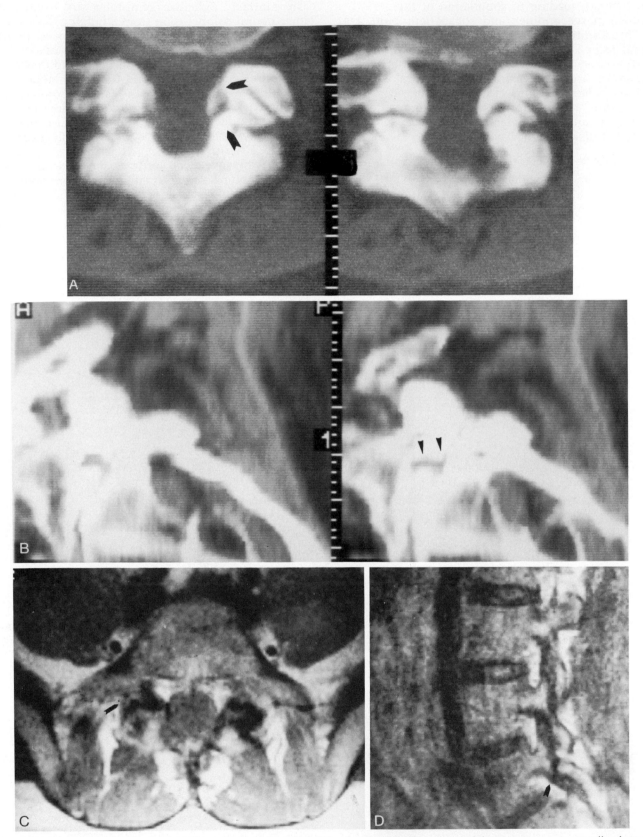

FIGURE 12–26 ■ Spondylolisthesis. Axial *(A)* and sagittal *(B)* reformations demonstrate bilateral pars defects. Note prominent callus from the pseudarthrosis *(arrows)*. Note also the characteristic deformity of the neural foramina. The foramina are horizontally oriented and flattened *(arrowheads)*. Axial *(C)* and sagittal *(D)* MR images of another patient demonstrate a region of low signal intensity in the area of the pars interarticularis *(arrows)*. (Courtesy of P. Berger, MD; W. Bradley, MD; and J. Amster, MD; Long Beach, CA.)

defects helps differentiate them from facets. Usually the transverse processes are visualized in the same scan slice as the pars defects, but are not seen at the level of the facet joints.

Spinal Neoplasia

The vast majority of neoplasms involving the spine are metastases or (less likely) primary tumors in patients who are neurologically intact. These patients are best evaluated with MRI.[18–21] A careful search for vertebral marrow replacement and extradural soft tissue masses using true T1-weighted images, as well as fat suppression MR techniques, should be made (Fig. 12–27). CT demonstrates bone destruction, as well as the tumor mass (see Fig. 12–27B,C).

Vertebral body compression as demonstrated on a conventional radiograph requires differentiation between compression resulting from trauma or osteoporosis and that caused by space-occupying lesions. The compressed vertebral body that retains a uniform MRI signal intensity can be presumed to be an old fracture of non-neoplastic origin. The vertebral body that demonstrates uniform low signal intensity or a mixed pattern of low and high signal intensities has a high probability of harboring a neoplasm, although this pattern is also compatible with an acute traumatic or osteoporotic fracture. Confirmation of abnormal findings and further delineation of bony detail with CT prior to instituting therapy may prove helpful (Fig. 12–28).

In those patients with neurologic symptoms, MRI is the study of choice. In difficult cases CT may provide additional information, such as the demonstration of tumor calcifications.

The most common benign spinal tumorous lesion is the vertebral hemangioma (Fig. 12–29).[22] It appears as a well-circumscribed, bright signal area within the marrow space, not only on T1- but also on T2-weighted images, thereby differentiating it from fat islands. It is very rare for a hemangioma to extend into the neural arch, except for the large cavernous hemangiomas. When this occurs, spinal compression may result.

Extradural lesions are well demonstrated by either CT or MRI. Lesions may be of high, intermediate, or low signal intensity, depending on the cell type and the presence of fat and calcium (Fig. 12–30).

Both intra- and extramedullary intradural tumors of the spinal cord should be evaluated first by MRI with the aid of gadopentetate dimeglumine. This should eliminate the need for myelography in nearly all patients (Fig. 12–31).

Multiple Sclerosis

On occasion, high-signal-intensity multiple sclerosis plaques may be identified in the cervical spinal cord (Fig. 12–32).[23] Real T2-weighted images, rather

Text continued on page 510

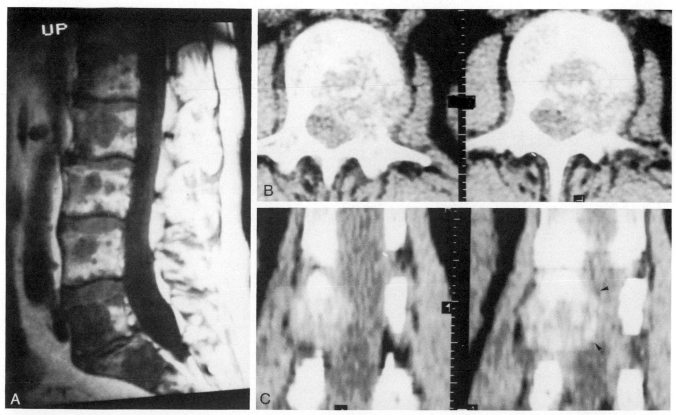

FIGURE 12–27 ■ Metastases to the spine. *A,* Sagittal T1-weighted MR image demonstrates replacement of the normal fatty marrow at multiple levels by low-signal-intensity tumor. Axial *(B)* and reformatted coronal *(C)* CT scans from a different patient demonstrate bone destruction and intraspinal tumor. (Courtesy of P. Berger, MD; W. Bradley, MD; and J. Amster, MD; Long Beach, CA.)

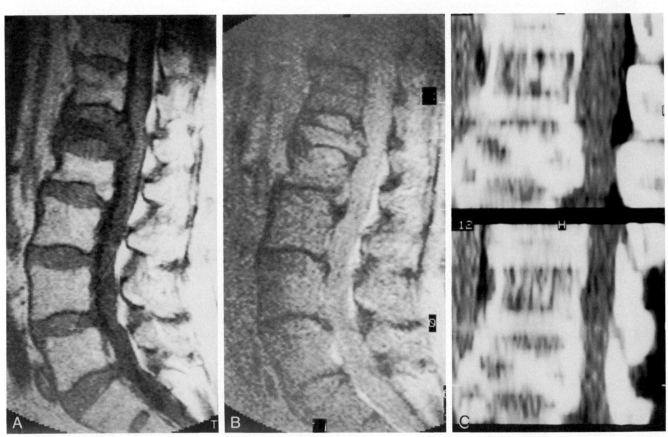

FIGURE 12–28 ■ Lateral T1- *(A)* and T2-weighted *(B)* images showing L1 and L2 vertebral compression. L2 is high in signal intensity, whereas L1 is low in signal intensity. Compression of both, however, is the result of severe osteoporosis. The upper fracture is more acute; the lower fracture was seen 1 year earlier. *C,* Sagittal reformatted CT scan demonstrates compression of the conus by bone rather than a soft tissue mass.

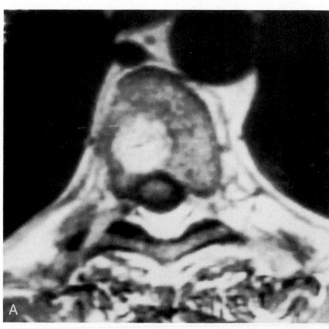

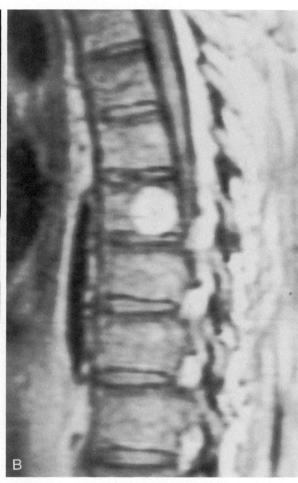

FIGURE 12–29 ■ Benign intraspinal hemangioma. Axial (A) and lateral (B) T1-weighted MR images.

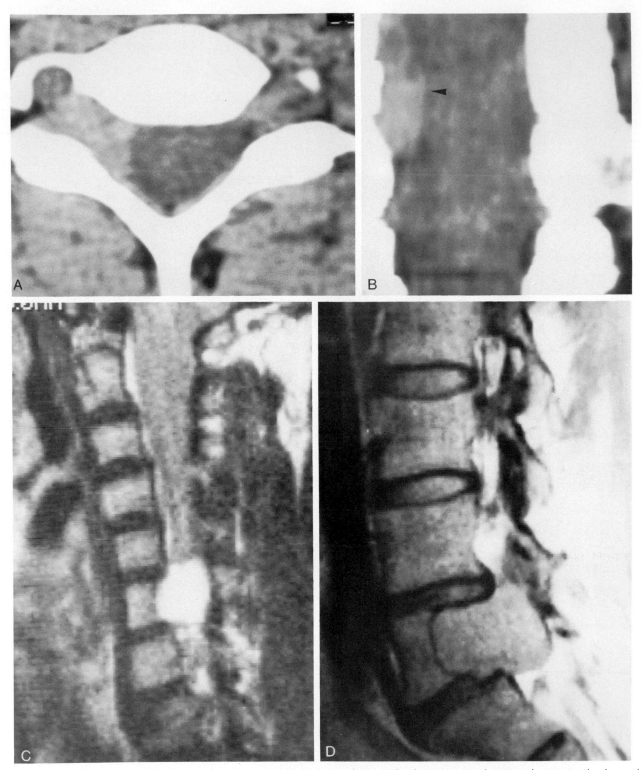

FIGURE 12–30 ■ Axial CT scan *(A)*, coronal reformation scan *(B)*, and sagittal T2-weighted MR scan *(C)* showing a large, extradural, very high signal tumor mass, cell type unproven. *D*, Scan from another patient with a large, intermediate-signal neurofibroma that caused erosion and modeling of the vertebral body. (Courtesy of P. Berger, MD; W. Bradley, MD; and J. Amster, MD; Long Beach, CA.)

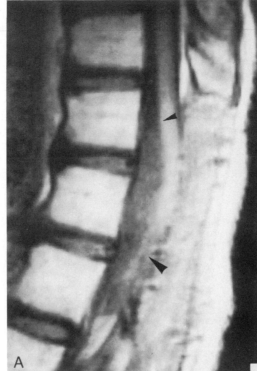
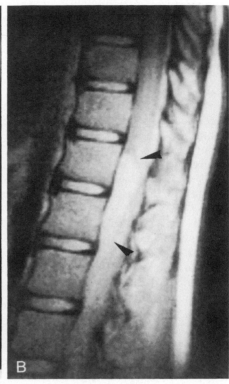

FIGURE 12–31 ■ Intrinsic glioma of the spinal cord. Lateral T1- *(A)* and T2-weighted *(B)* MR images demonstrate expansion of the spinal cord with exophytic tumor caused by ependymoma. (Courtesy of P. Berger, MD; W. Bradley, MD; and J. Amster, MD; Long Beach, CA.)

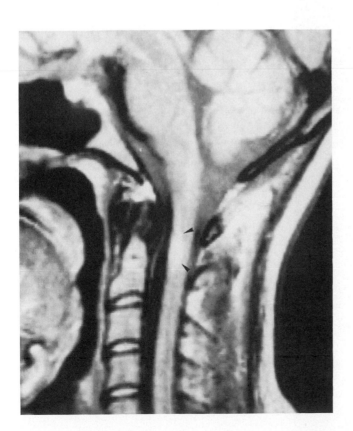

FIGURE 12–32 ■ Latent proton density MR scan reveals a localized swelling of the spinal cord at the C1 level. There is a zone of bright signal within the anterior portion of the cord *(arrows)*, indicating demyelination.

than gradient-echo images, are needed for evaluation of intrinsic spinal cord abnormality. Gadopentetate dimeglumine enhancement of multiple sclerosis lesions may enable easy identification of plaques undetected by routine MR.[24]

Inflammation

ARACHNOIDITIS

Arachnoidal adhesions are a nonspecific inflammatory response to a variety of infectious or chemical irritants. Blood and iophendylate (Pantopaque) are the most common causes, and together they have a synergistic effect in producing adhesions. Arachnoiditis is characterized by the deposition of immature collagen in the arachnoid and adjacent subarachnoid space.

MRI has replaced myelography and intrathecal contrast–assisted CT as the initial study of choice for the detection of arachnoiditis.[25] Both T1-[21] and T2-weighted images are routinely employed. The inflammatory tissue demonstrates a signal intensity that is higher than that of the surrounding cerebral spinal fluid on the T1-weighted images.

The T2-weighted images permit easier recognition of the distribution of the nerve roots within the thecal sac. Correlation with the T1-weighted images should prevent overlooking inflammatory tissues that are similar in signal intensity and therefore visually merge with the adjacent intrathecal spinal fluid.[26]

In this setting, MRI demonstrates, with progressively more advanced disease, clumps of nerve roots centrally positioned within the thecal sac (Fig. 12–33), peripheral adherence of nerve roots to the meninges, and in extreme cases, soft tissue masses replacing a majority of the subarachnoid space. These findings are usually noted below the L3 level and extend over at least two vertebral body segments. Rarely, calcification of the dura is seen in severe cases. Calcific arachnoiditis is often a severe symptomatic disorder with no surgical cure (Fig. 12–34). Arachnoiditis is considered to be absent if the nerve roots are well delineated and appear normal. If the MR examination fails to demonstrate the nerve roots

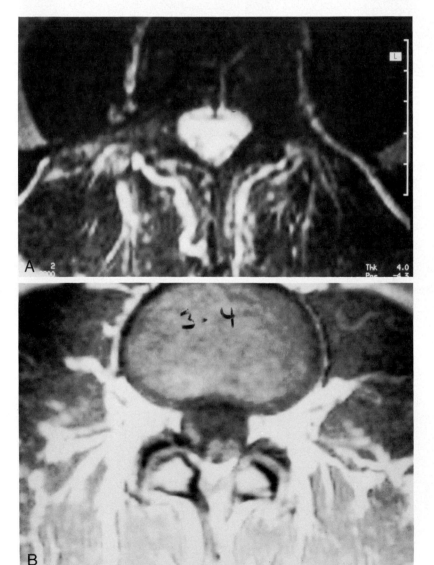

FIGURE 12–33 ■ *A*, Axial T2-weighted image demonstrates normal nerve roots floating within the cerebrospinal fluid at the dependent portion of the thecal sac. *B*, Axial T1-weighted MR images demonstrate posterior intrathecal clumping of nerve roots, indicative of arachnoiditis. (Courtesy of P. Berger, MD; W. Bradley, MD; and J. Amster, MD; Long Beach, CA.)

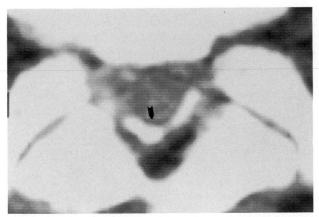

FIGURE 12–34 ■ Calcific arachnoiditis. Axial CT scan demonstrates the ringlike calcification within the dura *(arrow)*.

adequately and the patient is suspected of having arachnoiditis, then intrathecal contrast–assisted CT is the next appropriate step.

Disk Space Infection

Disk space infection is assessed by T1- and T2-weighted MRI images. The sagittal imaging plane usually proves to be the most helpful. Characteristically, T1-weighted images demonstrate diminished signal intensity of the vertebral disks and adjacent involved vertebral bodies. The additional finding of indistinct cortical end plates is helpful in identifying the presence of infection and differentiating it from degenerative disease. On the axial images, induration

or an indistinctness to the separation in soft tissue planes is another sign of infection. The T2-weighted images usually demonstrate, in the case of pyogenic infection, increased signal intensity in the vertebral disks and adjacent involved vertebral bodies (Fig. 12–35).

Spinal Abscess

A study by Post and co-workers has suggested that the use of intravenous gadopentetate dimeglumine will better define the limits of a spinal abscess already identified on precontrast T2-weighted images and will make the diagnosis and extent of a disk space infection and/or adjacent spinal abscess easier to diagnose (Fig. 12–36).[27]

The appearance of spinal infection with tuberculosis characteristically differs from that of pyogenic infection in that with tuberculosis no abnormal increased signal of the intervertebral disk space is observed on T2-weighted images.[28] With tuberculosis there is a predilection for involvement of the posterior elements and posterior aspects of the vertebral bodies and for involvement of more than two vertebral bodies. Additionally, large paraspinal soft tissue masses associated with tuberculosis are characteristically found (Fig. 12–37).

Computed tomography permits excellent study of involvement of the epidural and paraspinal regions, as well as the vertebrae and disks, by an infectious process. The distortion of fascial planes that is apparent in the immediate postspinal operation patient renders CT scan interpretation difficult. Soft tissue swelling often lasts 2 weeks. Postoperative infections

FIGURE 12–35 ■ Disk space infection. Lateral T1- *(A)* and T2-weighted *(B)* MR images demonstrate increased T2 intradiskal signal, indicating infection within the disk. Also demonstrated are a prevertebral abscess and vertebral osteomyelitis *(arrows)*. (Courtesy of P. Berger, MD; W. Bradley, MD; and J. Amster, MD; Long Beach, CA.)

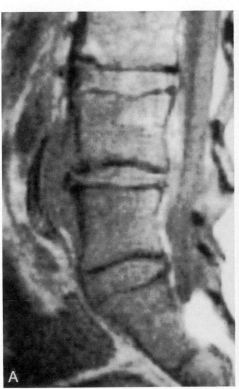
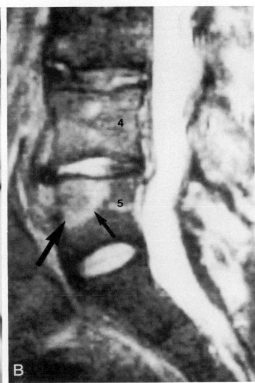

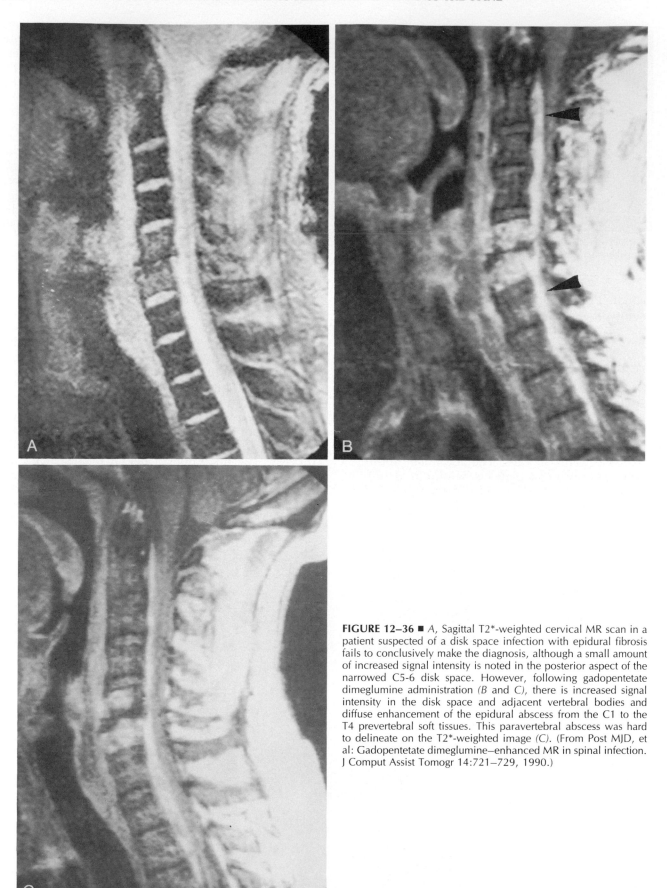

FIGURE 12–36 ■ *A,* Sagittal T2*-weighted cervical MR scan in a patient suspected of a disk space infection with epidural fibrosis fails to conclusively make the diagnosis, although a small amount of increased signal intensity is noted in the posterior aspect of the narrowed C5-6 disk space. However, following gadopentetate dimeglumine administration *(B* and *C),* there is increased signal intensity in the disk space and adjacent vertebral bodies and diffuse enhancement of the epidural abscess from the C1 to the T4 prevertebral soft tissues. This paravertebral abscess was hard to delineate on the T2*-weighted image *(C).* (From Post MJD, et al: Gadopentetate dimeglumine–enhanced MR in spinal infection. J Comput Assist Tomogr 14:721–729, 1990.)

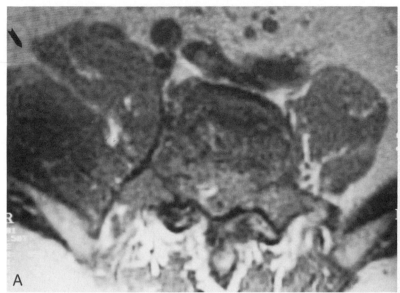
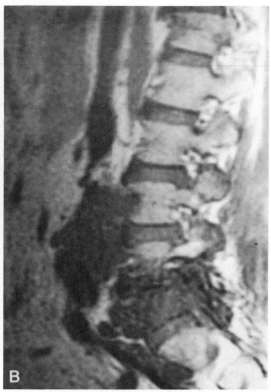

FIGURE 12–37 ■ Tuberculous osteomyelitis and diskitis. Axial *(A)* and sagittal *(B)* MR scans demonstrate low signal replacing the normal fatty marrow in the L5 vertebra. Note the large left psoas abscess and intraspinal mass.

generally become evident after this period. However, an increase in soft tissue swelling after the first postsurgical week may be regarded as suggestive of infection. Because both a resolving hematoma and an abscess can appear as a paraspinal mass with a central lucency, needle aspiration may be required for diagnosis. However, if at least 72 hours have elapsed since surgery, MRI is the modality of choice. In this setting the signal intensity of a hematoma is very bright on T1-weighted images, whereas the T1 signal intensity of an abscess is low to intermediate. On T2-weighted images, both abscesses and hematoma are bright in signal intensity and are therefore indistinguishable from one another.

Spinal Trauma

Proper treatment of the patient with an acutely traumatized spine rests on rapid, accurate, and thorough assessment of the injury.[29] Use of a high-resolution CT scanner for evaluation of the patient with a suspected spinal injury will expedite the institution of appropriate therapy.

Conventional radiographs remain the primary mode of examination following major spinal trauma. However, CT is the method of choice for studying integrity of the bony canal. If neurologic signs are present, MRI is the procedure of choice.

Spinal trauma may be thought of as having two components: orthopedic and neurologic. The orthopedic aspect of spinal trauma involves assessment of bony intregrity and both identification and localization of bony fragments. This orthopedic evaluation is best accomplished by CT with reformations (Fig. 12–38). The neurologic aspect of spinal trauma assessment refers to an assessment of the spinal cord and cauda equina. This evaluation is best performed by MRI (Figs. 12–39 and 12–40).

If a preoperative orthopedic decision is to be made, CT is the modality of choice. In the patient who has neurologic symptoms but normal plain films, MRI is the imaging modality of choice.

To reformat the axial CT scans into high-quality sagittal or coronal images, dynamic scanning with contiguous 1.5-mm-thick slices may be used. At the anatomically complex C1–2 level, the contiguous 1.5-mm slices are especially helpful, as correct diagnosis in this region often depends heavily on sagittal and coronal reformations (Fig. 12–41). This is particularly true for the nondisplaced transverse fracture of the dens. Sagittal reformations are routine in the remainder of the spine.

In this manner CT is an efficacious modality for the delineation of facet subluxation and fracture instability, the location of bony fragments within the spinal canal, and the existence of dural tears. Contrast-assisted CT provides the most accurate delineation of avulsion of a nerve root.

Failed Back Surgery Syndrome

The patient who is suffering from failed back surgery syndrome (FBSS) is likely to benefit from both modalities. MRI scans both prior and subsequent to the intravenous administration of gadopentetate dimeglumine are usually obtained first.

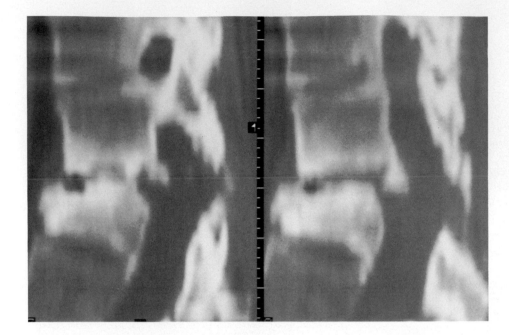

FIGURE 12–38 ■ Fracture of the lumbar spine. Lateral CT reformation reveals fracture-dislocation of the L1 vertebra.

FIGURE 12–39 ■ Sagittal craniocervical MR scan of a child who was born paraplegic. The differential diagnosis was between cerebral anoxia and spinal cord injury. The brain MR scan was normal. Craniocervical image demonstrates an atrophic area of the cervical-medullary junction resulting from birth trauma caused by hyperextension of the head (arrow).

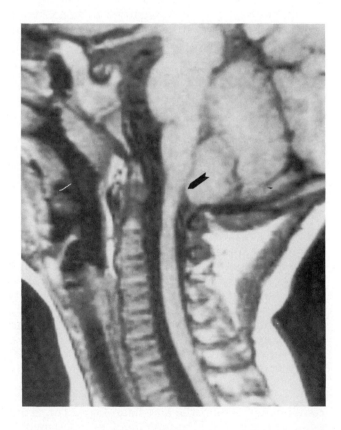

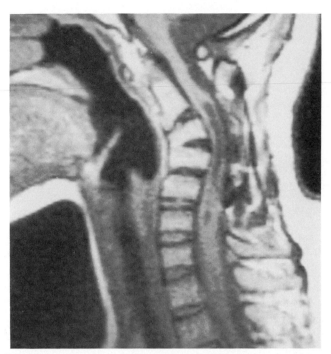

FIGURE 12–40 ■ Sagittal T1-weighted MR scan demonstrating a healed fracture of C3-4. There is a zone of low signal within the spinal cord, representing a posttraumatic syrinx.

The distinction between epidural fibrosis and recurrent disk herniation can often be made on unenhanced MR examination[3] on the basis of morphology, mass effect, and signal intensity. However, T1-weighted images taken immediately following intravenous injection of gadopentetate dimeglumine highlight the enhancement of the relatively vascular epidural fibrosis compared with the relatively avascular disk.[2] This method is currently considered the optimal way to differentiate scar from recurrent disk herniation. Gadopentetate dimeglumine permits easier recognition of the nerve roots and the contour of the thecal sac. This distinction between scar and disk can also be made on curved coronal CT reformations

by those experienced with this technique. The disk displaces neural elements as depicted on coronal reformations, whereas scar generally retracts the neural elements.

SPINAL FUSION

In the patient who is a candidate for fusion, the integrity of the disk above the planned levels of the fusion can be assessed by MRI. If the MRI scan shows the disk to be degenerated, an extension of the fusion can be considered.

Spinal instability is a frequent cause of pain in patients who have undergone surgical fusion. Fusion evaluation may be conceptually divided into evaluation of either structural or functional integrity. Structural integrity is indicated by firm attachment of an unbroken graft at each point of intended attachment. In contrast, functional stability implies that the surgically fused levels move together as one unit and no longer as separate segments. This must be evaluated with motion examinations.

The assessment of the patient suspected of having postfusion pseudarthrosis is optimally performed with CT, using complete multiplanar reformations extending in both the anteroposterior and transverse dimensions through the entire spinal fusion (Fig. 12–42). Both sagittal and curved coronal reformations are particularly helpful. In the patient studied solely for the purpose of structural fusion assessment, direct coronal CT images may be employed.[30] In the cervical spine, MRI often adequately depicts the structural integrity of an interbody fusion (Fig. 12–43). Occasionally the ferromagnetic material left behind from the surgical drill may cause severe artifacts (Fig. 12–44). Based on preliminary data, MRI appears to adequately assess functional stability after approximately 12 months have passed following surgical fusion.[31] Adjacent to the end plates of vertebral bodies included in the stable fusion on T1-weighted images are found subchondral bands of increased signal intensity, which on T2-weighted images are noted to be isointense or slightly hyperintense compared with normal marrow. In contrast, in fusion

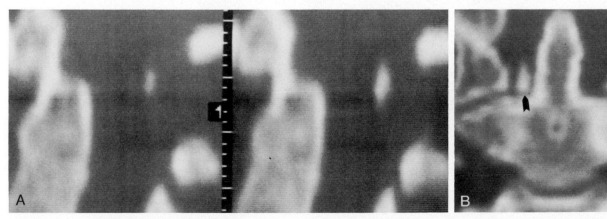

FIGURE 12–41 ■ *A*, Sagittal reformatted CT scan of a patient with a fracture through the base of the dens with near total dislocation. *B*, Coronal reformation demonstrating an avulsion fracture of the tubercle onto which the transverse ligament inserts. The tubercle and the end of the transverse ligament are displaced medially (*arrow*).

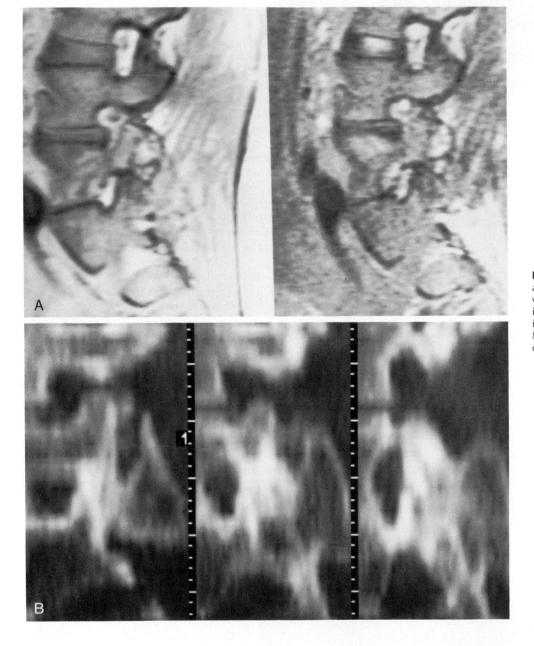

FIGURE 12–42 ■ Sagittal MR *(A)* and CT *(B)* scans from a patient with L5-S1 spine fusion. Note that it is very difficult to evaluate the integrity of the spine fusion on the MR image, but the sagittal CT scan clearly indicates solid fusion.

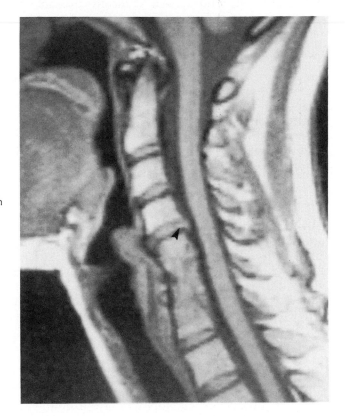

FIGURE 12–43 ■ Lateral T1-weighted MR scan showing solid C5 through C7 spine fusion with degenerative disk disease above the fusion.

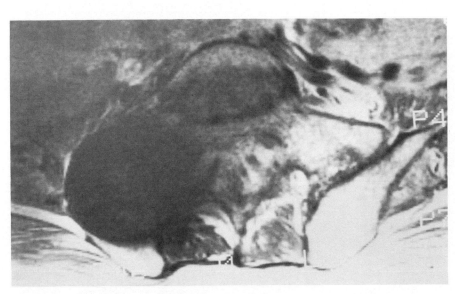

FIGURE 12–44 ■ Axial MR scan demonstrating metal artifacts in the area of the spine fusion.

instability, elements of low signal intensity on T1-weighted images become hyperintense on T2-weighted images. MRI is suggested for those post-fusion patients who appear clinically unstable but solidly fused on CT.

Postoperative Facet Fracture

Another cause of postoperative pain is the inferior articular process fracture, which occurs following laminectomy and medial facetectomy. This diagnosis is most easily made from sagittal or coronal CT reformatted images (Fig. 12–45). However, when carefully sought, the fracture can occasionally be identified on sagittal MR images (Fig. 12–46).

Spinal Dysraphism

In most patients MRI should follow conventional radiography in the assessment of a congenital spinal abnormality. Most dysraphic disorders are successfully evaluated on MRI. It is usually appropriate to obtain images in the coronal, sagittal, and axial planes to evaluate the vertebral abnormalities, intrathecal lipomata, and abnormal neural elements (Fig. 12–47).

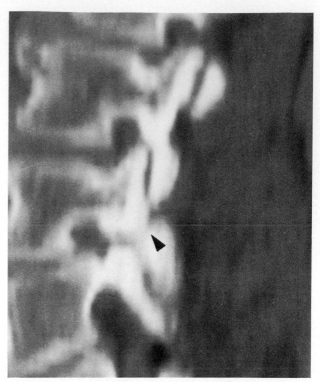

FIGURE 12–45 ■ Sagittal CT reformation demonstrates the fracture of an L4 inferior articular process *(arrowhead)*.

Medicolegal Aspects of Spinal Imaging

A large number of patients who are examined for spinal abnormalities are also involved in litigation. Millions of dollars are spent annually to evaluate claims of work-related injuries. Many patients also claim that they have sustained personal injuries in motor vehicle accidents and other non–work-related traumatic episodes. As with other patients, a precise anatomic diagnosis is a mandatory first step to permit the institution of appropriate treatment. It is also the task of the radiologist to determine whether the abnormalities objectively noted relate to the injury that is indicated to be the cause of the patient's clinical signs and symptoms. Our litigious society has strong incentives to claim illness and injury. Our newer and more sophisticated imaging methods pro-

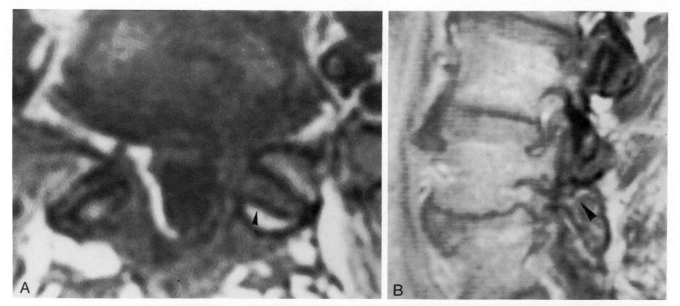

FIGURE 12–46 ■ *A*, T1-weighted axial MR image demonstrates the relative rotation of opposing facets on the left *(arrowhead)*, indicative of a fracture. *B*, The inferior articular process can be seen to be "free-floating" on the left parasagittal MR image *(arrowhead)*.

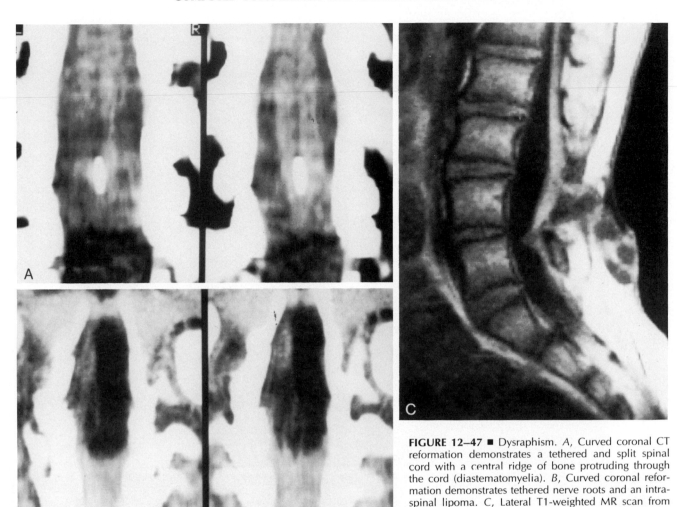

FIGURE 12–47 ■ Dysraphism. *A,* Curved coronal CT reformation demonstrates a tethered and split spinal cord with a central ridge of bone protruding through the cord (diastematomyelia). *B,* Curved coronal reformation demonstrates tethered nerve roots and an intraspinal lipoma. *C,* Lateral T1-weighted MR scan from another patient demonstrates meningomyelocele and a tethered cord. (Courtesy of P. Berger, MD; W. Bradley, MD; and J. Amster, MD; Long Beach, CA.)

vide excellent anatomic information that allows even those with the most rudimentary training to diagnose early degenerative abnormalities. Consequently MRI and CT scan reports of minor abnormalities are being presented on a routine basis to both judges and juries and are represented as hard evidence for traumatic injury and attendant monetary settlements. The "dark disk" of MRI has become the "bête noire" of defendants and insurance companies in many inappropriate law suits. Radiologists are responsible for much of this abuse, largely because of the absence of prior training and sensitivity to the specific problems involved in medical reporting in the medicolegal evaluation. When the radiologist uses the words *disk herniation* in a medicolegal report, a rather dramatic response by unsophisticated juries can be anticipated.

It may be difficult to precisely distinguish among a localized disk bulge, a disk protrusion, a disk herniation, and a disk extrusion on either MRI or CT. When unable to make a precise diagnosis, the physician may be tempted to use these terms interchangeably with no specific diagnostic implication in mind. However, the written words *disk herniation* used to describe a minor bulge or protrusion of the disk in a long-standing degenerated disk often is used in a court room or at a settlement conference to extract large settlements, because the jurors see the term as a familiar, painful, cataclysmic event to which they can relate. The amounts of money awarded are often disproportionately high when compared with those following similar cases in which the medical reports have used the words *disk bulge* or *degenerative disk.* It has been shown that by the age of 40 approximately one third of asymptomatic individuals have at least one abnormal disk apparent on MRI.[10] It is therefore incumbent on the radiologist to be anatomically precise when evaluating medicolegal patients and to correlate the abnormal disk with the timing of the injury if at all possible. True clinical correlation between the patient's symptoms and the findings on the examination should, however, be reserved for the clinician. MRI has become the plaintiff's examination of choice, because it is sensitive, is often abnormal, and demonstrates subtle bony abnormalities without difficulty. When looking at a T1-

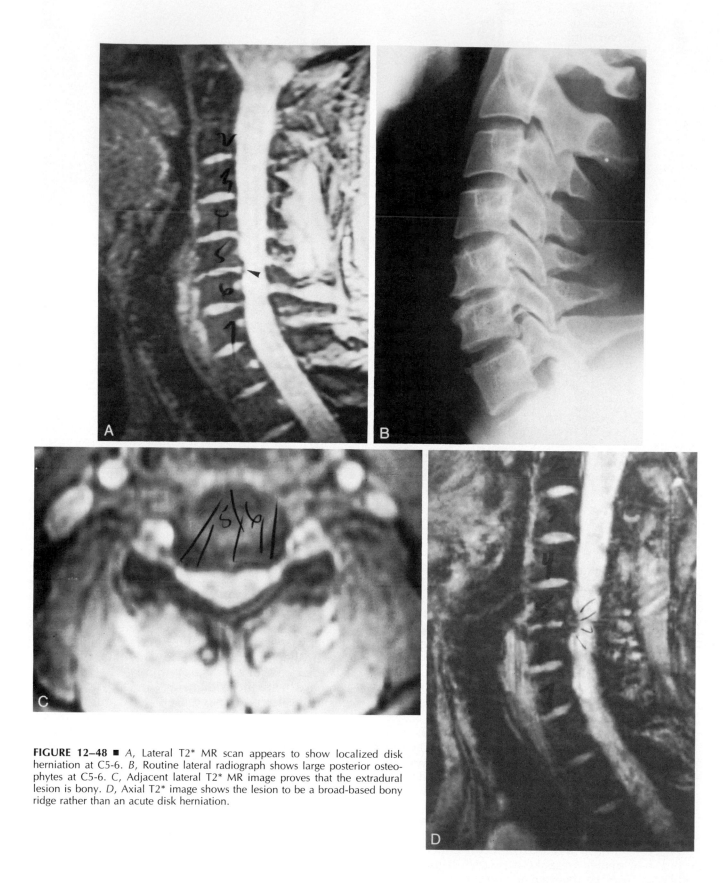

FIGURE 12–48 ■ *A,* Lateral T2* MR scan appears to show localized disk herniation at C5-6. *B,* Routine lateral radiograph shows large posterior osteophytes at C5-6. *C,* Adjacent lateral T2* MR image proves that the extradural lesion is bony. *D,* Axial T2* image shows the lesion to be a broad-based bony ridge rather than an acute disk herniation.

weighted lateral cervical spine MR image and noting 1 mm of bright signal projecting beyond the posterior border of the vertebral body, it is tempting for the radiologist to diagnose a 1-mm disk herniation. Often there are small osteophytes that, although present, are not readily apparent on MR images. These osteophytes frequently predate the accident in question. Furthermore, the annulus attaches to the osteophytes, and when bony ridges project posteriorly from the normal edge of the vertebra, the high-signal-intensity nuclear material must also appear to protrude posterior to the bone. This is in reality a bulge of the disk associated with the osteophyte (i.e., a degenerative rather than a traumatic condition) and not a disk herniation (Fig. 12–48). Using the term *protrusion* or *herniation* is doubly misleading. First, it suggests to the surgeon that surgery may be appropriate, and second, it suggests to lawyers and the jury that this may be traumatic in origin. Both assumptions are often wrong and lead to inappropriately large settlements. Radiologists must be cautious with what they say, as the medicolegal ramifications of their words may have profound and untoward consequences.

CT Versus MRI

When are CT and MR approximately equivalent examinations? When is CT the examination of choice? When is it appropriate to order MR? In this era of medical cost containment, it is important to assess which examination is appropriate for each patient. Computed tomography has distinct clinical advantages in assessing patients with spinal complaints. The standardization of the spine study and the ease of interpretation, accuracy, and confidence in diagnoses preclude the necessity of myelography.

MRI provides a delineation between the central portion of the disk, which contains the nucleus pulposus, and the outermost portion of the annulus. The loss of the normal water content that occurs with progressive degeneration of the disk is reflected in the MR image. This information is not apparent on CT. MR also provides, in a noninvasive manner, a myelogram-like view of the subarachnoid space. MR also has an advantage over CT in differentiating contained from noncontained herniations. MR also studies the entire lumbar spine; tumors of the conus medullaris are therefore far less likely to be overlooked by MR than by CT. Furthermore, MR provides an opportunity to identify pathologic processes in the medullary portion of the bone. The use of gadopentetate dimeglumine has provided further assistance in the assessment of the postoperative patient in whom the question of recurrent disk versus epidural fibrosis is raised.

CT Preferred

The patient who has spondylosis deformans or central or neural foraminal stenosis is generally better

understood with the use of CT. Although the presence of the central canal and neural foraminal stenosis is generally recognized by MRI, the identification of the precise cause is not always as clear with MRI as it is with CT. Small lesions are also best visualized by CT because of the availability of thin-slice CT with no data gaps between slices. CT is also preferred for the spinal trauma patient.

MRI Preferred

Young patients with radiculopathy who have not been previously operated on are especially good candidates for MRI. The young female patient is an especially ideal MRI candidate, as MRI can avoid exposing her to ionizing radiation during her childbearing years.

In the patient suspected of having a spinal cord tumor or multiple sclerosis, MRI should be the initial mode of examination. Similarly, if a patient is suspected of having a marrow-packing disease or metastatic disease to a portion of the lumbar spine, then MRI will prove to be superior to CT in demonstrating subtle lesions in the medullary space, as well as in better defining the extension of such tumors into the adjacent soft tissues. If the patient has a primary tumor with a propensity to spread to bone, but the patient does not have localized symptoms, then a nuclear bone scan (which, unlike MRI, will include all the bones in the body) should be the imaging modality of choice for pretherapeutic screening.

Both Modalities Preferred

The patient who has undergone spinal trauma and has neurologic symptoms is probably best served using both examinations. The CT examination demonstrates the position of bony fracture fragments, whereas MRI provides a better assessment of the impact of the fracture on the spinal cord. The complicated postoperative patient often should undergo both MRI and CT examinations.

Summary

The older patient with low back pain who generally has a significant degree of osteophytic changes as well as facet joint abnormalities should initially be scanned by CT.

When the primary problem is a disk, medullary space, soft tissue, or spinal cord abnormality, MRI is the most appropriate study. However, if the primary problem is likely to be a result of degenerative osteoarthritis or subluxation of the facet joints or osteophytes in the spine, then CT is the imaging modality of choice.

In the postoperative patient, MRI is often the most rewarding modality. However, CT is particularly helpful in the evaluation of surgical fusion integrity and the detection of postoperative facet fracture.

References

1. Parizel PM, Baleriaux D, Rodesch G, et al: Gd-DTPA-enhanced MR imaging of spinal tumors. AJNR 10:249–258, 1989.
2. Hueffle M, Modic MT, Ross JS, et al: Lumbar spine: postoperative MR imaging with Gd-DTPM. Radiology 167:817–824, 1988.
3. Bundschuh CV, Modic MT, Ross JT, et al: Epidural fibrosis and recurrent disc herniation in the lumbar spine: assessment with MR. AJNR 9:169–178, 1988.
4. Mcnab I: Backache. Baltimore, Williams & Wilkins, 1977.
5. Williams AL, Haughton VM, Daniels DL, Thornton RS: CT recognition of lateral lumbar disk herniation. AJR 139:345, 1982.
6. Yu S, Sether LA, Ho PSP, Wagner M, Haughton V: Tears of the annulus fibrous: correlation between MR and pathologic findings in cadavers. AJNR 9:367–370, 1988.
7. Ross JS, Modic MT, Masaryk TJ: Tears of the annulus fibrosis: assessment with Gd-DPTA-enhanced imaging. ASNR 10:1251–1254, 1989.
8. Modic MT, Masaryk TJ, Ross JS, Carter JR: Imaging of degenerative disc disease. Radiology 168:177–186, 1988.
9. Masaryk TJ, Ross JS, Boumphrey F, Bohlman H, Wilber G: High-resolution MR imaging of sequestered lumbar intervertebral disks. AJNR 9:351–358, 1988.
10. Boden SD, Davis DO, Dina TS, Patronas NJ, Wiesel SW: Abnormal magnetic resonance scans of the lumbar spine in asymptomatic subjects. J Bone Joint Surg 72-A(3):403–408, 1990.
11. Helms CA, Dorwart RH, Gray M: The CT appearance of conjoined nerve roots and differentiation from a herniated nucleus pulposus. Radiology 144:803, 1982.
12. Ullrich CG, Binet EF, Sanaecki MG, Kieffer SA: Quantitative assessment of the lumbar spinal canal by computed tomography. Radiology 134:137–143, 1980.
13. Mikhael MA, Ciric I, Tarkington JA, Vick NA: Neuroradiological evaluation of lateral recess syndrome. Radiology 140:97, 1981.
14. Ciric I, Mikhcal MA, Tarkington JA, Vick NA: The lateral recess syndrome: a variant of spinal stenosis. J Neurosurg 53:433, 1980.
15. Carrera GF: Lumbar facet joint injection in low back pain and sciatica. Radiology 137:665–667, 1980.
16. Dory MA: Arthrography of the lumbar facet joints. Radiology 140:23, 1981.
17. Carrera GF, Haughton VM, Syvertsen A, Williams AL: Computed tomography of the lumbar facet joints. Radiology 134:145, 1980.
18. Stimac GK, Porter BA, Olson DO, et al: Gadopentetate dimeglumine–DTPA enhanced MR imaging of spinal neoplasms: preliminary investigation and comparison with unenhanced spin-echo and STIR sequences. AJNR 9:839–846, 1988.
19. Modic MT, Masaryk TJ, Mulopulos GP, et al: Cervical radiculopathy: prospective evaluation with surface coil MR imaging, CT with metrizamide and metrizamide myelography. Radiology 161:753–760, 1986.
20. Sze G, Krol G, Zimmerman RD, Deck MDF: Intramedullary disease of the spine: diagnosis using gadopentetate dimeglumine DTPA–enhanced MR imaging. AJNR 9:848–858, 1988.
21. Post MJD, Quencer RM, Green BA, et al: Intramedullary spinal cord metastasis, mainly of non-neurogenic origin. AJNR 8:339–346, 1987.
22. Ross JS, Masaryk TJ, Modic MT, et al: Vertebral hemangiomas: MR imaging. Radiology 165:165–169, 1987.
23. Maravilla KR, Weinreb JC, Suss R, Nunnally RL: Magnetic resonance demonstration of multiple sclerosis plaque in the cervical spinal cord. AJR 144:381–385, 1985.
24. Grossman RI, Gonzales-Scarano F, Atlas SW, et al: Multiple sclerosis: gadopentetate dimeglumine enhancement in MR imaging. Radiology 161:721–725, 1986.
25. Ross JS, Masaryk TJ, Modic MT, et al: MR imaging of lumbar arachnoiditis. AJNR 8:885–892, 1987.
26. Reicher MA, Gold RH, Halboch VV, et al: MR imaging of the lumbar spine: anatomic correlations and the effects of technical variations. AJR 147:891–898, 1986.
27. Post MJD, Sze G, Quencer RM, Eismont FJ, Green BA, Gahbauer H: Gadopentetate dimeglumine enhanced MR in spinal infection. J Comput Assist Tomogr 14(5):721–729, 1990.
28. Smith AS, Weinstein MA, Mizushima A, et al: Tuberculous spondylos: a contradiction to the MR characteristics of vertebral osteomyelitis. AJNR 10:619, 1989.
29. Brant-Zawadski M, Jeffrey RB Jr, Minagi H, Pitts LH: High resolution CT of thoracolumbar fractures. AJR 138:699, 1982.
30. Chafetz N, Cann CE, Morris JM, Steinbach LS, Goldberg HI: Pseudarthrosis following lumbar fusion: detection by direct coronal CT scanning. Radiology 162:803–805, 1987.
31. Lang P, Chafetz N, Genant HK, Morris J: Lumbar spinal fusion assessment of functional stability with magnetic resonance imaging. Spine 15(6):581–588, 1990.

CHAPTER 13

QUANTITATIVE COMPUTED TOMOGRAPHY FOR THE ASSESSMENT OF OSTEOPOROSIS

HARRY K. GENANT ▪ *CLAUS-C. GLÜER* ▪ *PETER STEIGER* ▪ *KENNETH G. FAULKNER*

In recent years considerable effort has been expended in the development of methods for quantitatively assessing the skeleton so that osteoporosis can be detected early, its progression and response to therapy carefully monitored, and its risk effectively ascertained. However, there is not yet a consensus on which method or methods are most efficacious for diagnosing and monitoring of the individual patient or for extensive screening of large populations.[1] In this regard, the selection of anatomic sites and of methods for quantifying skeletal mass is of considerable importance.

The skeleton as a whole is composed of about 80 per cent cortical, or compact, bone and 20 per cent trabecular, or cancellous, bone.[2] The appendicular skeleton is composed of predominantly cortical bone, whereas the spine is composed of a combination of cancellous bone (predominantly in the vertebral bodies) and compact bone (mostly in the dense end plates and posterior elements). Trabecular bone, be-cause of its high surface-to-volume ratio, has a presumed turnover rate about eight times that of compact bone and is highly responsive to metabolic stimuli.[2, 3] This high turnover rate in trabecular bone makes it a prime site for detection of early bone loss, as well as for monitoring of response to various interventions. The clinical and epidemiologic observation that osteoporotic fractures occur first in the vertebral bodies or distal radius, areas of predominantly trabecular bone, substantiates physiologic studies showing a differential early loss from this bone compartment.[3]

Numerous methods have been used for quantitative assessment of the skeleton in osteoporosis, with variable resultant precision, accuracy, and sensitivity. The first methods to be developed were radiogrammetry[4] and photon absorptiometry,[5–8] which measure primarily cortical bone of the peripheral appendicular skeleton. Recently techniques have become available that can quantify bone mineral content in the spine, the site of early osteoporosis. Quantitative computed tomography (QCT)[9–41] provides a measure of purely trabecular bone of the vertebral spongiosum or other sites, whereas dual-photon absorptiometry (DPA) and dual-energy x-ray absorptiometry (DXA)[41–48] measure an integral of compact and cancellous bone of the spine, hip, or entire skeleton. The focus of this review is on the clinical application of QCT and its comparison with other methods commonly used to quantitatively assess the skeleton.

Computed Tomography for Bone Mineral Analysis

Computed tomography (CT) has been widely investigated and applied in recent years as a means for noninvasive quantitative bone mineral determination.[9–41] The usefulness of computed tomography for measurement of bone mineral lies in its ability to provide a quantitative image and thereby to measure trabecular, cortical, or integral bone centrally or peripherally. For measuring the spine, the potential advantages of QCT[21, 23, 35] are its capability for precise three-dimensional anatomic localization, providing a direct density measurement, and its capability for spatial separation of highly responsive cancellous bone from less responsive compact bone. The lumbar vertebrae contain substantial amounts of compact bone (60 per cent to 80 per cent), with only part of the spinal mineral (20 per cent to 40 per cent) being high-turnover trabecular bone.[29, 49, 50] The sensitivity of techniques measuring an integral of compact and cancellous bone (such as area projection with DPA or DXA) may be low when compared with QCT because of inclusion of low-turnover compact bone and extraosseous mineral such as osteophytes, sclerosis resulting from fractures and osteophytosis, or aortic calcification. The selective localization and the direct density measurement provided by QCT permit exclusion of these causes of low sensitivity or error and inclusion of purely trabecular bone.

QCT has been shown to measure changes in trabecular mineral content in the spine and in the radius and tibia with sensitivity and precision.[9–41] The extraction of this quantitative information from the CT image, however, requires sophisticated calibration and positioning techniques and careful technical monitoring. Specifically designed, small-scale CT scanners using isotope or x-ray sources have also been developed and applied, principally on a research basis, for measurement of the appendicular trabecular and cortical skeleton.[27, 37, 39]

Technical Considerations

Background

Since the discovery of x-rays by Roentgen in 1895, imaging techniques have steadily been refined and made more clinically useful. A major limitation of these techniques is their two-dimensional display of a three-dimensional structure, inevitably leading to a loss of sensitivity because of the superposition of all structures along the ray path. This limitation was finally overcome with the advent of computed tomography, which displays the three-dimensional structure of the object slice by slice. The cross-sectional slice under examination is irradiated subsequently from all directions by stepwise rotation of the x-ray source and the detector ($\phi = 0°$ to $360°$) around the object. For each step, the projected data p are stored digitally. If the section under examination is described by a density function $\mu(x,y)$ representing the linear attenuation coefficient, the projected data at an angle ϕ are given by a linear array of ray-sums p:

$$p(x',\phi) = \int \mu(x,y)\, dy' \qquad (13\text{–}1)$$

with x',y' describing the rotated coordinate system.

By inverting this equation we can compute the two-dimensional distribution of $\mu(x,y)$, and by repeating the measurement for adjacent slices we can calculate and display the complete three-dimensional information. Several techniques have been developed for this purpose, namely back-projection,[51, 52] iterative reconstruction,[53, 54] and analytical reconstruction methods as two-dimensional Fourier reconstruction[53] or filtered back-projection.[55] Brooks and Di Chiro describe the different methods in detail[56] and, in another paper, give a short overview and comparison.[57]

If the CT scanner were perfect, the reconstruction algorithm would yield a density function $\mu(x,y)$ that would accurately reflect the distribution of the attenuation and, if the linear attenuation coefficients of the materials within the field of view were known, give quantitative rather than just qualitative information about the density distribution of these structures. QCT techniques developed in the 1980s succeed in determining the density of a variety of clinically important substances, with remaining errors of (or sometimes lower than) the per cent level. A major step in overcoming imperfections of real CT scanners has been the introduction of calibration techniques that use calibration phantoms of a known element and density distribution.

Scanners

Scanner design has been altered considerably since the first studies were done on an EMI scanner. Third- and fourth-generation scanners are now predominantly used in clinical applications. Zatz[58] reviewed features of scanners of the first to the fourth generation. Most current whole-body scanners can be used for QCT. Unfortunately, there are still exceptions, and performance differs from scanner to scanner. Third-generation scanners have a relatively well-collimated detector aperture. Hence, when compared with fourth-generation scanners, they are less susceptible to quantification and calibration errors caused by scatter artifacts. Data about current scanner characteristics can be found in an article by Cann.[59]

Most current scanners can be operated at different voltages, thereby changing the energy spectrum of the emitted bremsstrahlung. The spectrum of the x-ray tube, with a maximum of the emitted energy (in keV) at about the voltage setting (in peak kilovolts, or kV[p]) and a bandwidth of tens of keV, can be characterized by its effective energy. It depends on the x-ray tube voltage, the beam filtration, the tube target angle and material, and the detector energy response. Moreover, as the beam passes through the patient, it gets increasingly harder (that is, its effective energy increases), because the lower energy components of the bremsstrahlung's spectrum are usually attenuated more than the high-energy components. Hence the effective energy of a measurement technique depends on both scanner characteristics and on the size of the patient and composition of the material being scanned.

Calibration

In determining the density function $\mu(x,y)$, most CT scanners calculate the CT number H rather than the linear attenuation coefficient μ. H, expressed in units of Hounsfield (HU) in honor of the developer of the first clinical CT scanner, is given by the equation:

$$H(E) = 1000 \cdot \left[\frac{\mu(E)}{\mu_W(E_0)} - 1 \right] \qquad (13\text{--}2)$$

where $\mu(E)$ is the linear attenuation coefficient at the effective energy E and $\mu_W(E_0)$ is the linear attenuation coefficient of water. For $E = E_0$ the CT number of water becomes zero; the CT number of air becomes -1000. Obviously the Hounsfield number is energy dependent. To determine bone mineral density, the CT number of the patient is compared with a reference standard of known composition and density.

Two different calibration methods are used: simultaneous and nonsimultaneous. Simultaneous calibration was introduced by Cann and Genant[60] and is used in most clinical applications; nonsimultaneous calibration was used with limited success[61] in some early studies,[62] and now there is renewed interest in this method.[63]

For simultaneous calibration the patient is placed on top of a calibration phantom that has inserts of known mineral density running perpendicular to the plane of the CT slices. The Cann-Genant phantom (Fig. 13–1),[60] which is in use at more than 1000 centers worldwide, has cylindrical channels of solute dipotassium hydrogen phosphate (K_2HPO_4) of 50 mg/mL, 100 mg/mL, and 200 mg/mL concentrations along with a water- and a fat-equivalent channel (60% ethanol). K_2HPO_4 has attenuation characteristics very similar to those of calcium hydroxyapatite ($Ca_{10}(PO_4)_6(OH)_2$), which closely represents the bulk of the mineral found in bone.

For calibration (CB) linear regression of CT number H versus mineral content MIN is performed for each individual slice:

$$H_{CB} = S_B \cdot MIN_{CB} + H_W \qquad (13\text{--}3)$$

With the slope S_B and intercept H_W being the CT number of water, the linear regression is very good ($r^2 \simeq 0.9999$), regardless of the shape of the object under study.[64]

Aqueous solutions, as are used in this phantom, have the potential drawback of limited long-term stability because of the production of gas bubbles, precipitation of the dissolved materials, and impurities.[65] Because of these drawbacks, solid-state reference phantoms have been developed. They are totally stable (i.e., their attenuating properties do not change with time), and they are sturdier and more resistant to damage.

Kalender and Süss[64] reported on a solid phantom with a small cross section ($2.5 \times 9\ cm^2$). This phantom incorporates only two samples, a 200 mg/mL calcium hydroxyapatite and a water equivalent. The density variations of this phantom were found to be better than 0.1 per cent, a tolerance that previously had been difficult to achieve with other solid phantoms.[66] Similarly, Arnold[67] has reported on a solid calcium hydroxyapatite–based phantom for simultaneous QCT calibration.

Simultaneous calibration corrects to a large extent for short- and long-term scanner instability. With

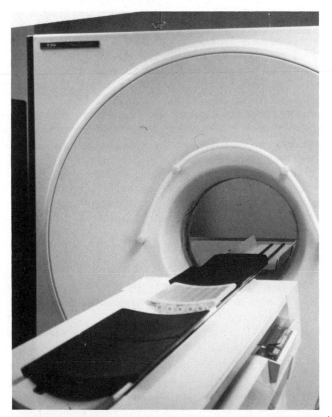

FIGURE 13–1 ■ Standardized version of Cann-Genant CT mineral calibration phantom[60] in use at more than 500 centers worldwide.

nonsimultaneous calibration techniques, which are generally used on fourth-generation scanners, a quasianthropomorphic tissue equivalent calibration phantom is scanned before and/or after the patient.[68, 69] By mounting one or two additional attenuator rings, the phantom can be matched approximately to the patient's size. Nonsimultaneous reference phantoms cannot correct for scanner instabilities between the calibration measurements, and the subjective choice of attenuator rings is only an approximation of patient size and composition. Moreover, it may lead to reproducibility errors if chosen differently.

Techniques

Four constituents of human bone contribute significantly to x-ray attenuation: bone mineral, organic bone matrix, hematopoietic (red) bone marrow, and fatty (yellow) bone marrow. As long as the ratio of inorganic (mineral) and organic bone tissue is constant (which holds true for healthy and osteoporotic but not for osteomalacic patients), it is possible to treat both constituents as one material and calculate their combined density. Because the x-ray attenuation of red marrow is very similar to that of water and because the sum of the volumes of all materials must equal the volume measured, it is possible to determine mineral content with one CT measurement at any energy. However, in the presence of yellow marrow, whose absorption properties are different from those of water, this single-energy (SE) technique underestimates the actual bone mineral content.

Because the energy dependence of x-ray attenuation of bone is different from that of fat, measurement of CT numbers at two different energies leads to two linear independent equations that can be solved for bone and for fat. In other words, this dual-energy (DE) technique allows for accurate determination of mineral content regardless of the amount of fat present, and it allows for accurate determination of fat content regardless of the amount of bone mineral present.

Although there is just one widely used SE approach,[60] a number of different DE techniques[20, 70–73] have been developed. In the following sections, the basic formulas are derived, including terms for the errors of each technique.

SINGLE-ENERGY QCT

The use of any calibration method leads to a calibration equation similar to (13–3) from which slope S_B and intercept H_W are determined.

If we assume trabecular bone (TB) tissue is composed only of bone- and water-equivalent tissue, the single-energy QCT (SEQCT) value, calculated from the measured CT number H_{TB} using the equation

$$\text{SEQCT} = (H_{TB} - H_W)/S_B \qquad (13–4)$$

is equal to the bone mineral density.

Because the vertebral body contains constituents other than bone tissue and water, however, the calculation of bone mineral density by (13–4) yields an error that can be calculated as follows. First,

$$f_B + f_W + \sum_{i=1}^{M} f_i = 1, \qquad (13–5)$$

where f_B is the volume fraction of bone tissue, f_W is the volume fraction of water equivalent tissue, and f_i is the volume fraction of other constituents.

The CT number of trabecular bone in the general case of more than two constituents is given by

$$H_{TB} = f_B \cdot H_B + f_W \cdot H_W + \sum_{i=1}^{M} f_i \cdot H_i. \qquad (13–6)$$

Substituting this equation for H_{TB} in (13–4) yields
SEQCT =

$$\left(f_B \cdot H_B + f_W \cdot H_W + \sum_{i=1}^{M} f_i \cdot H_i - H_W \right) \bigg/ S_B \qquad (13–7)$$

The water volume fraction f_W can be substituted using equation (13–5):

$$\text{SEQCT} = f_B \cdot (H_B - H_W) \bigg/ S_B$$
$$+ \sum_{i=1}^{M} f_i \cdot (H_i - H_W) \bigg/ S_B. \qquad (13–8)$$

The first term on the right of (13–8) represents the true mineral fraction of trabecular bone, and the second describes the error of SEQCT when calculated from (13–4) in the presence of materials other than bone or water-equivalent tissue.

When fat is the main component other than bone mineral and water-equivalent tissue, the error is

$$\text{SEQCT Fat Error} = f_F \cdot (H_F - H_W)/S_B. \qquad (13–9)$$

It should be noted that all calculations are made for a fixed effective energy and do not account for beam hardening or other nonlinear effects.

DUAL-ENERGY QCT

Single energy is all that is required to measure cortical bone. For trabecular bone, with its mixture of bone, red marrow, and yellow (fatty) marrow, measurements at two different energies are necessary to determine bone mineral density without fat-related error.

Two principal ways of performing dual-energy QCT (DEQCT) have been developed. One technique, called *preprocessing DEQCT*, yields results that are free of beam-hardening effects. It combines the two sets of projection raw data to derive a "fat-free" bone projection data set. (Alternatively, a "bone-free" fat projection data set could also be derived.) From this final projection data set, the CT image is calculated using standard reconstruction algorithms. In *postprocessing DEQCT*, by contrast, each of the two projection raw data sets is used to reconstruct a separate CT image. These two CT images can be processed to yield the final fat-free (or bone-free) image. For bone mineral determination, however, it is not necessary to calculate the complete image. Instead, just the region of interest (ROI) is evaluated on each CT image, leading to two average CT numbers H_B and H'_B. These can be used to calculate the "fat-free" bone mineral content, as shown later.

Preprocessing DEQCT ■ The concept of preprocessing dual-energy QCT was developed by Alvarez and Macovski.[71] It is commercially available on Somatom scanners (Siemens Inc.). Its fundamental underlying assumption is that the energy-dependent mass attenuation coefficient $\mu(E)/\rho$ of all materials can be expressed with sufficient accuracy as a linear combination of the Compton scatter and the photoelectric absorption coefficients:

$$\mu(E)/\rho \simeq a_c f_c(E) + a_p f_p(E), \qquad (13\text{–}10)$$

where a_c and a_p are characteristic constants of the materials, and f_c and f_p are the energy dependencies of Compton scatter (given by the Klein-Nishina function)[71] and photoelectric absorption (approximately $E^{-2.8}$).[72] This assumption holds true for basically all biologic materials for the diagnostic x-ray energy range, since their K edges are at much lower energies. In particular, this is a good approximation of the mass attenuation of bone, fat, and soft tissue.

Instead of using equation (13–10) we can conveniently express the attenuation coefficient of the materials of interest in relation to a pair of so-called basis materials:

$$\mu(E)/\rho = a_1 \cdot \mu_1(E)/\rho_1 + a_2 \cdot \mu_2(E)/\rho_2. \qquad (13\text{–}11)$$

Results of different sets of basis materials such as aluminum/lucite, calcium/water or calcium/lucite can be found in the literature.[73–76]

Using equation (13–11) we can express the ray-sum of equation (13–1) as

$$\int \mu(x,y,E)dy' = \mu_1(E)/\rho_1 \cdot \int \rho_1(x,y)dy'$$
$$+ \mu_2(E)/\rho_2 \cdot \int \rho_2(x,y)dy' \qquad (13\text{–}12)$$

with ρ_1 representing the pure and $\rho_1(x,y)$ the local density of basis material 1.

The reconstruction of $\rho_1(x,y)$ and $\rho_2(x,y)$ requires scanning at two energies to obtain two linear-independent sets of ray-sums $p(x', \phi, E_1)$ and $p(x', \phi, E_2)$. The calculation can be done conveniently by using lookup tables. Image reconstruction then yields a CT image of each of the basis materials.[73, 77]

It should be noted that when more than two materials other than water are present, their relative densities cannot be determined from two measurements. Even with more than two different measurements, this is not possible unless one of the measurements is carried out at an energy with measureable K-edge discontinuities.[74]

Postprocessing DEQCT ■ Postprocessing dual-energy techniques for bone mineral studies were initially proposed by Brooks[72] and also by Genant and Boyd.[20] Since then, additional postprocessing techniques have been described.[63] We will derive the formulas for a rigorous technique that theoretically allows for complete elimination of fat influence on

bone mineral density (called *exact dual-energy technique*) and for a simpler technique that reduces fat influences substantially (typically by a factor of two or three) but not completely. This "simplified" dual-energy technique is not as susceptible to errors in the fat calibration of the scanner and in practice yields results that are more reproducible.

In the dual-energy approach one gets two calibration equations:

$$H_{CB} = S_B \cdot MIN_{CB} + H_W \quad \text{(e.g., 80 kV[p])} \qquad (13\text{–}13a)$$
$$H'_{CB} = S'_B \cdot MIN_{CB} + H'_W \quad \text{(e.g., 140 kV[p])} \qquad (13\text{–}13b)$$

and (including specifically the fat term), two equations for determining the CT numbers at the two energies.

$$'H_{TB} = f_B \cdot H_B + f_W \cdot H_W + f_F \cdot H_F + \sum_{i=1}^{M} f_i \cdot H_i \qquad (13\text{–}14a)$$

$$H'_{TB} = f_B \cdot H'_B + f_W \cdot H'_W + f_F \cdot H'_F + \sum_{i=1}^{M} f_i \cdot H'_i \qquad (13\text{–}14b)$$

The water volume fraction f_W in equation (13–14) can be substituted using the following equation:

$$f_B + f_W + f_F + \sum_{i=1}^{M} f_i = 1 \qquad (13\text{–}15)$$

Combining equations (13–14a) and (13–14b) allows for elimination of the fraction f_F. Solving the derived equation for f_B yields:

$$f_B = \frac{(H_{TB} - H_W)(H'_W - H'_F) - (H'_{TB} - H'_W)(H_W - H_F) + \Delta_{RES}}{(H_B - H_W)(H'_W - H'_F) - (H'_B - H'_W)(H_W - H_F)} \qquad (13\text{–}16)$$

If no materials other than bone, water-equivalent tissue, and fat tissue contribute to the x-ray attenuation, the term

$$\Delta_{RES} = \sum_{i=1}^{M} f_i \cdot [(H'_i - H'_W)(H_W - H_F) \\ - (H_i - H_W)(H'_W - H'_F)] \qquad (13\text{–}17)$$

becomes zero.

Calibrating the scanner for fat in a similar way as for bone mineral density also yields two equations:

$$H_{CF} = S_F \cdot FAT_{CF} + H_W \qquad (13\text{–}18a)$$
$$H'_{CF} = S'_F \cdot FAT_{CF} + H'_W \qquad (13\text{–}18b)$$

Multiplying equation (13–16) by the density of bone ρ_B yields the "exact" dual-energy formula:

$$DEQCT_1 = \frac{(H'_{TB} - H'_W) \cdot S_F - (H_{TB} - H_W) \cdot S'_F + \rho_B \cdot \Delta_{RES}}{S'_B \cdot S_F - S_B \cdot S'_F} \qquad (13\text{–}19)$$

If the error caused by components other than bone, water-equivalent tissue, or fat is negligible, $DEQCT_1$ (as calculated from equation [13–19] without knowledge of the fat fraction) equals the true bone mineral density.

A disadvantage of this equation is the requirement of precise fat sensitivity calibration. Because of the subtraction in the denominator term, uncertainties in the determination of the slopes of fat or bone cause equation (13–19) to become unstable. To get better reproducibility, some accuracy can be sacrificed by assuming no change of fat sensitivity between energy 1 and 2, and the approximation

$$S_F \simeq S_F'$$ (13–20)

can be used. By disregarding any influence from constituents other than bone, water-equivalent tissue, or fat tissue, we arrive at the "simplified" DE formula:

$$DEQCT_2 \simeq \frac{(H_{TB}' - H_W') - (H_{TB} - H_W)}{S_B' - S_B}$$ (13–21)

Applying this equation to our DEQCT data, we could not expect the fat error to be eliminated completely. For a three-component system, the fat error can be calculated as the difference between equations (13–19) and (13–21):

$$DEQCT_2 \text{ Fat Error} = \frac{f_F \cdot \rho_F \cdot (S_F' - S_F)}{S_B' - S_B}$$ (13–22)

For a multicomponent system, the error caused by all constituents other than bone or water-equivalent tissue is

$$DEQCT_2 \text{ Error} = \sum_{i=1}^{M} f_i \cdot \rho_i \cdot (S_i' - S_i)/(S_B' - S_B)$$ (13–23)

Practical Considerations

QCT of the Spine

Vertebral mineral density is determined by measuring representative volumes (about 2 to 3 mL per vertebra) of purely trabecular bone. The ability to measure that area selectively is advantageous, because the turnover rate of trabecular bone is approximately eight times that of cortical bone of the spine.[78] The patient is positioned on top of the calibration phantom. To avoid artifacts, a bolus bag is used to fill the air gap between patient and phantom. Using a lateral computed radiograph (known as a *radiographic localizer*, a *scout view*, or a *topogram*) of the lumbar spine and cursor-determined coordinates, the midplanes of typically three to four vertebrae (T12 to L4) are identified. T12 may have to be excluded depending on the magnitude of superimposed lung tissue. Lordosis is reduced by elevating the knees with a pad. Slices of 8- to 10-mm thickness are taken parallel to the vertebral end plates by tilting the gantry appropriately (Fig. 13–2).

For SEQCT measurements, a low-dose, low-energy setting should be chosen if possible. This results in a skin dose of typically 200 to 300 mrem and essentially no gonadal exposure. (This is 1/10 the normal imaging dose per slice, 1/10 the usual number of slices per study, and therefore 1/100 the total integral dose of a routine abdominal CT imaging study.[18, 34, 79]) The low-voltage setting also provides a relatively high sensitivity of mineral to fat variations.[80] Care should be taken to ensure that the patient fits entirely in the field of view and does not move during the exposure. To check for any movement, a second localizer radiograph after the scan can be taken.

For DEQCT measurements, the lower energy setting should be as low as possible, with an optimum effective energy of about 40 keV[81] or a peak voltage setting of 65 kV(p).[66] Current scanners allow measurements to be taken at about 80 kV(p), which corresponds to about 55 keV effective energy. This setting is almost as good as 40 keV.[81] The upper energy should be as high as possible—typically 120 or 140 kV(p)—and the dose should be about equal at both energies.[81] For postprocessing DEQCT the skin dose is approximately 600 mrem. Preprocessing DEQCT usually requires higher milliampere settings.[61]

Automated evaluation optimizes reproducibility and simplifies the operator's task. Recent image evaluation software incorporating contour tracking techniques allows for anatomically adapted and automatically placed ROIs.[82, 83] Calibration is also performed automatically, with the option of operator interference in case the calibration ROIs are misplaced.[83] Calibrated bone mineral density can be averaged over all vertebrae to improve accuracy.[80]

Such automated image evaluation packages are already being offered commercially. Moreover, automated determination of the midvertebral CT slice,[84] may help to further reduce precision errors.

QCT of the Hip

There has been limited research on the clinical utility of QCT of the hip. The complex structural anatomy of the proximal femur makes it difficult to measure specific kinds of skeletal tissue selectively. Advances in image processing techniques, however, have opened up the possibility of performing site-specific QCT of the hip.[85]

Three different methods of calculating trabecular bone mineral density at the proximal femur have been reported.[86, 87] In each, the region to be examined must be scanned contiguously to obtain complete three-dimensional information. Also, in all of the techniques, the standard calibration phantom developed for spine scans is used.[60]

Using reformatting techniques, Reiser and Genant[86] calculated images of transverse slices perpendicular to the longitudinal axis of the proximal femur that had been defined by the center of the femoral head and the center of the femoral neck at its smallest width. The CT values of four to eight of these transverse slices of 5-mm thickness were integrated, thus covering 5 to 12 mL of bone volume in the femoral neck. The reproducibility of the quantitative measurements was found to be better than 3 per cent.

Results obtained with two other techniques have recently been published by Sartoris et al.[87] From a frontal localization image, they determined the region from the head-neck junction to the lesser trochanter and subsequently scanned it with contiguous 5- or 10-mm slices. The data were analyzed with ROI software, much as for quantitative vertebral bone analysis. Several nonoverlapping ROIs were chosen

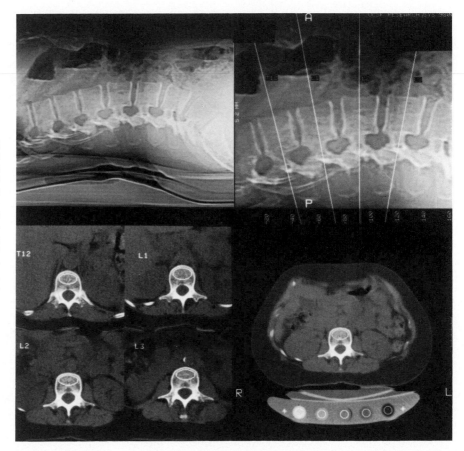

FIGURE 13–2 ■ QCT spine technique using GE 9800 scanner. Lateral scout view provides a rapid and simple localization approach in which the midplanes of four vertebral bodies are defined on the video monitor, and a single 10-mm-thick section is obtained at each level. An oval region of interest, centered in the midvertebral body, is used to determine cancellous bone mineral content (mg/mL), whereas circular regions of interest are used to quantify the K_2HPO_4 solutions in the calibration phantom. (From Genant HK, Steiger P, Block JE, Ettinger B, Harris ST: Calcif Tissue Int 41:174–186, 1987.)

to cover the maximum possible area of trabecular bone in each axial slice. From these data, the average trabecular bone density was calculated.

In the third approach, a threshold pixel value of 200 mg K_2HPO_4/mL was chosen to display the inner and outer contour of the cortical bone areas of each slice. Averaging over all pixels inside these areas yielded a mean value for trabecular bone density.

Comparing short-term reproducibility of the two latter techniques, three scans of the same cadaver yielded a coefficient of variation of 2.2 per cent for the axial slice technique and 0.7 per cent for the histogram analysis technique. The volume of interest was 14 to 19 mL and 33 to 37 mL, respectively.

A comparison of these techniques is difficult because of the limited number of observations. However, the histogram analysis technique has the advantages of reproducibility and simplicity, provided the necessary software is available.

When developing automated techniques for defining volumes of interest, reformatting techniques and three-dimensional representation[88–90] might be helpful in understanding which region of the bone is selected and which is excluded.

Validity of QCT

Functions Describing the Validity of QCT

QCT has the capability to provide exact results, but care must be taken to minimize several possible error sources. The specific functions chosen to describe the validity of the method depend on the question QCT is supposed to answer. Most basic research on the validity of QCT has focused on how well QCT can determine the true bone mineral density of an object. The answer usually is given in terms of two functions: *accuracy* and *precision*. In clinical practice these two functions can be used to describe the performance of QCT both for cross-sectional studies (using QCT to determine the degree of osteopenia) and for longitudinal studies (using QCT to quantify bone loss).

To describe the performance of QCT with respect to other techniques (e.g., its capability to discriminate between fractured and nonfractured patients), several concepts have been applied. The *sensitivity* of the techniques can be defined as the ratio of responsiveness (e.g., measured rate of bone loss at a given site) to precision of the measurement, or it can be used along with *specificity* in the context of relative (or receiver) operator characteristic (ROC) analysis.

Finally, there is the question of relevance for screening strategies. Is QCT a good risk predictor for bone diseases (e.g., hip fractures)? That answer could be given in terms of *relative risk factors*. Very little has been done so far to relate these three questions. The implicit assumption of most authors is that the best method of determining bone mineral density is also best suited for discriminating between diseased and nondiseased patients and in turn is the best predictor of risk; however, this has not been tested. Furthermore it does not follow that the best method for predicting risk is also the best method for studying the causes of bone metabolism. The following discussion is limited to the accuracy and precision of QCT.

ACCURACY

The accuracy of a bone mineral measurement technique is defined as the deviation of the results obtained with that technique from the true mineral content, usually expressed as a per cent. For QCT, bone mineral density in mg/mL of the calibration material (K_2HPO_4 or $Ca_{10}(PO_4)_6(OH)_2$) is usually compared with the results of some "gold standard," typically gravimetric or spectroscopic determination of the mineral in a sample following ashing at ~600°C for 48 to 96 hours. The results of that comparison are correct within 0.5 to 1 per cent if the ROI of the QCT measurement is thoroughly matched with the volume ashed during chemical analyses. If these analyses are not properly done, however, an error of up to 3 to 4 per cent may be introduced, falsely reflecting on accuracy of QCT.[61]

Results of accuracy of SEQCT and DEQCT are summarized in Table 13–1.[10, 20, 36, 76, 85, 91–94] Accuracy data for trabecular bone are usually determined by the coefficient of variation around the regression line of QCT versus ashweight; the assumption is that the average underestimation can be corrected for by using scanner-specific normative data. For SE techniques, and to some extent also for DE techniques, the accuracy error depends on the variability of the fat content of the specimens and the sensitivity of the scanner to fat changes. The data of Burgess and co-workers[76] and Glüer et al.[80] can be taken as an estimate for a population that covers a wide age range, excluding severe osteoporotic patients.

The physical and physiologic factors affecting accuracy are discussed after the next section.

PRECISION

The precision of a bone mineral examination technique is defined as the deviation of the outcome of a set of measurements about the expected value. The results of studies on the precision of QCT are summarized in Table 13–2.[20, 21, 31, 37, 60, 95–105] *Precision* and *reproducibility* are terms that are usually used synonymously. Clearly a precise measurement need not be accurate. Precision can be calculated in two ways:

1. If the bone mineral density of the object is kept unchanged, precision can be determined from n repetitive measurements by using

$$\text{prec} = \sqrt{\left[\sum_{i=1}^{n} (y_i - \bar{y})^2/(n - 1) \right]} \quad (13\text{–}24)$$

where y_i is the outcome of an individual measurement and

$$\bar{y} = \sum_{i=1}^{n} y_i /n \quad \text{(mean of } y_i) \quad (13\text{–}25)$$

2. If bone mineral density can be assumed to have changed in a linear way between subsequent measurements, precision equals the standard error of the estimate of linear regression on the data points, i.e.,

$$\text{prec} = \sqrt{\left(\sum_{i=1}^{n} (y_i - \hat{y}_i)^2/(n - 2) \right)} \quad (13\text{–}26)$$

$$\hat{y}_i = ax_i + b \quad \text{(estimate of } y_i) \quad (13\text{–}27)$$

where a is the slope and b is the intercept of the regression curve.

In view of dosage considerations, repetitive measurements on the same patient may be impossible, and method 2 is preferable for determining in vivo precision. It should be remembered that because there is no way of testing the assumption of linearity, the standard error of the estimate yields just an upper limit of precision.

The long-term reproducibility of a measurement technique defines its clinical utility, as it not only determines an upper limit for accuracy for single measurements, but also determines the validity of any change in the results of repeated measurements. For instance, if a method has a precision of ±2 mg, the change between two measurements must be 5.7 mg before there is 95 per cent confidence that the change is real.[106] This follows from the law of error propagation: the standard deviation of the difference

TABLE 13–1 ■ Accuracy of Bone Mineral Measurements by QCT

ACCURACY (%)	SITE	BONE	TECHNIQUE	AUTHOR	YEAR
1	Femur	C	SE (isotope)	Rüegsegger et al[91]	1974
~6[61]	Tibia/fibula	C	SE	Reich et al[92]	1976
3–4[61]	Dog bones	C	SE	Posner and Griffiths[93]	1977
1.9	Calcium phantom	C	SE	Genant and Boyd[20]	1977
8	Vertebra	T	SE	Rohloff et al[36]	1982
4.3	Distal femur	T	SE	Adams et al[9]	1982
26	Vertebra	T	SE	Laval-Jeantet et al[94]	1986
10.7	Vertebra	T	SE	Burgess et al[76]	1987
13.2	Vertebra	T	SE	Glüer et al[80]	1987
9.6	Vertebra	T	DE	Laval-Jeantet et al[94]	1986
7.3	Vertebra	T	DE	Burgess et al[76]	1987
7	Vertebra	T	DE	Glüer et al[80]	1987

Abbreviations: C = cortical; DE = dual energy; SE = single energy; T = trabecular.

TABLE 13–2 ■ Reproducibility of Bone Mineral Parameters Measured by CT

AUTHOR	BOND	SHORT-TERM (%) In vitro	SHORT-TERM (%) In vivo	LONG-TERM (%) In vitro	LONG-TERM (%) In vivo
Isherwood et al[95]	Radius	0.2	1.4–2		
Rüegsegger et al[37]	Radius		2		
Genant and Boyd[20]	Phantom	1			
Bradley et al[96]	Vertebra	25			
Liliequist et al[97]	Tibia		1.8		
Orphanoudakis et al[31]	Radius	2			
Cann and Genant[60]	Vertebra	1.5		2.8	
Rüegsegger et al[98]	Radius				0.3
Hangartner and Overton[99]	Radius		0.6		
Genant et al[21]	Vertebra		1.6		
Firooznia et al[100]	Vertebra	2–3			
Sashin et al[101]	Radius				0.5
Graves and Wimmer[102]	Vertebra			2.2	
Rosenthal et al[103]	Vertebra		1.6		
Meier et al[104]	Vertebra		4–5		
Cann et al[105]	Vertebra				0.8

of two measurements equals $\sqrt{2}$ times the standard deviation of a single measurement, and the 95 per cent confidence interval again is larger by about another factor of 2.

The physical and physiologic factors that limit precision are described in the following section.

Factors Influencing the Validity of QCT

Bone mineral density as calculated from CT scans differs from the actual density because of several factors. Understanding their origin helps to avoid or limit these error sources. Table 13–3 lists the most prominent factors and indicates whether these factors influence primarily accuracy or precision.

QUANTUM NOISE VERSUS DOSE

Like all other bone mineral measurement techniques, QCT requires the use of ionizing radiation. Compared with CT imaging techniques, QCT requires a relatively low dose (i.e., 1/100 of the integral and 1/10 of the skin dose for the spine technique described earlier). Imaging with a low dose is possible because just the mean CT number of a large area (typically 3 cm²) has to be calculated during evaluation, thereby averaging over the relatively high pixel-to-pixel variations. Two general physical laws describe quantum noise (natural statistical changes in x-ray intensity as described by the Poisson distribution):

1. Noise is reduced by a factor of r if the dose is increased by a factor of r^2.

2. Noise is reduced by a factor of s if the area of the ROI is enlarged by a factor of s^2.

In reality, additional error sources partly counterbalance or enhance this quadratic law. At very low doses (below about 100 mrem), noise caused by artifacts and inhomogeneities may dominate over quantum noise. Moreover, enlargement of ROIs does not always reduce noise. Because areas of great inhomogeneity are very susceptible to repositioning

errors, an enlargement of an ROI into such an inhomogeneous area might worsen the noise relations.

Following the law of quadratic error propagation, one usually needs to lower the dose to 20 to 30 per cent of the remaining precision error, thus compounding the precision error (i.e., 2 per cent) by about only 3 per cent (i.e., 2.06 per cent). In Cann's work on low-dose spinal SEQCT, a patient skin dose of 100 mrem was determined to be sufficient to provide useful quantitative vertebral mineral measurements.[79]

Unfortunately some manufacturers preprogram exposure settings so that doses cannot be reduced to this level. For this reason, doses quoted in the literature for QCT of the spine vary from a high of 2000 to 3000 mrem[107] to a low of less than 100 mrem.[79] A good rule of thumb for determining millirems for QCT is to multiply the milliampere setting by a factor of 7 for 120 to 130 kV(p) and by a factor of 1.7 for 80 kV(p).[61] Postprocessing DEQCT doubles radiation exposure, and preprocessing DEQCT increases dose requirements to a maximum skin dose of 2.7 to 4.1 rad.[108] Preprocessing requires a higher dose, because the dual-energy data must be separated on the projection raw data level. The noise must be sufficiently low to make the resulting line integral sets fall within

TABLE 13–3 ■ Factors Influencing the Validity of QCT

FACTOR	EFFECT	
Technique (SE, DE)	A	P
Quantum noise versus dose		P
Partial volume effects versus resolution	A	
Beam hardening effects	A	
Field inhomogeneity	A	P
Scanner stability		P
Interscanner differences		P
Positioning		P
Object size	A	
Material composition	A	(P)
Evaluation technique (automated)		P

Abbreviations: A = principally influences accuracy; DE = dual energy; P = principally influences precision; (P) = minor impact on precision; SE = single energy.

the limits of the basis set calibration data. If this requirement is not met, there will be artifacts in the reconstructed images.[61]

Because scanner images are mainly limited by factors other than quantum noise, reduction of these remaining error sources may further reduce the dose limits for all techniques.

PARTIAL VOLUME EFFECTS VERSUS RESOLUTION

QCT images are usually recorded, reconstructed, and presented in a digital and discrete pixel structure. Increasing the number of pixels increases resolution but also increases noise. Typically, pixel sizes of 0.25 × 0.25 mm² to 1.5 × 1.5 mm² and matrices of 256 × 256 or 512 × 512 are used for reconstructed CT images.

Objects that are larger than the pixel size of the projections (given by the detector element spacing) attenuate the beam corresponding to their linear attenuation coefficient. If they are smaller than the pixel size, however, the average attenuation is reduced, and the object appears to have a lower attenuation coefficient (partial volume effect). The situation is made even more complex because of the divergence of the x-ray beam, which leads to decreasing resolution with increasing distance between the x-ray source and the object. In addition, for any part of the object that is not centered in the scanning circle, the apparent attenuation in a given pixel differs even for two beams of opposite direction.[61] Finally, limitations of spatial resolution resulting from slice thickness have to be considered.

Slice thickness should be about two to four times greater than pixel size (e.g., 3-mm thickness with a size of 1 × 1 mm²). This is especially important if contiguous slices are taken to get the complete three-dimensional information of the object and if reconstruction in nonaxial slices is to be performed by means of reformation techniques.

BEAM-HARDENING EFFECTS

In practically all clinical QCT examinations, broadband (several tens of keV) bremsstrahlung x-ray spectra are used. As these x-rays pass through tissue, low-energy photons are absorbed with a greater frequency than high-energy photons because of the increased attenuation coefficient of matter at lower photon energies. For this reason the effective energy of the remaining spectrum increases as the beam passes through the object. As a result the effective energy of the radiation, after it has passed through an object, depends on both the composition of the object and its thickness.

This beam-hardening effect leads to shifts in the apparent CT numbers. Preprocessing dual-energy techniques allow for correction, but for single-energy and postprocessing dual-energy techniques, this would require perfect knowledge of both the composition and size of the object. Thus for patients only a partial correction is possible, as only general assumptions about the specific object can be made

(e.g., the abdomen is cylindrical in shape and uniform in density). These first-order corrections are performed automatically on current scanners.[61] Second-order beam-hardening corrections[109, 110] are necessary if a correction algorithm for one part of the body (e.g., the abdomen) is used for imaging other objects or parts of the body (e.g., the thigh).

FIELD INHOMOGENEITY

In an ideal scanner, the bone mineral density of an object could be determined accurately at any location within the scanning aperture and independently of patient size and the composition of surrounding tissue. However, older whole-body scanners (especially those using bowtie filters or reduced-field-of-view scanners) and even some newer scanners show severe nonuniformities in CT number for identical objects placed at various positions in the scanning field.[59, 61, 66] Therefore service personnel usually scan a reference phantom to adjust field uniformity. If the patient's size, shape, or density does not conform to this ideal phantom, field uniformity tends to deteriorate. CT scanners using low-energy beams tend to suffer more acutely from this problem.[66] Nonsimultaneous calibration phantoms with adjustable object size might be used to correct for this effect. Because precision is more important than accuracy in clinical practice, this dependence of field homogeneity on patient size might be of lesser importance as long as the patient's size does not vary too much between successive measurements.

When comparing field homogeneity on the scale of Hounsfield units, it is important to remember that the apparent per cent mineral changes caused by nonuniformity are generally smaller at lower energies. This might be explained in part by the greater calibration slope at lower energies, but Zamenhof[66] states that beam hardening, which is a major cause of field nonuniformities, depends less on the energy of the x-ray beam than on its energy spread. Low kV(p) x-ray spectra have a narrower energy spread and therefore result in greater field uniformity.[66]

Special care must be taken to avoid an air gap between the patient and the calibration phantom. Otherwise the algorithm designed to correct soft tissue beam-hardening effects may give misleading results, causing field inhomogeneity.

MATERIAL COMPOSITION

The CT number of a pixel represents the total x-ray attenuation in the corresponding voxel, given as the sum of the attenuation of all the different materials contained in that volume element. With SEQCT the densities of both materials of a two-component system can be calculated independently because of the known attenuation characteristics of the materials and the fact that the sum of their volumes must equal the volume measured (see equation [13–4]). DEQCT allows for independent determination of the densities of three materials. The formulas describing

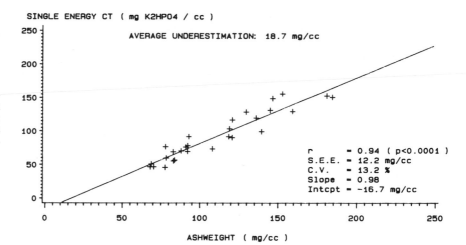

FIGURE 13–3 ■ Accuracy of SEQCT measurements of 80 kV(p) based on the averaged data obtained from two to three vertebrae each from 28 cadavers. (From Glüer CC, Reiser UJ, Davis CA, Rutt BK, Genant HK: J Comput Assist Tomogr 12(2):242–258, 1988.)

possible errors in SEQCT, simplified DEQCT, and exact postprocessing DEQCT are derived in an earlier section.

The composition of vertebral bodies can be described accurately with a three-component system: (1) bone (in a given ratio of mineral and organic collagen; this holds true for healthy as well as osteoporotic patients, but not for osteomalacic patients); (2) soft tissue (almost water equivalent); and (3) fat (mainly found in yellow marrow). In several studies QCT results for determination of vertebral bone mineral density are compared with chemical analysis, and the error introduced in SEQCT is reported.[76, 80, 94, 111–113] Figures 13–3 and 13–4 show results of Glüer et al. for SEQCT and (simplified) DEQCT versus chemical analysis.[80] They found that at 80 kV(p), the "true" bone mineral density is underestimated on the average by about 18 mg/mL. By analyzing fat content in the same specimens, they calculated that the underestimation resulted from a fat-related error of about 7 mg/mL per 10 per cent fat by volume increase (this is called the *fat-to-mineral sensitivity*, or simply the *fat sensitivity* of the scanner). Scanners that operate at a higher voltage setting (typically up to 120 to 140 kV[p]) have a greater fat-to-mineral

sensitivity (e.g., 12 mg/mL per 10 per cent fat by volume increase at 130 kV[p][94]), and consequently, fat-related underestimation of such scanners is also higher. Areas of great fat variability should be scanned at low kV(p) settings if possible. Cann determined the fat sensitivity of several newer scanners, and the results ranged from an apparent mineral decrease of 5 mg/mL to 11 mg/mL per 10 per cent fat by volume increase.[59, 114] To minimize fat-related errors, SEQCT measurements for a patient should be compared with normative SEQCT data obtained on the same scanner with an identical technique. On the average, this will eliminate the fat-induced underestimation. For the individual patient, however, some uncertainty remains because of the natural variability of fat content (e.g., 87.5 mg/mL as given by the standard error of the estimate of fat content versus age[80]). This uncertainty is given by the natural variability multiplied by the fat-to-mineral sensitivity. It is reduced by using DEQCT, but DEQCT provides less precision. Even with SEQCT, this uncertainty is much less than the natural variability of bone mineral content versus age. (Using the GE 9800 CT scanners, for example, the fat uncertainty is about one third of the natural biologic

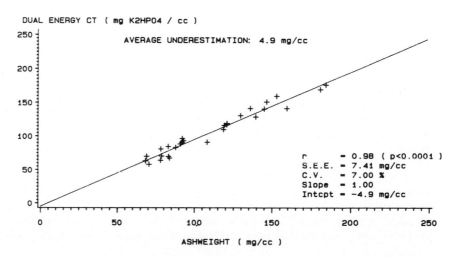

FIGURE 13–4 ■ Accuracy of DEQCT measurements at 80/140 kV(p) based on the averaged data obtained from two to three vertebrae each from the same 28 cadavers used for Figure 13–3. (From Glüer CC, Reiser UJ, Davis CA, Rutt BK, Genant HK: J Comput Assist Tomogr 12(2):242–258, 1988.)

variability for normal patients). A correction algorithm is available to reduce the average fat-related underestimation for SEQCT measurements of absolute bone mineral density.[80]

SCANNER STABILITY/INTERSCANNER DIFFERENCES

The mid- and long-term temporal stability of CT scanners is limited by a number of factors, including x-ray tube aging or changes, generator changes, and software updates. Short-term minute-to-minute, machine-dependent instabilities can also be observed. These errors are usually minimized by scanning a bone mineral calibration phantom simultaneously. The Cann-Genant phantom[60] is in widespread use and has been described previously. Even the use of a standardized calibration method, however, cannot completely eliminate differences among scanners.[59] In addition, the use of different calibration phantoms on the same scanner leads to changes in the measured CT numbers.[115] Although the expected differences can be estimated for most clinical applications,[59, 83] highly accurate interscanner cross calibration remains a challenge.

OBJECT SIZE AND COMPOSITION

Beam hardening increases or decreases according to the patient's size and affects the CT number. This phenomenon was studied using the Computerized Imaging Reference Systems (CIRS) spine phantom[68] as the "patient" and the Cann-Genant spine phantom for calibration. When researchers changed the "patient's" size from medium to large (about 3 cm additional thickness), they found a shift in the CT number of the calibration phantom of +6 mg/mL at 80 kV(p). At 140 kV(p) this effect is even more pronounced, and the shift is +9 mg/mL. No significant shift was observed in the CT number of the "patient," and no explanation was offered as to why the shift was not in the expected direction.[63]

This shift, which was found to be constant on an absolute scale independent of mineral density, does compound the accuracy error, but as long as a patient's size does not change between measurements, it does not limit precision. However, significant changes in body composition, such as body gas or lung air motion,[59] may produce errors in both accuracy and precision. Because these effects are hard to quantify, a measurement showing visible artifacts should be repeated.

REPOSITIONING

In longitudinal studies it is important to evaluate the same volume of interest in each measurement. Two principal repositioning methods have been reported:[15, 22, 24, 59, 60, 179] computed radiographs, generally used in clinical environments, and three-dimensional repositioning, the software for which is being developed for research purposes.[116] A method for automated determination of the midvertebral CT slice has also been reported.[84] Finally, an intermediate approach uses the radiograph for longitudinal-axis positioning and automated techniques for the definition of the ROI on the axial slices.

In computed radiographic localization systems (scout view, tomogram), lateral radiographs are usually taken for spinal measurements and anteroposterior radiographs for hip measurements. The operator can address the coordinate system that is logged to the image and uses trackballs to define the positions of the scans to be taken. Generally these systems are accurate to ±2 mm and reproducible to ±1 mm, which results in an error in the definition of the volume of less than 10 per cent.[59] Depending on the homogeneity of the area under study, a 2-mm repositioning error again results in a precision error of bone mineral content of 2 per cent for trabecular bone of the vertebrae.[60] The error is probably greater at sites of greater longitudinal inhomogeneity, such as the tibia,[117] distal femur,[10] and radius.[99] The new technique of automated determination of the midvertebral CT slice on the localization image promises reduction of errors resulting from operator influence.[84]

The localizer radiograph defines the region to be scanned, but the selection of the ROI in the transverse x-y plane is performed during the evaluation process and can be corrected if necessary. Automated selection of the ROI eliminates operator influence and is considered to offer better reproducibility, especially if different operators are involved.[60, 83, 118] In spinal studies contour tracking algorithms[82, 83, 108] trace the cortical walls of the vertebral body, the spinal canal, and other landmarks to select the optimum (no cortex) position and size (as large as possible[118]) of the ROI (Fig. 13–5). For hip studies, no automated procedure has been reported. For the spine, a one-pixel variation in the x-y plane introduces a variance of 0.8 HU in the measured area.[60] Automated selection of the ROI should yield even better results.[61] In studies of the knee bone, mineral density and shape measurements could be reproduced with 0.5 per cent and 1 per cent precision.[83] Hence ROI positioning errors are small compared with the errors introduced by the localizer radiograph.

Automated three-dimensional ROI positioning further reduces the repositioning error, as current scanners have resolving limits of 0.5 to 1 mm in all three axes. If a set of contiguous or overlapping slices is obtained, reconstruction in any plane of the scanned volume can be performed by means of multiplanar reformation techniques.[116] These techniques will be helpful for evaluation of nonaxial structures such as the femoral neck.[85, 86]

Clinical Applications of QCT

Background and Models of Bone Loss

QCT has been used to model patterns of vertebral bone diminution with aging, to evaluate skeletal status in health and disease, to predict subsequent

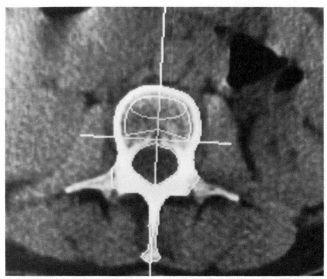

FIGURE 13–5 ■ The three different ROIs for lumbar vertebra (L2). The determination of the ROIs and their statistical analysis take 3 to 4 sec of a database VAX 11/780. (From Steiger P, Steiger S, Rüegsegger P, Genant HK: Two- and three-dimensional quantitative image evaluation techniques for densitometry and volumetrics in longitudinal studies. In Genant HK (ed): Osteoporosis Update 1987. Berkeley, CA: University of California Press, 1987, pp 171–180.)

fracture risk, and to monitor treatment interventions.[15, 21, 24, 100, 119] New data from the University of California San Francisco (UCSF) Osteoporosis Research Group indicate little skeletal involution of spinal trabecular bone prior to the onset of menopause in 538 healthy women between the ages of 20 and 80 (Fig. 13–6). Various statistical regressions were performed for the entire population to describe the general pattern of bone loss from the spine; linear, quadratic, cubic, and logarithmic models were found to be equally satisfactory in characterizing this pattern with r values of 0.65, 0.67, 0.68, and 0.67, respectively. QCT values were stratified into 5- and 10-year age brackets and analyzed separately for pre-

and postmenopausal women. The 5- and 10-year interval stratification revealed no identifiable bone mineral decrements prior to midlife; significant losses of bone mineral were noted to correspond with the usual time of menopause and to continue into old age. The statistical model of skeletal atrophy is best described as a two-phase regression consisting of a premenopausal period of skeletal consolidation followed by a period of exponential postmenopausal involution.

Discrimination Capability of QCT

Researchers using QCT have uniformly observed a statistically significant separation between patients with spinal compression deformities and age- and sex-matched comparison subjects without fractures.[15, 120] Cann and colleagues[15] found that female osteoporotic patients had a mean decrement in bone mineral values of 48 mg/mL (39 per cent) compared with normal subjects, whereas males with compression fractures had a mean decrement of 66 mg/mL (50 per cent) when compared with men of the same age without fractures. In general, vertebral deformities are absent in individuals with QCT mineral values above 110 mg/mL, whereas almost all patients with bone mineral values below 65 mg/mL have radiographic evidence of vertebral osteoporosis (Fig. 13–7). Although there is significant overlap in patients with intermediate values, it appears that QCT is useful in identifying those patients at increased risk of vertebral fracture. Firooznia and colleagues likewise found a moderate statistical separation between spinal osteoporotic patients and comparison subjects.[120] In a cohort of 96 women with evidence of vertebral compressions, 66 per cent had bone mineral values in the spine that were below the fifth percentile for age-matched normal subjects; 85 per cent of these same subjects had values below the fifth percentile for premenopausal women.

The QCT technique has been used less often to

FIGURE 13–6 ■ Statistical model of bone loss over lifetime, indicating insignificant premenopausal bone loss, a large decrement at the menopause, and rapid postmenopausal loss.

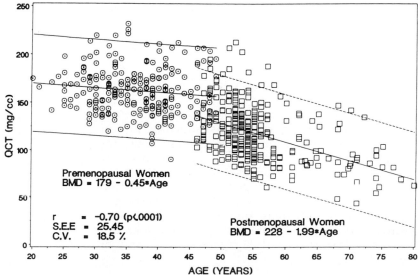

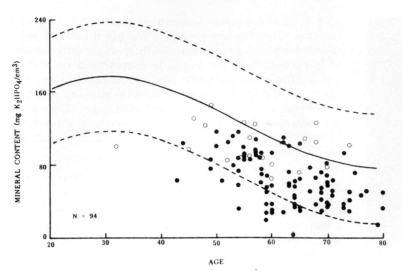

FIGURE 13–7 ▪ Vertebral mineral content in osteoporotic patients *(closed circles)* superimposed on mean and 95% confidence intervals for normal women. (Reprinted with permission from Bone, Volume 6, pp. 1–7, Cann CE, Genant HK, Kolb FO, Ettinger BF, Copyright 1985, Pergamon Press, plc.)

differentiate patients who have suffered spontaneous hip fracture from normal comparison subjects. In one study,[18] the trabecular bone mineral content of the lumbar spine was measured in 185 women age 47 to 84 years with vertebral fracture (n = 74), hip fracture (n = 83), and both vertebral and hip fracture (n = 28). Eighty-seven per cent of the vertebral fracture patients, 38 per cent of the hip fracture patients, and 82 per cent of the vertebral and hip fracture patients had spinal bone mineral content values below the fifth percentile for healthy premenopausal women and values 64 per cent, 9 per cent, and 68 per cent below the fifth percentile for age-matched control subjects, respectively. This study suggests that no preferential loss of spinal trabecular bone occurs in subjects with isolated hip fractures, whereas a significant difference can be observed between spine fracture and normal comparison subjects. Further studies utilizing direct hip measurements with QCT need to be undertaken to determine the degree to which bone loss occurring specifically at the hip affects the occurrence of fracture.

QCT and Osteoporosis Prophylaxis

Estrogen replacement therapy initiated soon after the cessation of ovarian function is universally accepted as an efficacious means of retarding bone loss and preventing fractures of the spine and hip.[121] QCT has been of great use in chronicling this period of rapid bone loss and substantiating the response to estrogen therapy. Genant and coworkers[21] serially assessed the bone mineral loss in 37 premenopausal women for a duration of 24 months following surgical oophorectomy and determined the dose-response for conjugated estrogen therapy in preventing this loss. Without intervention mean annual rates of loss from the spinal trabecular envelope were shown to be on the order of nine per cent (Fig. 13–8). An estrogen dose of 0.6 mg/day was found to be the lowest effective dose in abbreviating this rapid involution. In a later investigation of 73 women at the time of

menopause, slightly slower rates of loss, approximately five per cent/year, were observed in subjects on placebo and in those on 1500 mg of daily calcium supplementation.[119] However, a dose of 0.3 mg/day estrogen combined with 1500 mg daily calcium was found to be as effective as 0.6 mg/day estrogen alone. In both studies, bone was lost from the appendicular cortical skeleton at a significantly lower rate (one to three per cent annually) than from the vertebral spongiosum.

The effect of estrogen deprivation on younger premenopausal women has also been examined using QCT. Thirty-eight women (17 to 49 years of age) with hypothalamic and hyperprolactinemic amenorrhea and premature ovarian failure were studied.[12] The group with hypothalamic amenorrhea was made up primarily of athletes. Bone mass in the peripheral cortical skeleton was only slightly lower than values for age-matched normal subjects, but spinal trabecular bone was significantly lower (20 to

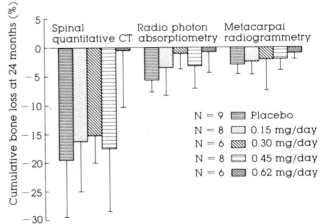

FIGURE 13–8 ▪ Cumulative bone loss 24 months after oophorectomy in 37 women as a function of quantitative technique and estrogen therapy. (From Genant HK, Cann CE, Ettinger B, Gordon GS: Ann Intern Med 97:699–705, 1982.)

25 per cent). A subpopulation of this study included both amenorrheic and exercise-matched eumenorrheic athletes.[122] In this study, eumenorrheic elite athletes had significantly more spinal mineral than sedentary controls, followed in order by amenorrheic elite athletes, amenorrheic casual athletes, and amenorrheic nonathletes. Thus the exercise effect is apparent in women but can be overridden by the strong effect of estrogen deprivation.

Types of exercise programs, as well as the intensity and duration of exercise, have not been well studied or described in research dealing with skeletal health. As a step toward elucidating the independent effects of exercise on the skeleton, the UC-SF group studied spinal bone mineral in 46 young men, 28 of whom engaged in regular and vigorous exercise programs.[123] Measurements of spinal trabecular bone mineral density (mg/mL) and vertebral integral bone mineral content (gm) were obtained for all subjects by QCT. Spinal trabecular bone density was greater by 14 per cent in the exercise group ($P = .0001$), and integral bone mineral was greater by ten per cent ($P = .04$). Subjects in the exercise group were further categorized to reflect their particular fitness regimen. Individuals who engaged in a program of both weight training and aerobic exercise had a mean value of trabecular bone density of 197.3 mg/mL; those who engaged in a weight training only regimen had a mean value of 183.1 mg/mL; and those who engaged in only aerobic exercise had a mean value of 172.9 mg/mL. Nonexercising control males had the lowest values, with a mean value for trabecular bone density of 161.3 mg/mL (Fig. 13–9). An analysis of variance across all four activity types indicated a significant difference among groups for trabecular bone density ($P = .0001$), although differences in total integral bone mineral were not significant.

QCT Versus Other Bone Density Techniques

A number of investigators have compared the various techniques of bone mineral assessment to quantify the effects of metabolic bone diseases on different skeletal compartments, to determine the fracture prediction value of each technique, and to assess each technique's usefulness for describing decrements observed from health to disease. Two of the most rigorous of these studies are presented in the sections that follow.

QCT VERSUS APPENDICULAR MEASUREMENTS IN METABOLIC BONE DISEASE

To investigate the effects of specific metabolic bone disorders on skeletal mass at different anatomic sites and to determine the associations among various methods for noninvasive measurement of bone mineral, the UCSF group studied 269 subjects.[35] The study group included 34 patients with hyperparathyroidism, 24 patients with steroid-induced osteoporosis, and 38 men with idiopathic osteoporosis. These subjects were compared with a group of 173 normal

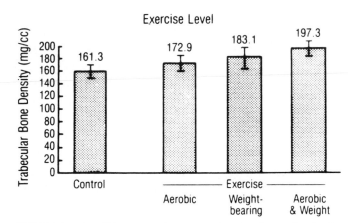

FIGURE 13–9 ■ Histogram of mean trabecular bone density by exercise level shows progressively greater vertebral trabecular bone mineral through each exercise type. (Reprinted by permission of Western Journal of Medicine from Block JE, Genant HK, Black D, 1986, Vol. 145, pp. 39–42.)

subjects representing the entire age range. The measurements taken included spinal QCT, Norland-Cameron single-photon absorptiometry of the radial diaphysis (NCD) and metaphysis (NCM) and divided by width (NCDW and NCMW), and combined cortical thickness (CCT) of the second metacarpal. Lateral thoracolumbar radiographs were evaluated semiquantitatively, and a spinal fracture index (FXI) was calculated.

The measurements of appendicular cortical bone correlated moderately well ($r = 0.54$ to 0.66) with each other (Table 13–4). The appendicular measurements correlated less well with spinal QCT measurements ($r = 0.33$ to 0.41). The spinal FXI correlated best with QCT ($r = -0.74$) and less well with the appendicular measurements ($r = -0.20$ to -0.33). A fracture threshold of approximately 110 mg/mL was noted for the group as a whole. Furthermore, below a level of 60 mg/mL, spinal deformities were common and absence of such abnormalities was uncommon.

The idiopathic osteoporotic men, the hyperparathyroid patients, and corticosteroid-treated patients differed significantly from age- and sex-matched comparison subjects ($P < .01$) (Fig. 13–10). The largest per cent decrements in the spine were seen in the idiopathic osteoporotic men and corticosteroid groups, reflecting the severity of the disease process on axial trabecular bone. The largest decrements in the appendicular indices were seen in the idiopathic osteoporotic men and the hyperparathyroid groups. It was concluded that knowledge of appendicular cortical mineral status is important in its own right but is not a valid predictor of axial trabecular mineral status, which may be disproportionately decreased in certain diseases. Furthermore, QCT provides a reliable means of assessing the latter region of the skeleton and correlates well with the spinal fracture index, a semiquantitative measurement of end-organ failure.

TABLE 13–4 ■ Spearman Correlation Matrix

	AGE	CT	CCT	NCD	NCDW	NCM	NCMW	NCDW/ NCMW	FXI
Age	1.00000*	−0.60972	−0.43969	−0.15230	−0.39689	−0.17956	−0.36982	0.03348	0.50067
	0.0000†	0.0001	0.0001	0.0127	0.0001	0.0051	0.0001	0.6050	0.0001
	267‡	259	266	267	266	242	242	241	255
CT	−0.60972	1.00000	0.38778	−0.00333	0.32837	0.10223	0.40685	−0.17430	−0.73982
	0.0001	0.0000	0.0001	0.9574	0.0001	0.1181	0.0001	0.0075	0.0001
	259	260	259	260	259	235	235	234	248
CCT	−0.43969	0.38778	1.00000	0.43558	0.63361	0.44808	0.54489	−0.07034	−0.32923
	0.0001	0.0001	0.0000	0.0001	0.0001	0.0001	0.0001	0.2757	0.0001
	266	259	268	268	268	242	242	242	256
NCD	−0.15230	−0.00333	0.43558	1.00000	0.75405	0.81586	0.42884	0.18566	0.04527
	0.0127	0.9574	0.0001	0.0000	0.0001	0.0001	0.0001	0.0037	0.4699
	267	260	268	269	268	243	243	242	257
NCDW	−0.39689	0.32837	0.63361	0.75405	1.00000	0.71001	0.65716	0.12875	−0.20359
	0.0001	0.0001	0.0001	0.0001	0.0000	0.0001	0.0001	0.0454	0.0011
	266	259	268	268	268	242	242	242	256
NCM	−0.17956	0.10223	0.44808	0.81586	0.71001	1.00000	0.60836	−0.05734	−0.03167
	0.0051	0.1181	0.0001	0.0001	0.0001	0.0000	0.0001	0.3745	0.6299
	242	235	242	243	242	243	243	242	234
NCMW	−0.36982	0.40685	0.54489	0.42884	0.65716	0.60836	1.00000	−0.59443	−0.24691
	0.0001	0.0001	0.0001	0.0001	0.0001	0.0001	0.0000	0.0001	0.0001
	242	235	242	243	242	243	243	242	234
NCDW/ NCMW	0.03348	−0.17430	−0.07034	0.18566	0.12875	−0.05734	−0.59443	1.00000	0.10042
	0.6050	0.0075	0.2757	0.0037	0.0454	0.3745	0.0001	0.0000	0.1264
	241	234	242	242	242	242	242	242	233
FXI	0.50067	−0.73982	−0.32923	0.04527	−0.20359	−0.03167	−0.24691	0.10042	1.00000
	0.0001	0.0001	0.0001	0.4699	0.0011	0.6299	0.0001	0.1264	0.0000
	255	248	256	257	256	234	234	233	257

*r value.
†P value.
‡number.

Abbreviations: CT = computed tomography; CCT = combined cortical thickness; FXI = spinal fracture index; NCD = Norland-Cameron single-photon absorptiometry of the radial diaphysis; NCDW = NCD divided by width; NCM = Norland-Cameron single-photon absorptiometry of the radial metaphysis; NCMW = NCM divided by width.

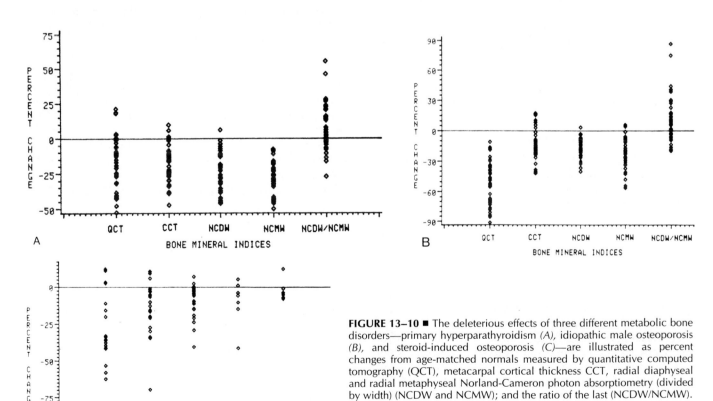

FIGURE 13–10 ■ The deleterious effects of three different metabolic bone disorders—primary hyperparathyroidism *(A)*, idiopathic male osteoporosis *(B)*, and steroid-induced osteoporosis (C)—are illustrated as percent changes from age-matched normals measured by quantitative computed tomography (QCT), metacarpal cortical thickness CCT, radial diaphyseal and radial metaphyseal Norland-Cameron photon absorptiometry (divided by width) (NCDW and NCMW); and the ratio of the last (NCDW/NCMW).

TABLE 13–5 ■ Pearson Correlation Coefficients in Early Postmenopausal Women (*n* = 40)

	SEQCT	DEQCT	DPA	SPA	SPA/W	CCT
SEQCT		0.9734	0.8661	0.3824	0.4874	0.5363
		0.0001	0.0001	0.0149	0.0014	0.0004
DEQCT	0.9734*		0.8156	0.3716	0.4345	0.5345
	0.0001†		0.0001	0.0182	0.0051	0.0004
DPA	0.8661	0.8156		0.4673	0.5396	0.5029
	0.0001	0.0001		0.0024	0.0003	0.0009
SPA	0.3824	0.3716	0.4673		0.7307	0.3650
	0.0149	0.0182	0.0024		0.0001	0.0206
SPA/W	0.4874	0.4345	0.5396	0.7307		0.5466
	0.0014	0.0051	0.0003	0.0001		0.0003
CCT	0.5363	0.5345	0.5029	0.3650	0.5466	
	0.0004	0.0004	0.0009	0.0206	0.0003	

Abbreviations: CCT = combined cortical thickness; DEQCT = dual-energy QCT; DPA = dual-photon absorptiometry; SEQCT = single-energy QCT; SPA = single-photon absorptiometry; SPA/W = SPA divided by width. *r value. †p value.

QCT VERSUS OTHER TECHNIQUES IN NORMAL AND OSTEOPOROTIC WOMEN

To investigate the associations among the principal methods for the noninvasive measurement of spinal and appendicular bone mass, the UC-SF group studied 40 normal early postmenopausal women and 68 older postmenopausal women with osteoporosis.[34] The methods of determining bone mineral content included single- and dual-energy QCT and dual-photon absorptiometry (DPA) of the lumbar spine, single-photon absorptiometry (SPA) of the distal radius, and CCT measurements of the second metacarpal shaft. Lateral thoracolumbar radiography was also evaluated, and a spinal fracture index was calculated. The correlation coefficients and levels of significance for both patient groups are shown in Tables 13–5 and 13–6. SEQCT showed a good correlation (*r* = 0.87) with DPA for early postmenopausal women and a moderate correlation (*r* = 0.53) for postmenopausal osteoporotic women (Fig. 13–11). DEQCT did not improve these correlations with DPA. Appendicular measurements correlated only modestly among themselves, as well as with the axial measurements by either QCT or DPA. The severity of spinal fracture correlated highly with QCT (*r* = −0.91) but only moderately with DPA (*r* = −0.44)

(Fig. 13–12). Reinbold and co-workers[34] also showed a small but significant decrease in the correlation between SEQCT and DEQCT from the younger to the older population (Fig. 13–13). Although this decrease is presumably caused by age-related increases in marrow fat, generally excellent correlations were observed between DEQCT and SEQCT regardless of the age group. Moreover, it was found that the use of DEQCT failed to improve the correlation with DPA, to reduce the normal biologic variation found with QCT in general, or to enhance the discrimination between normal and osteoporotic women. These facts suggest that in most circumstances DEQCT is unnecessary in the assessment of postmenopausal women and that SEQCT, with its lower radiation dose, is adequate. However, for special research purposes or when highly accurate assessments are needed, the use of DEQCT may be necessary.

Widely differing correlations between QCT and DPA have been reported in apparently similar groups of patients (Table 13–7).[15, 25, 32, 34, 35, 38, 124, 125] Some reported correlations may be poor because of inadequate sample sizes; however, in our large cohort good correlation (*r* = 0.87 and 0.82) is shown between either SEQCT or DEQCT, respectively, and

TABLE 13–6 ■ Pearson Correlation Coefficients in Postmenopausal Osteoporotic Women (*n* = 68)

	SEQCT	DEQCT	DPA	SPA	SPA/W	CCT	FXI
SEQCT		0.9482	0.5310	0.2005	0.2390	0.2285	−0.9102
		0.0001	0.0001	0.1012	0.0497	0.0609	0.0001
DEQCT	0.9482*		0.4245	0.2005	0.2133	0.2366	−0.8817
	0.0001†		0.0003	0.1012	0.0809	0.0521	0.0001
DPA	0.5310	0.4245		0.3633	0.1622	0.2522	−0.4399
	0.0001	0.0003		0.0023	0.1864	0.0380	0.0002
SPA	0.2005	0.2005	0.3633		0.4021	0.5788	−0.0775
	0.1012	0.1012	0.0023		0.0007	0.0001	0.5316
SPA/W	0.2390	0.2133	0.1622	0.4021		0.2522	−0.2195
	0.0497	0.0809	0.1864	0.0007		0.0381	0.0720
CCT	0.2285	0.2366	0.2522	0.5788	0.2522		−0.1720
	0.0609	0.0521	0.380	0.0001	0.0381		0.1610
FXI	−0.9102	−0.8817	−0.4399	−0.0775	−0.2195	−0.1720	
	0.0001	0.0001	0.0002	0.5316	0.0720	0.1610	

Abbreviations: CCT = combined cortical thickness; DEQCT = dual-energy QCT; DPA = dual-photon absorptiometry; FXI = spinal fracture index; SEQCT = single-energy QCT; SPA = single-photon absorptiometry; SPAW = SPA divided by width. *r value. †p value.

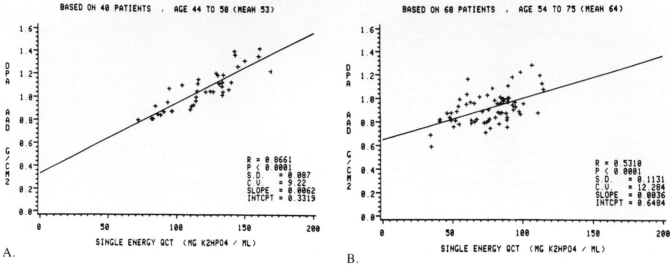

FIGURE 13–11 ■ Moderately good correlation is shown for DPA versus SEQCT for normal early postmenopausal women *(A)*. Modest correlation is shown for DPA versus SEQCT for postmenopausal osteoporotic women *(B)*.

DPA in early postmenopausal women, and moderate correlation ($r = 0.53$ and 0.42) is shown in post-menopausal osteoporotic women. The modest correlation observed in osteoporotic women, although statistically significant, shows sufficient dispersion that a reliable prediction of QCT value from DPA value or vice versa is precluded for the individual patient.

Some authors[25, 112] have tried to improve the correlation between QCT and DPA by measuring the same bone envelopes with both methods and expressing the quantities measured in dimensionally similar units. The UC-SF Osteoporosis Research group previously found, in a mixed group of 52 patients, that the modest correlation ($r = 0.67$) between the anatomically and dimensionally dissimilar integral DPA in gm/cm² and trabecular QCT in mg/mL was significantly improved when both techniques

measured the same parameters. For example, integral mass (gm) assessed by DPA correlated well ($r = 0.88$) with integral mass as determined by QCT; likewise, integral density (mg/mL) assessed by DPA correlated well ($r = 0.84$) with integral density assessed by QCT. Nevertheless, the strongest correlation ($r = 0.91$) was observed between trabecular and integral density when both were measured by QCT. Thus the differences observed between QCT and DPA were not explained entirely by anatomic considerations. This finding suggests that residual fundamental differences exist between these techniques and are perhaps related to their respective abilities to define bone edges, regions of interest, baseline measurements, and volumes and their respective other sources of error.

Mazess and Vetter[112] used QCT and DPA to examine comparable bone envelopes in ten excised

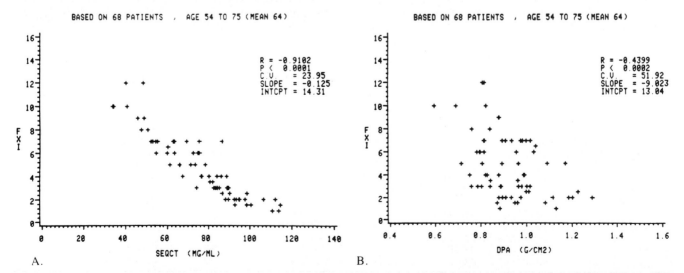

FIGURE 13–12 ■ High correlation is shown for SEQCT versus spinal fracture index *(A)*. Modest correlation is shown for DPA versus spinal fracture index in the same patients *(B)*.

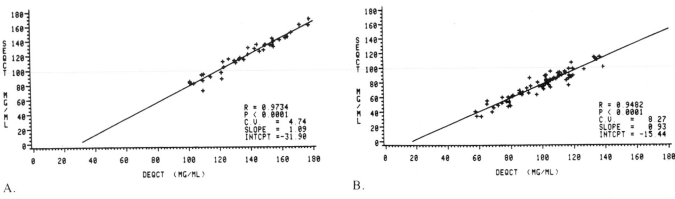

FIGURE 13–13 ■ High correlation is shown for SEQCT versus DEQCT for *(A)* normal early postmenopausal and *(B)* postmenopausal osteoporotic women.

vertebrae. They found that the mineral mass obtained by integrating all bone voxels by DEQCT correlated highly (r = 0.97) with the mass determined by DPA. The mineral density of the total vertebra, including all processes, as determined by DPA correlated highly (r = 0.87) with the density as assessed by DEQCT, whereas the correlation with the density of the body was lower (r = 0.82) and even lower (r = 0.79) with the density of a section from the spongiosum of the anterior vertebral body. In other words, correlations between DPA and QCT weakened when integral density was compared with the more labile trabecular density.

The study of early postmenopausal and older osteoporotic females showed that the older women have less bone mineral than younger postmenopausal women and that the magnitude of the difference depends on the method used for measurement. The mean differences observed were 35.6 per cent by SEQCT, 28.2 per cent by DEQCT, 13.7 per cent by DPA, 13.7 per cent by SPA, and 15.1 per cent by CCT. The substantial decrement observed by QCT suggests that measurements of spinal trabecular bone density by QCT discriminate those women with spinal osteoporosis from younger postmenopausal normals better than does DPA or measurements of appendicular cortical bone mass by SPA or CCT. This observation is supported by the work of Jones et al.,[49] which showed disproportionate loss of trabecular bone relative to compact bone in the spine, both in aging and in osteoporosis. Furthermore, two recent studies have compared the differences between young normals and osteoporotic patients measured by QCT and DPA. Sambrook et al.[38] found a 54 per cent (P = .01) decrement by QCT and a 23 per cent (P = .05) decrement by DPA, whereas Gallagher and colleagues[19] found a 65 per cent (P = .001) decrement by QCT and 16 per cent (P = NS) decrement by DPA. Finally, Raymakers et al.[33] tested the ability of these two techniques to differentiate between women with crush fractures and age-matched normals. QCT was slightly better, showing a sensitivity and specificity of 83 per cent and 83 per cent, respectively, compared with 73 per cent and 76 per cent for DPA.

The UC-SF group concluded that although measurements of bone mineral content by QCT, DPA, SPA, and CCT are positively correlated, their relationships are not strong enough and their dispersions are too large to predict one measure by another for the individual patient. SEQCT was determined to be adequate and perhaps preferable for assessing postmenopausal women. Measurements of spinal trabecular bone density by QCT can also discriminate osteoporotic women from younger normal women more sensitively than can measurements of spinal integral bone by DPA or appendicular cortical bone by SPA or CCT. Table 13–7[15, 25, 32, 34, 35, 38, 124, 125] summarizes the results of previous similar studies comparing QCT, DPA, and SPA in different population groups, and Table 13–8[25, 30, 32, 34, 35, 126] indicates correlations between QCT or DPA and the severity of vertebral fracture.

TABLE 13–7 ■ Correlations Among QCT, DPA, and SPA

AUTHOR	SEQCT/DPA	SEQCT/SPA	DPA/SPA
Cann et al[15]	—	0.48	—
Genant et al[25]	0.67–0.88	0.40–0.476	0.47–0.55
Kilcoyne et al[124]	0.32	—	—
Ott et al[125]	0.26–0.46	0.44–0.51	0.54–0.60
Powell et al[32]	0.40	0.48	0.56
Richardson et al[35]	—	0.33–0.41	—
Sambrook et al[38]	0.65–0.80	0.30	0.38
Reinbold et al[34]	0.53–0.87	0.20–0.49	0.16–0.54

Abbreviations: DPA = dual-photon absorptiometry; SEQCT = single-energy QCT; SPA = single-photon absorptiometry.

TABLE 13–8 ■ Correlations Among FXI, SEQCT, and DPA

AUTHOR	FXI/SEQCT		FXI/DPA	
	r	P	r	P
Genant et al[25]	−0.83	0.0001	−0.47	0.0006
Mack et al[30]	−0.45	0.001	−0.023	NS
McBroom et al[126]	−0.91	0.061	—	—
Powell et al[32]	−0.83	0.01	−0.50	0.02
Richardson et al[35]	−0.74	0.0001	—	—
Reinbold et al[34]	−0.91	0.0001	−0.44	0.0002

Abbreviations: DPA = dual-photon absorptiometry; FXI = spinal fracture index; SEQCT = single-energy QCT.

Recommended Clinical Applications

The question remains whether bone densitometry, by any method, should be recommended widely and become standard medical practice. We know more about each technique's advantages and shortcomings than we ever have, and there is continuing rapid improvement of technology and development of exciting new modalities. However, in the midst of this development and improvement and while we await the results of numerous ongoing and future clinical and epidemiologic investigations, we are faced with important management decisions involving the current population of women already afflicted with osteoporosis or at risk for developing it. We must therefore rely on sound expert opinion and available technology to guide a clinical approach to patient management.

Previously it was thought that osteoporosis, by clinical definition, could be reduced to a simple distinction between atraumatic fracture and nonfracture. Indeed, this philosophy led some researchers[127-130] to suggest that bone density per se is not a sensitive predictor of fracture risk, because only a modest difference was observed between fracture patients and nonfracture comparison subjects of the same age. The suggestion was based in part on early densitometry studies[131-133] showing considerable overlap between hip fracture subjects and matched controls. A more recent study, in which the Ward's triangle region of the hip was evaluated using newer techniques, suggests better hip fracture discrimination with bone density measurements.[134] Moreover, those studies[135, 136] that have assessed the contribution of absolute bone density for fracture risk have shown a strong predictive ability for a variety of techniques. Certainly many investigators have shown that direct quantitative assessment of the spine by QCT or DPA satisfactorily discriminates spine fracture from nonfracture subjects.[34, 120, 137] Additionally, all bone densitometry techniques illustrate a progressive and substantial loss of bone over the life span from all skeletal sites (albeit at different rates),[24, 138, 139] and it is this systematic bone loss that contributes most significantly to fractures in the elderly. In fact, several studies[15, 140-142] have shown that osteoporotic fractures do not become likely until a certain threshold of bone density is crossed, and that higher density values, independent of age, confer significant protection against fracture. Most importantly, these recent findings have convinced many researchers to no longer consider osteoporosis as a fracture/nonfracture dichotomy but rather to redefine osteoporosis as the lower part of a continuum of bone density, with the greatest fracture risk existing in those with lowest absolute density values. Wasnich[143] draws a parallel to the use of blood pressure monitoring to predict stroke risk. Bone mass, he points out, like blood pressure, must be treated as a continuous variable, with fracture, analogous to stroke, as a primary outcome. Indeed, most individuals with hyperten-

TABLE 13-9 ■ Clinical Applications of Bone Densitometry

Assessment of patients with metabolic disorders known to affect the skeleton
Assessment of perimenopausal women for initiation of estrogen replacement therapy
Establishing a diagnosis of osteoporosis or assessing its severity in context of clinical care
Serial assessment to monitor disease progression or therapeutic response

sion have not suffered a stroke, but they are nonetheless at great risk. Similarly, because of the probabilistic nature of fractures, many individuals with low bone density have not experienced a fracture, but they should not be considered normal or free of osteoporosis.

Although controversy exists with regard to the appropriate use of bone densitometry,[128, 129, 143-146] we currently consider a number of clinical applications valid (Table 13–9).[147] Only the first of these, however, could be said to be supported by all investigators in the field. Nonetheless, a growing body of literature supports wider applications for the individual patient.[143-145] Each of the four recommendations listed in Table 13–9 will be discussed separately.

Assessment of Patients With Metabolic Diseases Known to Affect the Skeleton

Many metabolic disorders—including hyperparathyroidism, renal insufficiency, Cushing's syndrome, chronic immobilization, amenorrhea (among premenopausal women), and chronic steroid or thyroid therapy—have profound influences on calcium metabolism and may adversely affect the skeleton. Some of these secondary forms of osteoporosis, such as Cushing's syndrome, preferentially affect the trabecular bone envelope, with relative sparing of cortical bone, making assessment of trabecular sites advisable.[35, 148-150] On the other hand, diseases such as renal osteodystrophy may cause dramatic appendicular cortical demineralization in the presence of low, normal, or even high spinal trabecular bone density.[151] Therefore assessment by a combination of techniques may be appropriate in some instances. In these secondary forms of osteoporosis, bone density measurements have importance in the overall clinical evaluation, as they may influence therapy decisions (e.g., the reduction of corticosteroids in the case of steroid-induced osteoporosis,[148-150] subtotal parathyroidectomy in hyperparathyroid bone disease,[152-154] or initiation of estrogen replacement therapy in the case of amenorrhea/oligomenorrhea[12, 21, 144]).

Assessment of Perimenopausal Women for the Initiation of Estrogen Replacement Therapy

The loss of bone as a result of accelerated resorption in women at the menopause is a universally accepted phenomenon. However, the magnitude of this loss is dependent on the site and specific bone envelope measured. Typically one to two per cent per year is lost from appendicular cortical regions and 4 to 6 per cent from spinal trabecular regions.[21, 119, 155] This finding has led some investigators[156] to differentiate between a form of osteoporosis (type I) specifically associated with this rapid, menopause-related, preferential loss of trabecular bone and a relatively slower, age-related loss of both cortical and trabecular bone (type II). Despite this distinction, it is clear that the loss of ovarian function has a profound influence on the risk for the development of osteoporosis.

Most women who initiate estrogen replacement therapy at the time of menopause or soon thereafter are spared the normal skeletal degradation that would otherwise occur at this point in the life cycle.[119] Discontinuation of therapy results in resumption of the normal menopausal bone loss phase.[157] Perhaps more important, long-term estrogen replacement therapy reduces the likelihood of fracture twofold.[121]

Although estrogen replacement therapy is known to decrease bone loss, it does have side effects and is unacceptable to many women.[144-158] Decisions about the initiation of estrogen therapy may be contingent on a number of factors, including the current level of bone density, severity of menopausal symptoms, patient or physician preferences, laboratory evidence of rapid bone loss, and possibly the long-term risk of cardiovascular disease.[159] Many experts would agree that compliance with estrogen therapy may be enhanced by quantitative information concerning fracture risk and efficacy of treatment.

The absolute level of bone density at the menopause and the magnitude of subsequent bone loss are important considerations in assessing the risk for future fracture. Even considering menopausal and subsequent age-related decrements in bone mass, the subgroup of women who have high bone density at the menopause will most likely be conferred significant protection by virtue of their relatively dense skeleton and may not require estrogen or any other intervention. By the same token, women with low-to-moderate levels of bone density appear to be at increased risk for fracture if therapy is not initiated early.[141, 143, 144] The decision to begin prophylaxis against osteoporosis, therefore, can most appropriately be made with knowledge of the woman's bone density.

Establishing a Diagnosis of Osteoporosis or Assessing its Severity

A growing number of individuals are concerned about their current skeletal status and their future risk of fracture. Some authorities[144, 158, 160] have recommended a comprehensive approach for managing these patients in which clinical risk factors (Table 13-10) are assessed and bone densitometry is performed if a number of risk factors are found. We agree that

TABLE 13–10 ■ Clinical Risk Factors for Osteoporosis

Female	Petite frame
White/Asian	Family history
Menopausal	Dietary deficiency of calcium
Elderly	Alcohol or tobacco consumption
Atraumatic fracture	
Inactivity	

bone density should be measured if factors predisposing to secondary forms of osteoporosis are found (see Assessment of Patients With Metabolic Diseases Known to Affect the Skeleton). However, evidence[161, 162] suggests that historically based risk factors (e.g., low calcium diet, smoking, family history of osteoporosis, petite frame), taken either singularly or in combination, have limited predictive value for fracture risk or for bone density in the individual patient, but some factors (e.g., female, postmenopausal, white, and elderly) may be helpful in targeting certain populations for study. Similarly, it is generally acknowledged that conventional spinal radiography is neither highly sensitive nor highly specific for detecting osteoporosis, particularly in its early stages. Substantial bone loss may precede radiographically detectable osteoporosis or fracture, and radiographic evidence of vertebral deformity or fracture may result from causes other than osteoporosis. Furthermore, even the presence of osteoporotic fracture may confer variable and uncertain future fracture risk. Finally, the use of biochemical analysis, although helpful in excluding secondary forms of osteoporosis, is of limited value in diagnosing osteoporosis or assessing its severity.

In contrast, evidence now supports the concept that the absolute level of bone density is predictive of future fracture risk. First, most of the variance in bone strength is attributable to bone density.[126, 163, 164] Second, recent studies suggest a gradient of increasing fracture risk corresponding to declining levels in bone density.[140, 141, 165-168] Third, prophylactic agents, such as estrogen, that reduce the occurrence of hip and spine fractures undoubtedly do so by retarding bone loss. Thus bone density per se provides the principal standard of osteoporosis risk.

Therefore it should be recommended that quantitative evaluation of the skeleton be performed in individuals in whom there is concern for osteoporosis or in whom there is radiographic suggestion or confirmation of atraumatic fracture. If fracture risk assessed by bone densitometry is low, then conservative management, perhaps with calcium and exercise, should be employed. If fracture risk is high, however, more aggressive treatment, perhaps with estrogen or calcitonin, should be prescribed.

Serial Assessment to Monitor Disease Progression or Therapeutic Response

In the past, bone density measurement techniques were associated with high precision errors relative to estimated rates of change and were therefore criticized for their inability to monitor individual patient changes in bone density. In response to this criticism, substantial improvements have been made in the past few years. SPA with rectilinear scanning; the new high-speed, x-ray–based DPA; and QCT with automatic image analysis have precision errors that approach one to two per cent. To achieve precision levels of this degree, however, adherence to strict quality assurance measures and careful technical monitoring are necessary.

Several authors[128, 169] have appropriately advised caution in interpretation of serial bone density measurements. Based on two-point measurements and two percent precision error, they showed that bone density changes in individual patients must be greater than 5.5 per cent to be detected with 95 per cent confidence. It should be noted, however, that these authors used a two-tailed estimation of confidence intervals, which may be inappropriate for assessing individual changes in bone density. The important clinical questions under consideration are (1) whether an individual is losing bone at a rate considered clinically significant (e.g., at the time of menopause); (2) whether the individual is gaining bone as a result of some treatment intervention (e.g., calcitonin therapy in osteoporotic patients); or (3) whether the individual is stable relative to an expected loss or an expected gain. Effects to the contrary are of limited clinical importance, and monitoring bone mass changes in the individual patient can be satisfactorily accomplished using a one-tailed test of significance. In addition, 90 per cent confidence is most probably adequate for purposes of clinical decision making.[170] As indicated in Tables 13–11 and 13–12, if two-point serial measurements are used, a technique with a two per cent precision error can detect changes in bone mass greater than 3.6 per cent with 90 per cent confidence. Similarly, with 1.5 per cent precision, changes of 2.7 per cent can be detected. The measurement time intervals should be appropriately spaced and the measurement sites appropriately selected such that the changes to be detected match the precision and sensitivity capabilities of the technique. Numerous studies have shown that large annual losses (of 5 to 20 per cent) from sites rich in trabecular bone can be observed in women undergoing surgical or natural menopause,[21, 119, 155] in patients initiating high-dose corticosteroid treatment,[35, 149] and in individuals who are completely immobilized.[171, 172] Similarly, large annual gains of 5

TABLE 13–12 ■ Bone Density Measurements to Monitor Progress of Disease or Therapeutic Response

	SPA (%)	DPA (%)	QCT (%)
Average annual losses (after menopause)	1–3	2–4	4–6
Average annual gains (after treatment with calcitonin, sodium fluoride, diphosphonates, or parathyroid hormones)	0–1	2–10	4–20

Abbreviations: DPA = dual-photon absorptiometry; SPA = single-photon absorptiometry.

to 15 per cent have been observed in osteoporotic patients receiving calcitonin treatment[173, 174] or investigational agents such as sodium fluoride,[175] diphosphonates,[176] or parathyroid hormone.[177]

Given the marked effect of some interventions and the continued improvements in measurement precision, the speed at which bone density measurements can be performed, and the reduced cost, it is difficult to pose convincing arguments against monitoring individual patients when important therapeutic decisions are to be made.

The Dilemma of Mass Screening

The purpose of any screening instrument is to identify individuals at risk who should receive further assessment or treatment. The technique should be a reliable, easily administered, and inexpensive measure of a variable that has practical significance. In general, bone density measurements qualify on all these counts. The term *mass screening,* however, has a negative connotation among researchers and clinicians. As an alternative, many experts have recommended so-called "selective screening" for white and Asian women, at the age of menopause and beyond, who have several presumed risk factors for osteoporosis, and in consultation with their physicians.[144, 158, 160, 178] Of course, certain prerequisites must be achieved before these recommendations could be realistically followed.

Knowledge about the proper use and interpretation of bone densitometry studies and an understanding of appropriate medical interventions are not universal among physicians, nor is instrumentation and technical performance of bone density studies of uniformly high quality. Indeed, this deficiency of medical and technical expertise is the principal deterrent to widespread implementation of these recommended clinical applications. However, given the current impetus to disseminate information about osteoporosis, to make newer instrumentation more readily available, and to limit the cost of these techniques, these recommendations may become standard medical practice.

References

1. National Institutes of Health. Osteoporosis consensus conference. JAMA 252:199–802, 1984.

TABLE 13–11 ■ Bone Density Changes Based on Two Measurements: Two-Tailed Versus One-Tailed Estimation of Confidence Limit

PRECISION ERROR (%)	95%/TWO-TAILED CONFIDENCE LIMIT (%)	90%/ONE-TAILED CONFIDENCE LIMIT (%)
1	±2.8	1.8
2	±5.5	3.6
3	±8.3	5.4

2. Snyder W: Report of the task group on reference man. Oxford, England, Pergamon Press, 1975.
3. Frost HM: Dynamics of bone remodeling. In: Frost HM (ed): Bone Biodynamics. Boston, Little, Brown, 1964, pp 315–334.
4. Garn SM: The Earlier Gain and Later Loss of Cortical Bone. Springfield, IL, Charles C Thomas, 1970.
5. Cameron JR, Mazess RB, Sorenson JA: Precision and accuracy of bone mineral determination by direct photon absorptiometry. Invest Radiol 3:141–145, 1968.
6. Mazess RB, Cameron JR: Bone mineral content in normal U.S. whites. In Mazess RB (ed): Proceedings of the International Conference on Bone and Mineral Measurement, October, 1973, Chicago, IL. Washington, DC, US Government Printing Office, 1974. DHEW publication no. (NIH) 75-683.
7. Sorenson JA, Mazess RB: Effects of fat on bone mineral measurements. In Cameron JR (ed): Proceedings of the Bone Measurement Conference. (US Atomic Energy Commission (USAEC) Conference 700515). Washington, DC, USAEC, 1970, pp 255–262.
8. Wahner HW, Eastell R, Riggs BL: Bone mineral density of the radius: where do we stand? J Nucl Med 26(11):1339–1341, 1985.
9. Adams JE, Chen S, Adams PH, Isherwood I: Dual energy computed tomography (CT) and the estimation of bone mass. J Comput Assist Tomogr 6:204, 1982.
10. Adams JE, Chen SZ, Adams PH, Isherwood I: Measurement of trabecular bone mineral by dual energy computed tomography. J Comput Assist Tomogr 6:601–607, 1982.
11. Burgess AE, Colborne B, Zoffmann E: Vertebral bone mineral content. Proceedings of the 5th International Workshop on Bone and Soft Tissue Densitometry, Bretton Woods, NH, October 14–18, 1985.
12. Cann CE, Martin MC, Genant HK, Jaffe RB: Decreased spinal mineral content in amenorrheic women. JAMA 251:626, 1984.
13. Cann CE, Genant HK: Cross-sectional studies of vertebral mineral content using quantitative computed tomography. J Comput Assist Tomogr 6:216, 1982.
14. Cann CE, Rutt BK, Genant HK: Effects of extraosseous calcification on vertebral mineral measurement. Presented at the annual meeting of the American Society of Bone and Mineral Research, Detroit, MI, April 9–12, 1983.
15. Cann CE, Genant HK, Kolb FO, Ettinger BF: Quantitative computed tomography for prediction of vertebral fracture risk. Bone 6:1–7, 1985.
16. Cann CE, Ettinger B, Genant HK: Normal subjects versus osteoporotics: no evidence using dual energy computed tomography for disproportionate increase in vertebral marrow fat. J Comput Assist Tomogr 9:617–618, 1985.
17. Faul DD, Couch JL, Cann CE, Boyd DP, Genant HK: Composition-selective reconstruction for mineral content in the axial and appendicular skeleton. J Comput Assist Tomogr 6:202, 1982.
18. Firooznia H, Rafii M, Golimbu C, Schwartz MS, Ort P: Trabecular mineral content of the spine in women with hip fracture: CT measurement. Radiology 159:737–740, 1986.
19. Gallagher JC, Gogar D, Mahoney P, McGill J: Measurement of spine density in normal and osteoporotic subjects using computed tomography: relationship of spine density to fracture threshold and fracture index. J Comput Assist Tomogr 9:634, 1985.
20. Genant HK, Boyd D: Quantitative bone mineral analysis using dual energy computed tomography. Invest Radiol 12(6):545–551, 1977.
21. Genant HK, Cann CE, Ettinger B, Gordan GS: Quantitative computed tomography of vertebral spongiosa: a sensitive method for detecting early bone loss after oophorectomy. Ann Intern Med 97:699–705, 1982.
22. Genant HK, Boyd DP, Rosenfeld D, Abols Y, Cann CE: Computed tomography. In Cohn SH (ed): Non-invasive measurements of bone mass and their clinical application. Boca Raton, FL, CRC Press, 1981, pp 121–149.
23. Genant HK, Cann CE, Boyd DP, Kolb FO, Ettinger B, Gordan GS: Quantitative computed tomography for vertebral mineral determination. In Frame B, Potts JT (eds): Clinical Disorders of Bone and Mineral Metabolism: Proceedings of the Frances and Anthony D'Anna Memorial Symposium (International Congress Series no 617), May 9–13, 1983, Detroit, MI. Amsterdam, Excerpta Medica, 1983, pp 355–359.
24. Genant HK, Cann CE, Pozzi-Mucelli RS, Kantner AS: Vertebral mineral determination by QCT: clinical feasibility and normative data. J Comput Assist Tomogr 7:554, 1983.
25. Genant HK, Powell MR, Cann CE, Stebler B, Rutt BK, et al: Comparison of methods for in vivo spinal bone mineral measurement. In Christiansen C, Arnaud CD, Nordin BEC, Parfitt AM, Peck WA, Riggs BL (eds): Osteoporosis. Proceedings of the Copenhagen International Symposium on Osteoporosis, June 3–8, 1984, Copenhagen, Denmark. Copenhagen, Aalborg Stiftsbogtrykkeri, 1984, pp 97–102.
26. Genant HK, Cann CE, Ettinger B, Gordan GS, Kolb FO, et al: Quantitative computed tomography for spinal mineral assessment. J Comput Assist Tomogr 9:602–604, 1985.
27. Hangartner TN, Overton TR: The Alberta gamma CT system. J Comput Assist Tomogr 6:1156, 1983.
28. Laval-Jeanet AM, Cann CE, Roger B, Dallant P: A postprocessing dual energy technique for vertebral CT densitometry. J Comput Assist Tomogr 8(6):1164–1167, 1984.
29. Laval-Jeanet AM, Jones CD, Bergot C, et al: Comparison of bone loss from spongiosa and from compact vertebral bone in the aging process and in osteoporotics. Proceedings of the 5th International Workshop on Bone and Soft Tissue Using Computed Tomography, Bretton Woods, NH, October 14–18, 1985.
30. Mack LA, Hanson JA, Kilcoyne RF, Oh SM, Gallagher JC, et al: Correlation between fracture index and bone densitometry by CT and dual photon absorptiometry. J Comput Assist Tomogr 9:635–636, 1985.
31. Orphanoudakis SC, Jensen PS, Rauschkolb EN, Lang R, Rasmussen H: Bone mineral analysis using single energy computed tomography. Invest Radiol 14:122–130, 1979.
32. Powell MR, Kolb FO, Genant HK, Cann CE, Stebler BG: Comparison of dual photon absorptiometry and quantitative computed tomography of the lumbar spine in the same subjects. In Frame B, Potts JT (eds): Clinical Disorders of Bone and Mineral Metabolism. Amsterdam, Excerpta Medica, 1983, pp 58–61.
33. Raymakers JA, Hoekstra O, Van Puten J, Kerkhoff H, Duursma SA: Osteoporotic fracture prevalence and bone mineral mass measured with CT and DPA. Skeletal Radiol 15:191, 1986.
34. Reinbold WD, Genant HK, Reiser UJ, Harris ST, Ettinger B: Bone mineral content in early-postmenopausal and postmenopausal osteoporotic women: comparison of measurement methods. Radiology 160(2):469–478, 1986.
35. Richardson ML, Genant HK, Cann CE, Ettinger B, Gordan GS, et al: Assessment of metabolic bone diseases by quantitative computed tomography. Clin Orthop 185:224–238, 1985.
36. Rohloff R, Hitzler H, Arndt W, Frey W: Vergleichende Messungen des Kalksalzgehaltes spongioeser Knochen mittels Computertomographie und J-125-Photonen-Absorptionsmethode. In Lissner J, Doppman JL (eds): CT'82, Konstanz, Schnetztor Verlag, 1982, pp 126–130.
37. Rüegsegger P, Elsasser U, Anliker M, Gnehm H, Kind HP, Prader A: Quantification of bone mineralization using computed tomography. Radiology 121:93–97, 1976.
38. Sambrook PN, Bartlett C, Evans R, Hesp R, Kaltz D, Reeve J: Measurement of lumbar spine bone mineral: a comparison of dual-photon absorptiometry and computed tomography. Br J Radiol 58:621, 1985.
39. Stebler BG, Rutt BK, Hosier K, Cann CE, Boyd DP, Genant HK: Signal system and data acquisition system for multielement germanium detectors. Proceedings of CT densitometry workshop. J Comput Assist Tomogr 9:610–611, 1985.
40. Cann CE: Quantitative bone mineral analysis using dual energy computed tomography. Radiology 152:257–261, 1987.
41. Dalen N, Lamke B: Bone mineral losses in alcoholics. Acta Orthop Scand 47:469–471, 1976.
42. Krolner B, Pors-Nielsen S: Measurement of bone mineral content of the lumbar spine: theory and application of a new two-dimensional dual photon attenuation method. Scand J Clin Lab Invest 40:485–487, 1980.

43. Madsen M, Peppler W, Mazess RB: Vertebral and total body bone mineral content by dual photon absorptiometry. Calcif Tissue Res 2:361–364, 1976.
44. Nilas L, Borg J, Gotfredsen A, Christiansen C: Comparison of single and dual photon absorptiometry in postmenopausal bone mineral loss. J Nucl Med 26:1257–1262, 1985.
45. Peppler WW, Mazess RB: Total body bone mineral and lean body mass by dual-photon absorptiometry. Calcif Tissue Int 33:353, 1981.
46. Riggs BL, Wahner HW, Dunn WL, Mazess RB, Offord KP, Melton LJ III: Differential changes in bone mineral density of the appendicular and axial skeletal with aging. J Clin Invest 67:328–335, 1981.
47. Roos B, Rosengren B, Skoldborn H: Determination of bone mineral content in lumbar vertebrae by a double gamma-ray technique. In Cameron JR (ed): Proceedings of the Bone Measurement Conference: USAEC Conf-700515. Springfield, VA, Clearinghouse for Federal Scientific and Technical Information, National Bureau of Standards, US Dept of Commerce, 1970, pp 243–254.
48. Wahner HW, Dunn WL, Mazess RB, Towsley M, Lindsay R, et al: Dempster: Dual-photon Gd-153 absorptiometry of bone. Radiology 156:203–206, 1985.
49. Jones CD, Laval-Jeantet AM, Laval-Jeantet MH, Genant HK: Importance of measurement of spongious vertebral bone mineral density in the assessment of osteoporosis. Bone 8(4):201–206, 1987.
50. Nottestad SY, Baumel JJ, Kimmel DB, Recker RR, Heaney RP: The proportion of trabecular bone in human vertebrae. J Bone Miner Res 2:221–229, 1987.
51. Kuhl DE, Edwards RQ: Image separation radioisotope scanning. Radiology 80:653–661, 1963.
52. Kuhl DE, Hale J, Eaton WL: Transmission scanning: a useful adjunct to conventional emission scanning for accurately keying isotope deposition to radiographic anatomy. Radiology 87:278–284, 1966.
53. Bracewell RN: Strip integration in radioastronomy. Aust J Phys 9:198–217, 1956.
54. Gordon R, Bender R, Herman GT: Algebraic reconstruction techniques (ART) for three-dimensional electron microscopy and x-ray photography. J Theor Biol 29:471–481, 1970.
55. Bracewell RN, Riddle AC: Inversion of fan-beam scans in radio astronomy. Astrophys J 150:427–434, 1967.
56. Brooks RA, Di Chiro G: Principles of computer assisted tomography (CAT) in radiographic and radioisotopic imaging. Phys Med Biol 21(5):689–732, 1976.
57. Brooks RA, Di Chiro G: Theory of image reconstruction in computed tomography. Radiology 117:561–572, 1975.
58. Zatz LM: General overview of computed tomography instrumentation. In Newton TH, Potts DG (eds): Radiology of the Skull and Brain. Technical Aspects of Computed Tomography. St Louis, CV Mosby, 1981, pp 4025–4057.
59. Cann CE: Quantitative CT applications: comparison of current scanners. Radiology 162:257–261, 1987.
60. Cann CE, Genant HK: Precise measurement of vertebral mineral content using computed tomography. J Comput Assist Tomogr 4(4):493–500, 1980.
61. Cann CE: Quantitative computed tomography for bone mineral analysis: technical considerations. In Genant HK (ed): Osteoporosis Update 1987. Berkeley, CA, University of California Press, 1987, pp 131–145.
62. Abols Y, Genant HK, Rosenfeld D, Boyd DP, Ettinger B, Gordon GS: Spinal bone mineral determination using computerized tomography in patients, control and phantoms. In Mazess RB (ed): Proceedings of the Fourth International Conference on Bone Measurement. NIH 80-1928. Washington, DC, US Government Printing Office, 1979.
63. Goodsitt MM, Rosenthal DI: Quantitative computed tomography scanning for measurement of bone and bone marrow fat content: a comparison of single and dual energy techniques using a solid synthetic phantom. Invest Radiol 22:799–810, 1987.
64. Kalender WA, Süss C: A new calibration phantom for quantitative computed tomography. Med Phys 9:816–819, 1987.
65. Reiser U, Heuck F, Faust U, Genant HK: Quantitative Computertomographie zur Bestimmung des Mineralgehalts in Lendenwirbeln mit Hilfe eines Festkoerper-Referenzsystems. Biomed Tech (Berlin) 30:187–188, 1985.
66. Zamenhof RGA: Optimization of spinal bone density measurement using computerized tomography. In Genant HK (ed): Osteoporosis Update 1987. Berkeley, CA, University of California Press, 1987, pp 145–169.
67. Arnold B: Solid phantom for QCT-bone mineral analysis. Proceedings of the 7th International Workshop on Bone Densitometry, Sept. 17–21, 1989, Palm Springs, California.
68. Computerized Imaging Reference Systems: CIRS Model IV Lumbar Reference Simulator Technical Manual. Norfolk, VA, CIRS, 1986.
69. Computerized Imaging Reference Systems: CIRS Model V Femoral Neck Reference Simulator Technical Manual. Norfolk, VA, CIRS, 1987.
70. Rutherford RA, Pullan BR, Isherwood I: Measurement of effective atomic number and electron density using an EMI scanner. Neuroradiology 11:15–21, 1976.
71. Alvarez RE, Macovski A: Energy-selective reconstructions in x-ray computerized tomography. Phys Med Biol 21(5):733–744, 1976.
72. Brooks RA: A quantitative theory of the Hounsfield unit and its application to dual energy scanning. J Comput Assist Tomogr 1(4):487–493, 1977.
73. Kalender WA, Perman WH, Vetter JR, Klotz E: Evaluation of a prototype dual-energy computed tomographic apparatus. I. Phantom studies. Med Phys 13(3):334–339, 1986.
74. Lehmann LA, Alvarez RE, Macovski A, Brody WR: Generalized image combinations in dual-kVp digital radiography. Med Phys 8:659–667, 1981.
75. Vetter JR, Kalender WA, Mazess RB, Holden JE: Evaluation of a prototype dual-energy computed tomographic apparatus. II. Determination of vertebral bone mineral content. Med Phys 13(3):340–343, 1986.
76. Burgess AE, Colborne B, Zoffman E: Vertebral trabecular bone: comparison of single and dual-energy CT measurements with chemical analysis. J Comput Assist Tomogr 11:506–515, 1987.
77. Kalender WA: Dual Energy Methods for SOMATON DR. No. A 19100-M2112-A114-01-7600. Erlangen, Germany, Siemens Incorporated, 1984.
78. Report of the Task Group on Reference Man. ICRP publication no. 23. Oxford, England, Pergamon Press, 1975.
79. Cann CE: Low-dose CT scanning for quantitative spinal mineral analysis. Radiology 140:813–815, 1981.
80. Glüer CC, Reiser UJ, Davis CA, Rutt BK, Genant HK: Vertebral mineral determination by quantitative computed tomography (QCT): accuracy of single and dual energy measurements. J Comput Assist Tomogr 12(2):242–258, 1988.
81. Talbert AJ, Brooks RA, Morgenthaler DG: Optimum energies for dual-energy computed tomography. Phys Med Biol 25(2):261–269, 1980.
82. Sandor T, Kalender WA, Hanlon WB, Weissman BN, Rumbaugh C: Spinal bone mineral determination using automated contour detection: application to single and dual energy CT. Proceedings of SPIE: The International Society for Optical Engineering, 555:188–194, 1985.
83. Steiger P, Steiger S, Rüegsegger P, Genant HK: Two- and three-dimensional quantitative image evaluation techniques for densitometry and volumetrics in longitudinal studies. In Genant HK (ed): Osteoporosis Update 1987. Berkeley, CA, University of California Press, 1987, pp 171–180.
84. Kalender WA, Brestowsky H, Felsenberg D: Bone mineral measurements: automated determination of the midvertebral CT section. Radiology 168:219–221, 1988.
85. Glüer CC, Genant HK: Quantitative computed tomography of the hip. In Genant HK (ed): Osteoporosis Update 1987. Berkeley, CA, University of California Press, 1987, pp 187–195.
86. Reiser UJ, Genant HK: Determination of Bone Mineral Content in the Femoral Neck by Quantitative Computed Tomography. Washington, DC, Radiological Society of North America, 1984.
87. Sartoris DJ, Andre M, Resnick C, Resnick D: Trabecular bone

density in the proximal femur: quantitative CT assessment. Radiology 160:707–712, 1986.

88. Steiger P, Rüegsegger P, Felder M: Three-dimensional evaluation of bone changes in joints of patients who have rheumatoid arthritis. J Comput Assist Tomogr 9(3):622–623, 1985.

89. Sartoris DJ, Resnick D, Bielecki D, Andre M, Gershuni D, Meyers M: A technique for multiplanar reformation and three-dimensional analysis of computed tomographic data: application to adult hip disease. J Can Assoc Radiol 37:69–72, 1986.

90. Gillespie JE, Isherwood I: Three-dimensional anatomic images from computed tomographic scans. Br J Radiol 59:289–292, 1986.

91. Rüegsegger P, Niederer P, Anliker M: An extension of classical bone mineral measurements. Ann Biomed Eng 2:194, 1974.

92. Reich NE, Seidelmann FE, Tubbs RR: Determination of bone mineral content using CT scanning. AJR 127:593, 1976.

93. Posner I, Griffiths HJ: Comparison of CT scanning with photon absorptiometric measurement of bone mineral content in the appendicular skeleton. Invest Radiol 12:545, 1977.

94. Laval-Jeantet AM, Roger B, Bouysse S, Bergot C, Mazess RB: Influence of vertebral fat content on quantitative CT density. Radiology 159:463–466, 1986.

95. Isherwood I, Rutherford RA, Pullan BR, Adams PH: Bone mineral estimation by computer assisted transverse axial tomography. Lancet II:712–715, 1976.

96. Bradley JG, Huang HK, Ledley RS: Evaluation of calcium concentration in bones from CT scans. Radiology 128:103–107, 1978.

97. Liliequist B, Larsson SE, Sjogren I, Wickman G, Wing K: Bone mineral content in the proximal tibia measured by computed tomography. Acta Radiol Diagn 20:957–966, 1979.

98. Rüegsegger P, Anliker M, Dambacher M: Quantification of trabecular bone with low dose computed tomography. J Comput Assist Tomogr 5:384–390, 1981.

99. Hangartner TN, Overton TR: Quantitative measurement of bone density using gamma-ray computed tomography. J Comput Assist Tomogr 6:1156, 1982.

100. Firooznia H, Golimbu C, Rafii M, Schwartz MS, Alterman ER: Quantitative computed tomography assessment of spinal trabecular bone: age-related regression in normal men and women. J Comput Assist Tomogr 8:91–97, 1984.

101. Sashin D, Sternglass EJ, Sandler RB, Slasky BS, Herbert DL, et al: The development and evaluation of a CT technique for measurement of the density of cortical bones in the appendicular skeleton. J Comput Assist Tomogr 7:552, 1983.

102. Graves VB, Wimmer R: Long term reproducibility of quantitative computed tomography vertebral mineral measurements. CT 9:73–76, 1985.

103. Rosenthal DI, Ganott MA, Wyshak G, Slovik DM, Doppelt SH, Neer RM: Quantitative computed tomography for spinal density measurement factors affecting precision. Invest Radiol 20:306–310, 1985.

104. Meier DE, Orwoll ES, Jones JM: Marked disparity between trabecular and cortical bone loss with age in healthy men. Ann Intern Med 101:605–612, 1984.

105. Cann CE, Henzi M, Burry K, Andreko J, Hanson F, et al: Reversible bone loss is induced by GnRH agonists. Presented at the 68th Annual Meeting of the Endocrine Society, Anaheim, CA, June 25–27, 1986, p 37.

106. Heaney RP, Recker RR: Distribution of calcium absorption in middle-aged women. Am J Clin Nutr 43:299–305, 1986.

107. Mazess RB: Measurement of skeletal status by noninvasive methods. Calcif Tissue Int 28:89, 1979.

108. Kalender WA, Klotz E, Süss C: Vertebral bone mineral analysis: an integrated approach with CT. Radiology 164:419–423, 1987.

109. Joseph PM, Spital RD: A method for correcting bone-induced artifacts in computed tomography scanners. J Comput Assist Tomogr 2:100, 1978.

110. Robertson DD, Huang HK: Quantitative bone measurements using x-ray computed tomography with second-order correction. Med Phys 13:474, 1986.

111. Mazess RB: Errors in measuring trabecular bone by computed tomography due to marrow and bone composition. Calcif Tissue Int 35:148–152, 1983.

112. Mazess RB, Vetter J: Comparison of dual-photon absorptiometry and dual-energy computed tomography for vertebral mineral. J Comput Assist Tomog 9:624–625, 1985.

113. Rohloff R, Hitzler H, Arndt W, Frey KW: Experimentelle Untersuchungen zur Genauigkeit der Mineralsalzgehaltsbestimmung spongioeser Knochen mit Hilfe der Quantitativen CT (Einenergiemessung). Fortschr Roentgenstr 143:692–697, 1985.

114. Cann CE: Erratum. Radiology 164(3):879, 1987.

115. Steiger P, Glüer CC, Genant HK: Simultaneous calibration in QCT: a comparison of commercial calibration phantoms. Abstract. Calcif Tissue Int 44(2):147, 1989.

116. Cann CE, Heller M, Skinner HB: A functional presentation format for 3-D bone images. Radiology 153P:311, 1984.

117. Helms CA, Cann CE, Brunelle FO, Gilula FA, Chafetz N, Genant HK: Detection of bone marrow metastases using quantitative CT. Radiology 140:745, 1981.

118. Banks LM, Stevenson JC: Modified method of spinal computed tomography for trabecular bone mineral measurements. J Comput Assist Tomogr 10:463–467, 1986.

119. Ettinger B, Genant HK, Cann CE: Postmenopausal bone loss is prevented by treatment with low-dosage estrogen with calcium. Ann Intern Med 106:40–45, 1987.

120. Firooznia H, Golimbu C, Rafii M, Schwartz MS, Alterman ER: Quantitative computed tomography assessment of spinal trabecular bone in osteoporotic women with and without vertebral fractures. J Comput Assist Tomogr 8:99–103, 1984.

121. Ettinger B, Genant HK, Cann CE: Long-term estrogen replacement therapy prevents bone loss and fractures. Ann Intern Med 102:319–324, 1985.

122. Marcus R, Cann CE, Madvig P, Minkoff J, Goddard M, et al: Menstrual function and bone mass in elite women distance runners. Ann Intern Med 102:158–163, 1985.

123. Block JE, Genant HK, Black D: Greater vertebral bone mineral mass in exercising young men. West J Med 145:39–42, 1986.

124. Kilcoyne RF, Hanson JA, Ott SM, Mack L, Chesnut CH: Vertebral bone mineral content measured by two techniques of computed tomography and compared with dual photon absorptiometry. J Comput Assist Tomogr 8:1164–1167, 1984.

125. Ott SM, Chesnut CH, Hanson JA, Kilcoyne RF, Murano R, Lewellen TK: Comparison of bone mass measurements using different diagnostic techniques in patients with postmenopausal osteoporosis. In Christiansen C, Arnaud CD, Nordin BEC, Parfitt AM, Peck WA, Riggs BL (eds): Osteoporosis. Proceedings of the Copenhagen International Symposium on Osteoporosis, June 3–8, 1984, Copenhagen. Copenhagen, Aalborg Stiftsbogtrykkeri, 1984, pp 93–96.

126. McBroom RJ, Hayes WC, Edwards WT, Goldberg RP, White III AA: Prediction of vertebral body compressive fracture using quantitative computed tomography. J Bone Joint Surg 67A:1206–1214, 1985.

127. Aitken JM: Relevance of osteoporosis in women with fractures of the femoral neck. Br J Med 288:1084–1085, 1984.

128. Cummings SR, Black D: Should perimenopausal women be screened for osteoporosis. Ann Intern Med 104:817–823, 1986.

129. Hall FM, Davis MA, Baran DT: Bone mineral screening for osteoporosis. N Engl J Med 316:212–214, 1987.

130. Ott SM: Should women get screening bone mass measurements? Ann Intern Med 104:874, 1986.

131. Bohr H, Schaadt O: Bone mineral content of femoral bone and the lumbar spine measured in women with fracture of the femoral neck by dual photon absorptiometry. Clin Orthop 179:240–245, 1983.

132. Krolner B, Pors Nielsen S: Bone mineral content of the lumbar spine in normal and osteoporotic women: cross-sectional and longitudinal studies. Clin Sci 62:329–336, 1982.

133. Riggs BL, Wahner HW, Seeman E, Offord KP, Dunn WL, et al: Changes in bone mineral density of the proximal femur and spine with aging: differences between the postmenopausal and senile osteoporosis syndromes. J Clin Invest 70:716–723, 1982.

134. Mazess RB, Barden H, Ettinger M, Schultz E: Bone density of the radius, spine, and proximal femur in osteoporosis. J Bone Miner Res 3:13–18, 1988.

135. Ross PD, Wasnich RD, MacLean CJ, Vogel JM: Prediction of individual lifetime fracture expectancy using bone mineral measurements. In Christiansen C, Johansen JS, Riis BJ (eds): Osteoporosis 1987. Proceedings of the International Symposium on Osteoporosis, September 27–October 2, 1987, Aalborg, Denmark. Copenhagen, Osteopress ApS 1987, pp 288–293.

136. Melton LJ, Kan SH, Wahner HW, Riggs BL: Lifetime fracture risk: an approach to hip fracture risk assessment based on bone mineral density and age. J Clin Epidemiol 41(10):985–994, 1988.

137. Mazess RB, Barden HS, Ettinger M, Johnston C, Dawson-Hughes B, et al: Spine and femur density using dual-photon absorptiometry in US white women. Bone Miner 2:211–219, 1987.

138. Garn SM, Rohmann CG, Wagner B: Bone loss as a general phenomenon in man. Fed Proc 6:1729–1736, 1967.

139. Mazess RB: On aging bone loss. Clin Orthop 165:239–252, 1982.

140. Ross PD, Wasnich RD, Vogel JM: Detection of prefracture spinal osteoporosis using bone mineral absortiometry. J Bone Miner Res 3(1):1–11, 1988.

141. Melton LJ III, Wahner HW, Richelson LS, O'Fallon WM, Riggs BL: Osteoporosis and the risk of hip fracture. Am J Epidemiol 124:254–261, 1986.

142. Odvina CV, Wergedal JE, Libanati CR, Schulz EE, Baylink DJ: Relationship between trabecular vertebral body density and fractures: a quantitative definition of spinal osteoporosis. Metabolism 37(3):221–228, 1988.

143. Wasnich RD: Fracture prediction with bone mass measurements. In Genant HK (ed): Osteoporosis Update 1987. Berkeley, CA, University of California Press, 1987, pp 95–101.

144. Riggs BL, Wahner HW: Bone densitometry and clinical decision-making in osteoporosis. Ann Intern Med 108(2):293–295, 1988.

145. Riis BJ, Christiansen C: Measurement of spinal or peripheral bone mass to estimate early postmenopausal bone loss? Am J Med 84:646–653, 1988.

146. Slemenda CW, Johnston C: Bone mass measurement: which site to measure. Am J Med 84:643–645, 1988.

147. Genant HK, Block JE, Steiger P, Glüer CC, Ettinger B, Harris ST: Appropriate use of bone densitometry. In Kleerekoper M, Krane S (eds): Clinical Disorders of Bone and Mineral Metabolism. New York, Mary Ann Liebert, Inc, 1989, pp 153–161.

148. Rickers H, Deding AA, Christiansen C, Rodbro P: Mineral loss in cortical and trabecular bone during high-dose prednisone treatment. Calcif Tissue Int 36:269–273, 1984.

149. Montag M, Belter SV, Meyer-Galander HM, Peters PE: BMC of the spongiosa in lumbar spine, measured by QCT: follow-up study in patients suffering from pemphigus and treated with high doses of cortisone. Presented at the Sixth International Workshop on Bone and Soft Tissue Densitometry, September 22–25, 1987, Buxton, England.

150. Gennari C, Imbimbo B: Effects of prednisone and deflazacort on vertebral bone mass. Calcif Tissue Int 37:592–593, 1985.

151. Meema HE, Oreopoulos DG, Rabinovich S, Husdan H, Rapoport A: Periosteal new bone formation (periosteal neostosis) in renal osteodystrophy: relationship to osteosclerosis, osteitis fibrosa and osteoid excess. Radiology 110:513, 1974.

152. Genant HK, Heck LL, Lanzl LH, Rossmann K, Vander Horst J, Paloyan E: Primary hyperparathyroidism. Radiology 109(3):513–519, 1973.

153. Kochersberger G, Buckely NJ, Leight GS, Martinez S, Studenski S, et al: What is the clinical significance of bone loss in primary hyperparathyroidism? Arch Intern Med 147:1951–1953, 1987.

154. Richardson ML, Pozzi-Mucelli RS, Kanter AS, Kolb FO, Ettinger B, Genant HK: Bone mineral changes in primary hyperparathyroidism. Skeletal Radiol 15:85–95, 1986.

155. Riis B, Thomsen K, Christiansen C: Does calcium supplementation prevent postmenopausal bone loss? N Engl J Med 316:173–177, 1987.

156. Riggs BL, Melton LJ: Evidence for two distinct syndromes of involutional osteoporosis. Am J Med 75:899–901, 1983.

157. Lindsay R, Hart DM, Forrest C, Baird C: Prevention of spinal osteoporosis in oophorectomized women. Lancet 2:1151–1153, 1980.

158. Tohme JF, Lindsay R: Bone mineral screening for osteoporosis. Letter. N Engl J Med 317:316, 1987.

159. Hillner BE, Hollenberg JP, Pauker SG: Postmenopausal estrogen in the prevention of osteoporosis: a benefit that is virtually without risk if cardiovascular effects are considered. Am J Med 80:1115, 1986.

160. Raisz LG, Lorenzo JA, Smith JA: Bone mineral screening for osteoporosis. Letter. N Engl J Med 317:315, 1987.

161. Citron JT, Ettinger B, Genant HK: Prediction of peak premenopausal bone mass using a scale of weighted clinical variables. In Christiansen C, Johansen JS, Riis BJ (eds): Osteoporosis 1987. Proceedings of the International Symposium on Osteoporosis, September 27–October 2, 1987, Aalborg, Denmark. Copenhagen, Osteopress ApS, 1987, pp 146–152.

162. Wasnich RD: Screening for osteoporosis: pro. In Genant HK (ed): Osteoporosis Update 1987. Berkeley, CA, University of California Press, 1987, pp 123–127.

163. Hansson T, Roos B, Nachemson A: The bone mineral content and ultimate compressive strength of lumbar vertebrae. Spine 5:46–55, 1981.

164. Melton LJ, Riggs BL: Risk factors for injury after a fall. Clin Geriatr Med 1:525–536, 1985.

165. Wasnich RD, Ross PD, Heilbrun LK, Vogel JM: Prediction of postmenopausal fracture risk with bone mineral measurements. Am J Obstet Gynecol 153(7):745–751, 1985.

166. Ross PD, Wasnich RD, Vogel JM: Definition of a spine fracture threshold based upon prospective fracture risk. Bone 8:271–278, 1987.

167. Ross PD, Wasnich RD, Vogel JM: Sources of accuracy and precision errors in dual photon absorptiometry. Abstract. Calcif Tissue Int 44(2):148, 1989.

168. Melton LJ III, Wahner HW, Riggs BL: Bone density measurement. J Bone Miner Res 3(1):ix–x, 1988.

169. Heaney RP: En recherche de la différence (P<0.05). Bone Miner 1:99–114, 1986.

170. Steiger P, Glüer CC, Black DM, Block JE, Smith R, et al: Monitoring change in bone mineral content: using the dispersion around the regression line as an estimate of precision. In Christiansen C, Johansen JS, Riis BJ (eds): Osteoporosis 1987. Proceedings of the International Symposium on Osteoporosis, September 27–October 2, 1987, Aalborg, Denmark. Copenhagen, Osteopress ApS 1987, pp 396–398.

171. Krolner B, Toft B: Vertebral bone loss: an unheeded side effect of therapeutic bed rest. Clin Sci 64:537–549, 1983.

172. Mazess RB, Whedon GD: Immobilization and bone. Calcif Tissue Int 35:265–267, 1983.

173. Gruber HF, Ivey JL, Baylink DJ, Matthews M, Nelp WB, et al: Long-term calcitonin therapy in postmenopausal osteoporosis. Metabolism 33:295, 1984.

174. Gennari C, Chierichetti SM, Bigazzi S, Fusi L, Gonnelli S, et al: Comparative effects on bone mineral content of calcium and calcium plus salmon calcitonin given in two different regimens in postmenopausal osteoporosis. Curr Ther Res 38(3):455–464, 1985.

175. Duursma SA, Glerum JH, Van Dijk A, Bosch R, Kerkhoff H, et al: Responders and non-responders after flouride therapy in osteoporosis. Bone 8:131–136, 1987.

176. Genant HK, Harris ST, Steiger P, Davey PF, Block JE: The effect of etidronate therapy in postmenopausal women: preliminary results. In Christiansen C, Johansen JS, Riis BJ (eds): Osteoporosis 1987. Proceedings of the International Symposium on Osteoporosis, September 27–October 2, 1987, Aalborg, Denmark. Copenhagen, Osteopress ApS, 1987, pp 1177–1181.

177. Slovik DM, Rosenthal DI, Doppelt SH, Potts JT, Daly MA, et al: Restoration of spinal bone in osteoporotic men by treatment with human parathyroid hormone (1-34) and 1,25-dihydroxyvitamin D. J Bone Miner Res 1(4):377–381, 1986.

178. Chesnut CH: Report from the NIH consensus conference, 1984, and the NIH/NOF Workshop, 1987. In Genant HK (ed): Osteoporosis Update 1987. Berkeley, CA, University of California Press, 1987, pp 3–6.

179. Genant HK, Steiger P, Block JE, Ettinger B, Harris ST: Quantitative computed tomography: update 1987. Editorial. Calcif Tissue Int 41:174–186, 1987.

CHAPTER 14

MUSCULOSKELETAL TUMORS

LYNNE S. STEINBACH ▪ *HARRY K. GENANT* ▪ *CLYDE A. HELMS*

The role of imaging in the evaluation of musculoskeletal tumors has increased with the development of computed tomography (CT) and magnetic resonance imaging (MRI). These imaging techniques provide improved tissue contrast and additional tissue planes for assessment of the anatomic extent of neoplasm. There is also a trend toward limb-sparing surgery for malignant musculoskeletal tumors, which creates a demand for more accurate preoperative assessment and follow-up for recurrence and complications such as hemorrhage and infection. Tumor response to radiation and chemotherapy protocols can also be evaluated by CT and MRI. The most important contributions of imaging to the assessment of a musculoskeletal tumor are its detection, characterization, staging, and follow-up; CT and MRI substantially aid in this quest, particularly in the latter two categories.

Detection

Detection of a pathologic condition by CT depends on differences in the linear attenuation coefficients between normal and abnormal tissue. MRI provides more contrast between background tissue and tumor when using pulse sequences designed to maximize differences in signal intensity. Neoplasms tend to have T2 and proton density values that are significantly greater than background tissues and T1 values that exceed those of fat.

Most musculoskeletal tumors occur in the extremities. To evaluate their extent by CT, multiple axial images are required. MRI allows for direct sagittal and coronal demonstrations of tumor extent, facilitating evaluation of longitudinal extent. Direct sagittal and coronal MR images have a spatial resolution superior to that of reformatted sagittal and coronal images by CT.[1]

Staging

The prognosis and treatment of a tumor is influenced by its anatomic location and extent, as well as its histologic grade. These criteria form the basis of staging of musculoskeletal tumors. Current management of malignant musculoskeletal tumors emphasizes limb-salvaging procedures, which may utilize prosthetic implants and allograft replacements. These procedures offer wide but local enbloc resection of tumor followed by reconstructive surgery to restore function. This approach requires more precise knowledge of the extent of tumor, which can be provided by CT and MRI.

Important anatomic considerations for local staging include the intra- and extramedullary boundaries, as well as involvement of cortical bone, neurovascular structures, and neighboring joints.

Intramedullary Extent

MRI is superior to CT and scintigraphy in defining tumor spread within the marrow.[2, 3] On CT scans, abnormal tissue displays higher attenuation values than does fatty marrow. Normal marrow ranges between −100 and −120 Hounsfield units (H). When the medullary cavity is infiltrated by tumor the attenuation is usually more than 15 H. Tumors that show minimal or normal findings by conventional radiographic techniques can be demonstrated by CT (Figs. 14–1 and 14–2).[4–6] When the tumor is osteoblastic, the intramedullary extent is easily identified, whereas at other times the invasion may be more subtle. The extent of marrow involvement is more readily determined by MRI. MRI provides greater contrast with sharper demarcation between normal and abnormal tissue. Contrast differences also facilitate determination of marrow invasion in smaller bones.

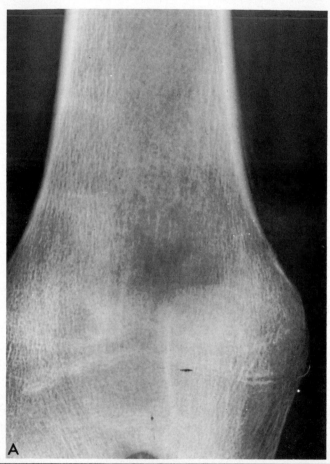

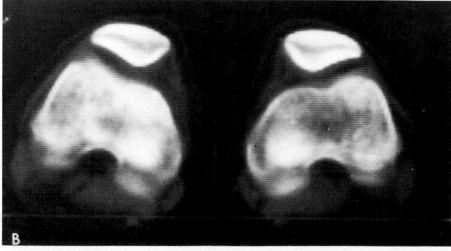

FIGURE 14–1 ■ Osteosarcoma. *A*, In this adolescent with a painful right knee, minimal, patchy sclerosis is noted in the distal end of the femur, and a subtle periosteal reaction is seen medially. *B*, CT scan demonstrates osteosclerosis of the medullary space of the right knee, indicating a central osteosarcoma but showing no evidence of any extraosseous soft tissue mass.

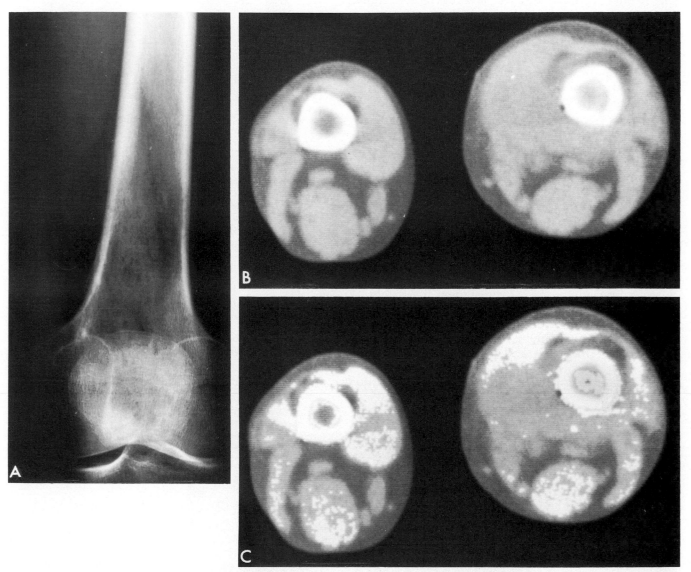

FIGURE 14–2 ■ Intramedullary involvement by fibrous histiocytoma. *A,* A plain radiograph of the left femur shows an ill-defined permeative lesion with minimal periostitis. This 35-year-old man had pain and a large soft tissue mass in the left thigh. *B,* CT scan through this region shows a large soft tissue mass with an increase in the intramedullary density on the left side. *C,* The "blink mode" confirms the increased intramedullary density on the left side. A biopsy showed this mass to be a malignant fibrous histiocytoma. The CT scan showed the extent of the intramedullary involvement and influenced therapy.

CT is limited to the axial plane unless reformations are attempted. This limitation is not ideal for evaluation of intramedullary extent in the extremities. However, direct coronal, sagittal, axial, and oblique planes can be utilized with MRI, thus facilitating determination of intraosseous extent.

The T1-weighted spin-echo MR technique (short repetition time [TR] and echo time [TE]) is best for evaluating the intraosseous extent of tumor. Using this sequence, most tumors have decreased signal intensity when compared with high-signal marrow (Figs. 14–3 and 14–4). These differences in signal intensity produce sharp contrast at the tumor margin. T1-weighted images in the coronal or sagittal plane are best for the evaluation of intramedullary extent in the long bones. This sequence also aids in the identification of skip metastases, which are seen in two to ten per cent of osteosarcomas (Fig. 14–5).[7, 8] Skip metastases are separate lesions of a tumor in the same bone or in the opposing side of a joint. Knowledge of their existence can alter patient prognosis and treatment.

Edematous or reactive marrow, which frequently surrounds a tumor, may simulate tumor by bone scintigraphy, CT, or MRI.[9–17] The edematous or reactive marrow demonstrates increased uptake on bone scan, high marrow density on CT, low signal within the marrow on T1-weighted MR images, and high signal on T2-weighted MR images. Although surrounding edema may overestimate the extent of tumor, it often contains microscopic neoplastic foci that should be resected. Nevertheless, a strong correlation has been shown between the boundary of tumor as seen by MRI and that seen on pathologic specimens.[3, 18, 19]

Osseous invasion by a primary soft tissue tumor

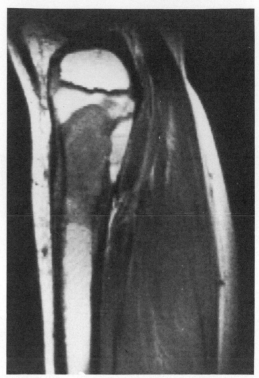

FIGURE 14–3 ■ High contrast between the intermediate-signal osteosarcoma and the surrounding marrow is shown on this T1-weighted sagittal MR image (TR, 500; TE, 40).

is rare.[13, 20, 21] If there is bone destruction and a soft tissue mass, the tumor is most likely to have originated in the bone. If soft tissue tumors lie close to bone, a wide resection may lead to excision of a portion of the bone.

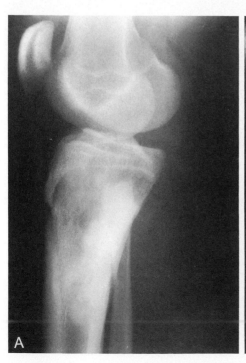

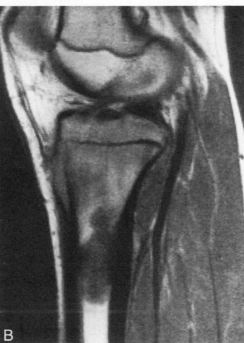

FIGURE 14–4 ■ A, Conventional lateral view of the proximal tibia reveals a sclerotic osteosarcoma with surrounding periosteal reaction. B, T1-weighted sagittal MR image demonstrates the extent of the tumor in the medullary cavity. The less sclerotic component extends to the tibial epiphysis. Low-intensity periosteal reaction blends imperceptibly into the cortex, giving it a thickened appearance.

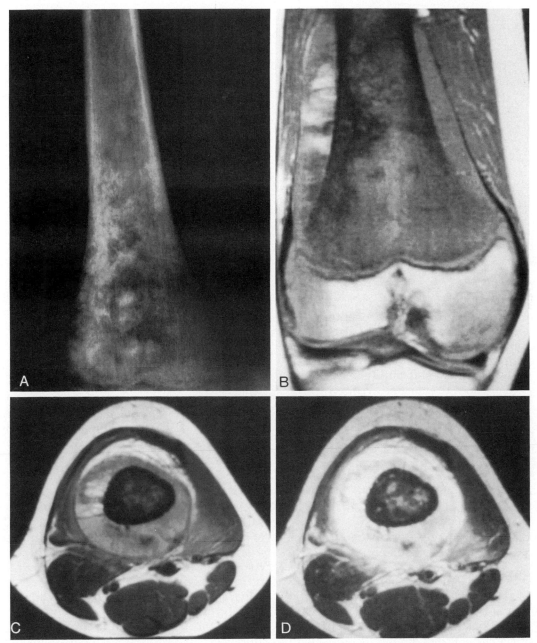

FIGURE 14–5 ■ *A,* Conventional radiograph of an osteosarcoma demonstrates foci of high density within the distal femoral diametaphysis. *B,* The sclerotic foci have low signal intensity on this T1-weighted coronal MR image of the femur. There is also intermediate signal intensity in the rest of the femoral diametaphysis consistent with tumor invasion. The tumor does not extend into the epiphysis. Soft tissue extension of the tumor is bordered by a low signal margin. There is a region of high signal in the soft tissue component of the tumor that represents hemorrhage.

T1- *(C)* and T2-weighted *(D)* axial MR images of this osteosarcoma reveal low-signal sclerotic tumor in the medullary region on both sequences. The tumor spreads radially into the soft tissues, with high contrast on the T2-weighted image. Tumor new bone is well seen as scattered low-signal areas within the soft tissue.

Illustration continued on following page

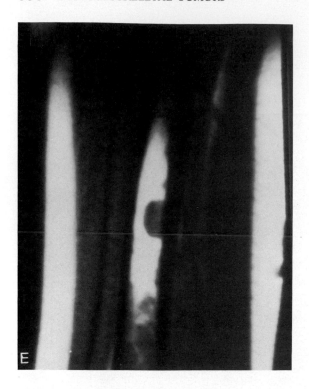

FIGURE 14–5 *Continued E,* Normal high-signal marrow separates the primary osteosarcoma in the distal femur and a more proximal skip metastasis on this sagittal T1-weighted MR image.

Extramedullary (Soft Tissue) Extent

MRI is frequently superior to CT in defining the extraosseous extent of a tumor.[2, 9, 18, 21–26] The role of CT in evaluation of soft tissue masses related to primary bone and soft tissue tumors has been elucidated.[5, 27–29] On CT scans, soft tissue masses are delineated by distortion of normal architecture or alteration in attenuation of the involved tissue (Figs. 14–6 through 14–8). Most soft tissue masses have an attenuation range of between −20 and +50 H—somewhat lower than adjacent muscle. Density differences may be sufficiently similar as to make detection of tumor boundaries very difficult.[30] In those cases, intravenous contrast enhancement often increases detection of the soft tissue component of the tumor (Figs. 14–9 and 14–10).[13, 31]

T2-weighted axial MR images (long TR and TE) are best for evaluating extraosseous extent of musculoskeletal tumors. On these images, the greatest contrast is achieved between high-signal tumor and muscle (Fig. 14–11). The axial plane allows for evaluation of the radial spread of tumor into the soft tissues. MRI is particularly helpful in evaluating the extent of tumor in the upper extremity and lower leg, where there is a paucity of fat and the muscles are smaller in size.[32] A study by Bloem and co-workers[2] evaluated 515 muscular compartments in 53 patients with tumors localized in the knee, pelvis, or shoulder region. Twenty-eight per cent of the compartments contained tumor. MRI was more sensitive (96 versus 71 per cent), more specific (99 versus 93 per cent), and more accurate (97 versus 80 per cent) in detecting muscular invasion than was CT.[2] Demas and colleagues also concluded that evaluation of the anatomic compartment and individual muscle involvement was more accurately accomplished with MR imaging than with CT.[22] Because of its high soft tissue contrast, MRI is also capable of distinguishing between pathologic soft tissue masses and hypertrophy or prominence of normal tissues.

Tumor extension to fat in the soft tissues can be assessed by both CT and MRI. Tumor has higher attenuation than does fat on CT scans, and its margin is easily seen (Fig. 14–12). The T1-weighted MR sequence is best when evaluating tumor invasion of fat by MRI, as this sequence provides the greatest contrast at the tumor margin.

Cortical Invasion

Investigations that have utilized high-resolution MRI techniques demonstrate MRI to be as accurate as CT in evaluating cortical invasion by tumor.[2, 14, 25, 33] Cortical bone has a very high attenuation coefficient on CT scans, thus facilitating identification of infiltration and destruction (Fig. 14–13). Cortical bone has low proton density, which produces a signal void on MRI scans, and invasion of cortical bone is most easily identified on axial T2-weighted spin-echo images.[34] High-signal tumor may be identified within low-signal cortex in the shafts of long bones on T2-weighted images (Figs. 14–14 and 14–15). The axial plane is favored, because it eliminates partial volume averaging of signal intensity in cortical bone, something that is often seen on coronal and sagittal MR images. One advantage of MRI over CT is that there are no streak artifacts from cortical bone to disrupt the image. MRI is helpful in identifying cortical invasion by highly aggressive malignant tumors with subtle permeative patterns of destruction (e.g., Ewing's sarcoma).[10]

Text continued on page 564

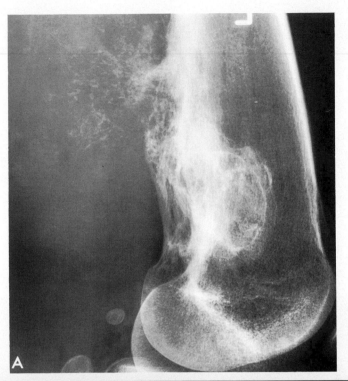

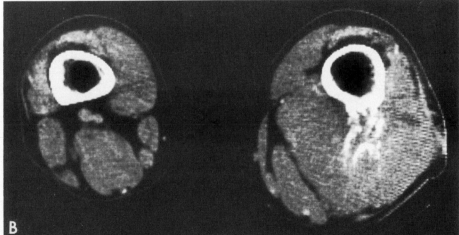

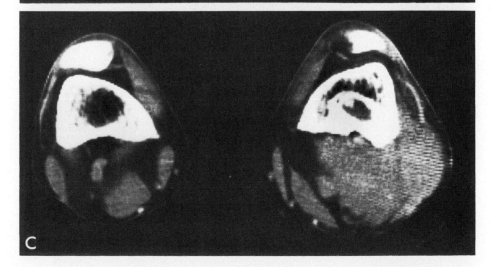

FIGURE 14–6 ■ Osteosarcoma. *A,* Lateral magnification radiograph of the left knee demonstrates a blastic sclerotic process involving the distal femoral metaphysis associated with aggressive periosteal reaction and a large soft tissue mass. *B,* CT scan defines the borders of the large soft tissue component. *C,* The CT scan was also useful in defining the intraosseous extent of the osteosarcoma.

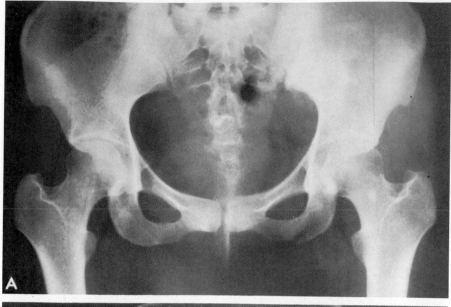

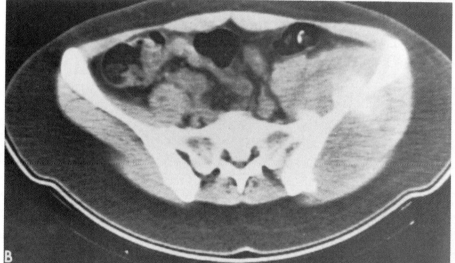

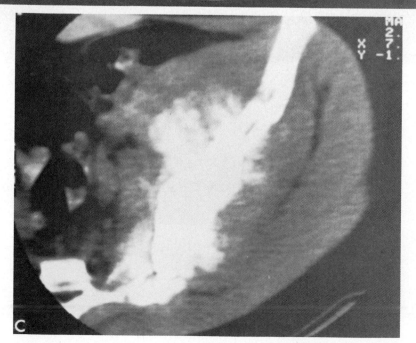

FIGURE 14–7 ■ Osteosarcoma of ilium. *A,* Conventional radiograph of the pelvis of a young adult reveals mixed sclerosis and destruction of the left ilium. *B* and *C,* CT scans reveal osteoblastic activity with destruction of the ilium. This activity is accompanied by a large soft tissue mass, suggesting osteosarcoma. In this case, the CT study yielded important diagnostic, prognostic, and therapeutic information.

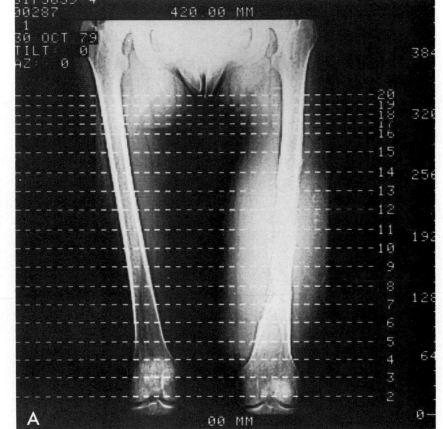

FIGURE 14–8 ■ Malignant fibrous histiocytoma. A, Scout view of the left thigh demonstrates the planes of sections obtained every 2 cm distally and through the main portion of the tumor and every 1 cm proximally to evaluate the extent of tumor.

Illustration continued on following page

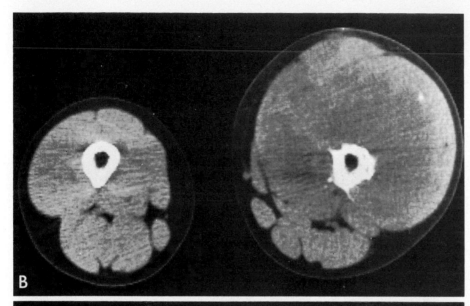

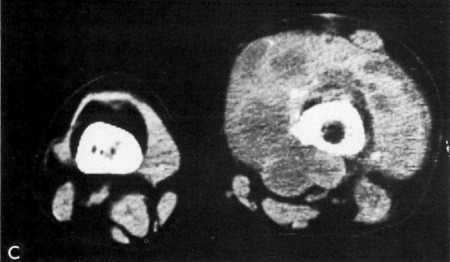

FIGURE 14–8 *Continued B* and *C,* CT scans with wide and narrow windows show a multilobulated, mixed-density soft tissue mass with underlying bone involvement. The proximal borders of the tumor were identified in other planes, facilitating surgical planning.

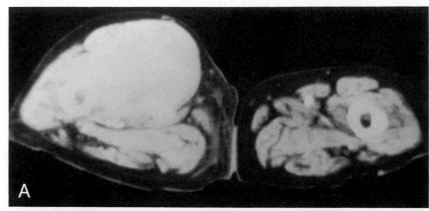

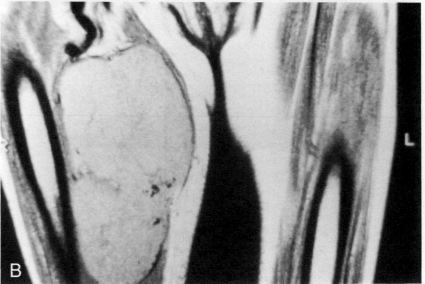

FIGURE 14–9 ■ *A,* A large enhancing mass anteromedial to the right femur is evident on this CT scan obtained with intravascular contrast. The borders of this malignant fibrous histiocytoma are difficult to distinguish relative to muscle.

B, The extent of this tumor in the thigh is better demonstrated on a coronal MR scan (TR, 1000; TE, 40).

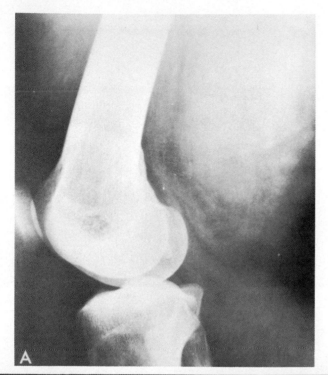

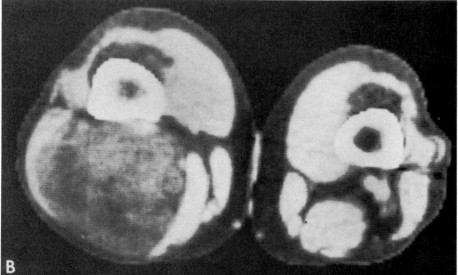

FIGURE 14–10 ■ Liposarcoma. *A,* Radiograph demonstrates a bulky mass with areas of low density in the right popliteal fossa. *B,* CT scan (without contrast) reveals a large, inhomogeneous mass of overall low density located between the semimembranosus and semitendinosus muscles.

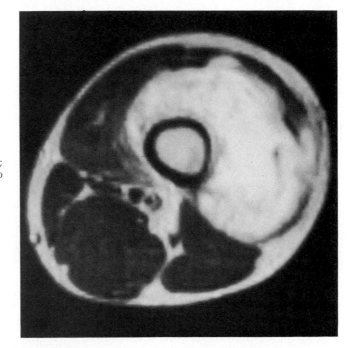

FIGURE 14–11 ■ Axial MR image of a myxoid liposarcoma (TR, 2000; TE, 60) demonstrates its extent in the soft tissues. The tumor extends into the quadriceps muscle and invades the subcutaneous fat medially.

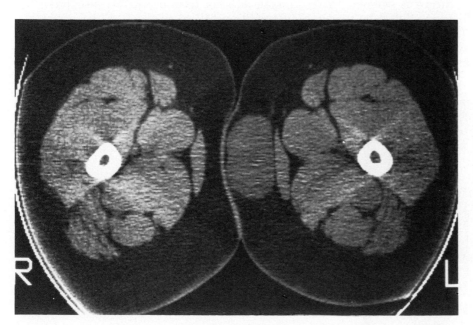

FIGURE 14–12 ■ Fibrous histocytoma. CT scan through the proximal thighs demonstrates a well-defined, smoothly marginated, homogeneous soft tissue mass of the left thigh. The mass has a density slightly lower than that of adjacent muscle but well above that of subcutaneous fat. Precise localization by CT was helpful in planning surgical excision.

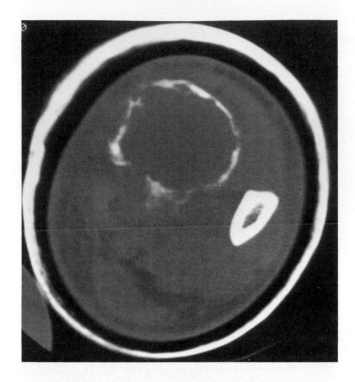

FIGURE 14–13 ■ Malignant fibrous histiocytoma presents on CT as an expansile lesion in the tibia that has destroyed and eroded the surrounding cortex. The cortical damage is easily assessed by CT because of the high attenuation of cortical bone.

Calcification, Ossification, and Periosteal Reaction

Calcification, ossification, and periosteal reaction associated with musculoskeletal tumors are more specifically identified using conventional radiographs and CT, in which the high density in the tissues is sharply contrasted against all background tissues except cortical bone.[18, 21, 25, 35, 36] If a tumor is osteoblastic, cortical invasion will be difficult to detect by both CT and MRI, as the density (i.e., intensity) is similar between tumor and cortical bone. There may be a subtle increase in signal intensity of osteosclerotic tumor when compared with cortical bone on T2-weighted MR images.

Calcified and ossified structures do not contain signal on MRI scans. Because visibility depends on the signal intensity in the surrounding tissues, the low signal is more difficult to detect, and calcification is not consistently identified (Fig. 14–16). The low signal is also nonspecific, as some vascular structures, metal, fibrous tissue, and air also have low signal intensity on MRI scans.[35]

Periosteal reaction that runs parallel and close to the cortical margin is more difficult to identify by MRI than periosteal reaction that courses at oblique

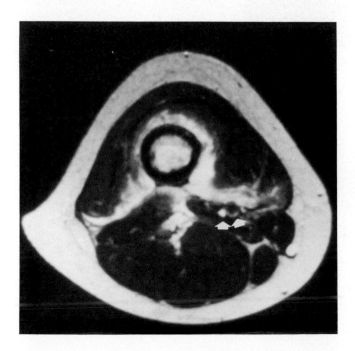

FIGURE 14–14 ■ High-intensity osteosarcoma invading cortex, marrow, and soft tissues on a T2-weighted axial MR image (TR, 2000; TE, 60). Tumor is easily identified within the low-intensity cortex. The tumor abuts but does not surround the femoral artery and vein (arrows).

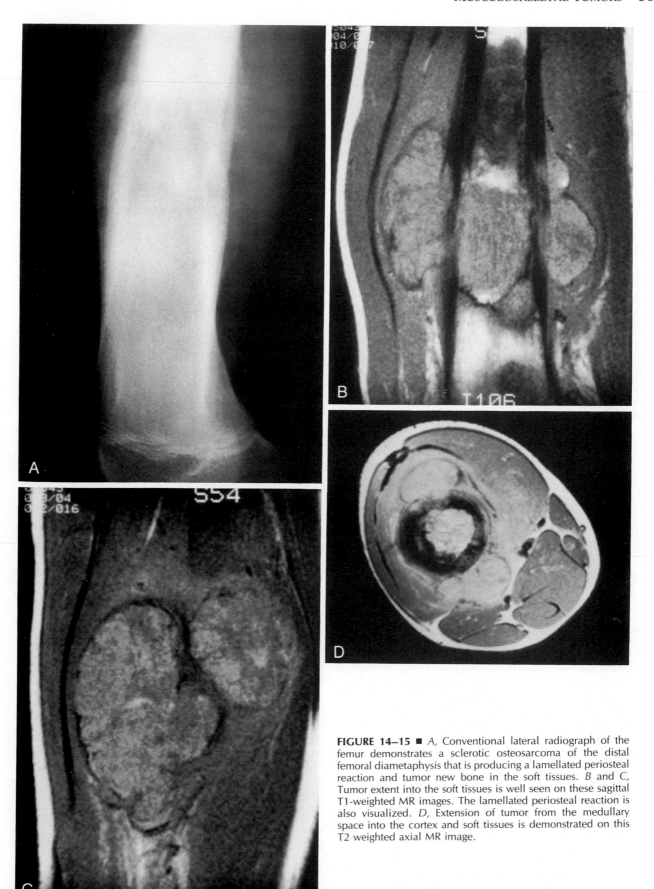

FIGURE 14–15 ■ *A,* Conventional lateral radiograph of the femur demonstrates a sclerotic osteosarcoma of the distal femoral diametaphysis that is producing a lamellated periosteal reaction and tumor new bone in the soft tissues. *B* and *C,* Tumor extent into the soft tissues is well seen on these sagittal T1-weighted MR images. The lamellated periosteal reaction is also visualized. *D,* Extension of tumor from the medullary space into the cortex and soft tissues is demonstrated on this T2 weighted axial MR image.

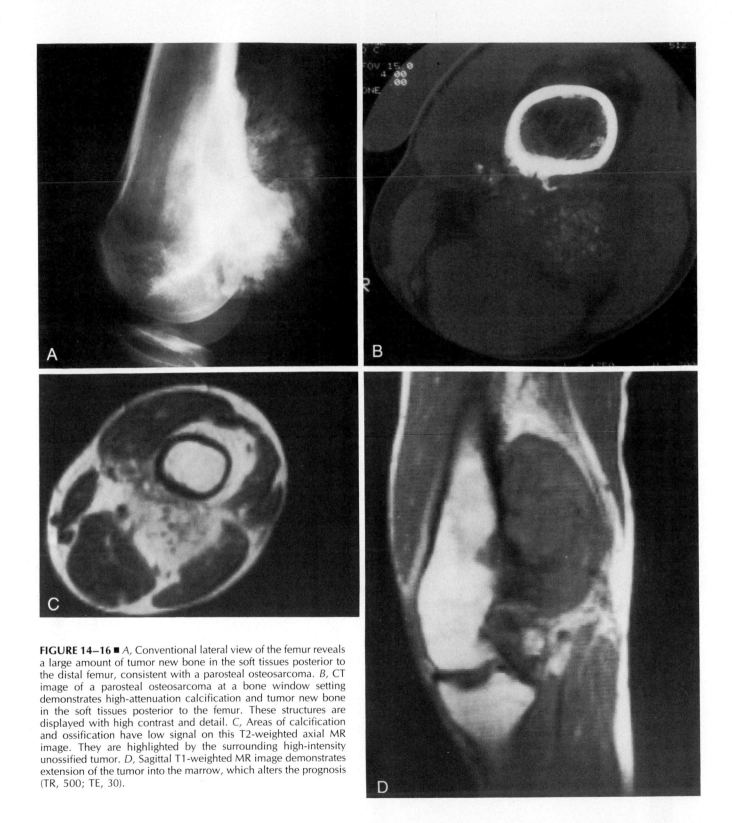

FIGURE 14–16 ■ *A,* Conventional lateral view of the femur reveals a large amount of tumor new bone in the soft tissues posterior to the distal femur, consistent with a parosteal osteosarcoma. *B,* CT image of a parosteal osteosarcoma at a bone window setting demonstrates high-attenuation calcification and tumor new bone in the soft tissues posterior to the femur. These structures are displayed with high contrast and detail. *C,* Areas of calcification and ossification have low signal on this T2-weighted axial MR image. They are highlighted by the surrounding high-intensity unossified tumor. *D,* Sagittal T1-weighted MR image demonstrates extension of the tumor into the marrow, which alters the prognosis (TR, 500; TE, 30).

or right angles to the cortex (Figure 14–17; also see Figs. 14–4 and 14–5). A rim of increased signal intensity may be seen at the periphery of periosteal reaction on T2-weighted images. This is thought to represent unmineralized thickened periosteum and associated edema and may be mistaken for a soft tissue mass.[30]

Neurovascular Invasion

Tumor extension into neurovascular structures worsens patient prognosis and alters treatment. When using CT, the vascular structures must be opacified with intravenous contrast, which introduces some risk and invasiveness. Most CT images are obtained perpendicular to the plane of the neurovascular structures. On MRI scans, larger vascular structures are low in signal intensity on T1-weighted images (see Fig. 14–4B), unless there is slow-flowing blood, as in smaller arteries and veins. There is often high contrast between the tumor and blood vessels on T2-weighted images (see Fig. 14–14). Ideally, at least one imaging plane should be parallel to the vascular structures to facilitate evaluation. Some studies have shown MRI to be superior to CT in demonstrating arterial involvement by tumor, whereas others show both to be equally accurate in the assessment of tumor relationships with neurovascular structures.[2, 25, 32, 35, 36] Neither MRI nor CT can be used to determine whether there is tumor invasion of neurovascular structures, except when there is complete encasement by the tumor.[20, 22]

Peripheral nerves are poorly visualized by all imaging techniques, including CT and MRI. However, larger nerves such as the sciatic nerve may be identified and are of intermediate signal intensity on spin-echo MR images.

Joint Invasion

Extension of tumor to a joint worsens patient prognosis and usually alters therapy.[37–40] In fact, it may be the deciding factor between a limb-salvaging procedure and amputation. If a tumor at the end of a long bone does not invade the joint capsule or synovium, an intraarticular resection can usually be done without risk of seeding the tumor elsewhere in the soft tissues. If the tumor does extend into the synovium, more extensive extraarticular resection is usually required.

CT and MRI are equally accurate in demonstrating or excluding the presence of tumors in major joints.[2] The advantages of MRI include direct multiplanar imaging, improved soft tissue contrast, and the use of surface coils, which provide more detail of the smaller structures within a joint (Figure 14–18; also see Fig. 14–3).[26, 35] MRI allows for noninvasive visualization of the hyaline cartilage, fibrocartilage, synovium, ligaments, tendons, effusions, and intraarticular masses.

Suggested Protocols for Staging

Optimum technical factors for the staging of musculoskeletal tumors by CT or MRI vary with the individual tumor, but some general guidelines can be followed. Precise localization of extremity neoplasms by CT usually requires 5- to 10-mm-thick sections from the joint above through the joint below the tumor, including normal areas on both sides of the lesion. Intravenous contrast is not usually required, but contrast administration can be tailored to the individual case. If a lesion is found to be isodense with muscle or if there is difficulty in identifying vascular structures, then intravenous contrast can be

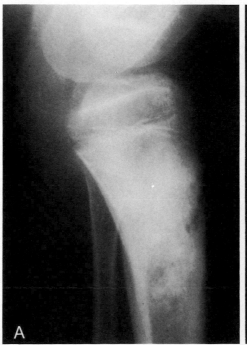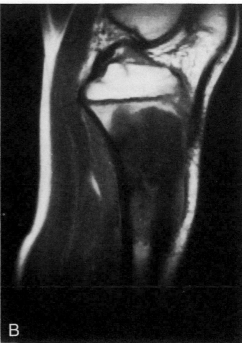

FIGURE 14–17 ■ A, Conventional lateral radiograph of an osteosarcoma of the tibia reveals an osteoblastic tumor with thick periosteal reaction parallel to the posterior tibial cortex. B, On a sagittal T1-weighted MR image, the periosteal reaction is again identified as a low signal band parallel to the posterior tibial cortex. The tumor is well seen as a region of low attenuation within the marrow.

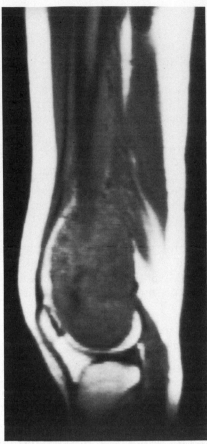

FIGURE 14–18 ■ Sagittal T1-weighted MR image shows that there is intervening normal marrow between this osteosarcoma and the knee joint (TR, 500; TE, 20).

administered by either constant infusion or bolus injection. If the lesion is in an extremity, then the contrast should be infused into a distal vein of the involved extremity. The contralateral extremity should be included in the field of view for baseline comparison. The lesion should be imaged using both bone and soft tissue window settings.

The recommended protocol for evaluation of musculoskeletal tumors in the extremities using spin-echo MRI includes images in multiple planes with both T1- (TR, <600 ms; TE, <40 ms) and T2- (TR, >1500 ms; TE >60 ms) weighted pulse sequences for evaluation of marrow and soft tissue extent.[10, 26, 37, 41] Surface coils should be used when possible to improve signal-to-noise ratio and spatial resolution. Slice thickness can range from 5 to 10 mm depending on the size of the tumor. At least one coronal or sagittal T1-weighted and one axial T2-weighted sequence should be included in the MR examination. Using the coronal T1-weighted sequence, the intramedullary extent of tumor is seen directly on a few slices and facilitates planning of surgical techniques. Skip metastases are also well visualized in this plane. The best demonstration of circumferential tumor spread into the soft tissues is seen on axial T2-weighted sequences. Additional sequences as appropriate may include a coronal T2-weighted sequence to demonstrate the longitudinal extent of tumor in the soft tissues and the relationship of tumor to neighboring vascular structures.

Gradient-echo techniques are being increasingly utilized in musculoskeletal MR imaging.[42] Gradient-echo sequences produce multiplanar T2 (T2*) images in a shorter time period than conventional spin-echo sequences by using a short TR and a flip angle with a theta value of less than 90°. Most musculoskeletal tumors have high signal intensity on gradient-echo images that is similar to that on T2-weighted images. Such fast scanning techniques can be added to a conventional spin-echo protocol in a plane other than that obtained by conventional spin echo or as a substitute for T2 weighting if there are time constraints.

Another sequence that is being investigated for tumor MR imaging is the short T1 inversion recovery (STIR) sequence.[43, 44] This sequence facilitates detection and localization of tumor by making the effects of prolonged T1 and T2 times on signal intensity additive and by nulling the signal from fat, which increases contrast at the tumor-fat interface. A study by Shuman and co-workers[43] of STIR technique versus spin echo in 45 patients with extremity tumors concluded that STIR is a useful adjunct in the imaging of musculoskeletal tumors. Three of the lesions missed on spin echo were detected on STIR images. In 77 per cent of cases, lesions were more conspicuous on the STIR images.

The addition of gadolinium DTPA to T1-weighted spin-echo sequences for tumor imaging is being widely investigated. Advantages of T1-weighted gadolinium images include the increased signal-to-noise ratio when compared with a T2-weighted image, the decreased acquisition time when compared with T2 weighting, and the observation that gadolinium usually increases the signal intensity of the tumor relative to necrosis.[45–50]

Characterization

In general, CT and MRI are nonspecific in differentiating among tumor, inflammation, and edema and often cannot distinguish benign from malignant tumors. Specific diagnoses are provided, however, in some instances. Morphologic criteria used to separate benign from malignant neoplasms are occasionally helpful. The hallmark of a benign tumor is a lesion with uniform density or signal intensity and with sharp, well-defined margins. Malignant musculoskeletal tumors are usually inhomogeneous because of internal necrosis, hemorrhage, or calcification. They often have indistinct borders extending into surrounding marrow, fat, and musculature. T1 and T2 measurements are of limited value for histologic characterization of musculoskeletal tumors. No correlation has been found between relaxation values of tumors and tumor type.[9, 51, 52]

Tumors with Osteoid Matrix

Osteoid osteomas contain a vascular osteoid nidus that is lucent on CT scans (Figs. 14–19 and 14–20). Within the nidus there may be an area of calcification, and sclerosis is frequently seen surrounding the nidus, except when the lesion is intraarticular. Synovitis with joint effusion is also seen when osteoid osteomas occur in a joint. When using MRI, the nidus has low signal on T1- and varying signal on T2-weighted images. A low signal on T2 weighting may be related to the osteoid matrix, central calcification, or extremely rapid regional blood flow within the nidus.[53] The marrow surrounding an osteoid osteoma may have low signal on T1 and T2 weighting if sclerotic, and high signal on T2 weighting if there is hyperemia and a surrounding inflammatory response.

Osteoblastomas occur predominantly in the spine and are larger and more aggressive than osteoid osteomas. Their extent is well seen by CT and MRI, particularly in the spine, where the degree of involvement of the osseous structures and spinal canal can be determined. Density and signal intensity vary, depending primarily on the amount of calcified osteoid in the osteoblastoma.

Osteosarcomas vary in their osteoid, cartilaginous, vascular, and fibrous content and are subdivided into osteoblastic, chondroblastic, telangiectatic, and fibroblastic types. Most osteosarcomas contain osseous matrix, which is of higher density than marrow on CT scans (see Fig. 14–1). When using MRI, the osteoblastic component will have low signal on both T1- and T2-weighted images, whereas unossified components will have high signal on T2 weighting (see Fig. 14–5).[19] Telangiectatic osteosarcomas are angiomatous lesions with large, cystic, blood-filled spaces that may mimic aneurysmal bone cysts, although they are less well defined. They frequently contain focal areas of high signal on T1- and T2-weighted images secondary to subacute hemorrhage, similar to aneurysmal bone cysts (Fig. 14–21).[54]

Parosteal osteosarcomas are rare primary bone tumors that usually occur posterior to the distal femur (Figure 14–22; also see Fig. 14–16). They are seen in the third and fourth decades and have a better patient prognosis than do central osteosarcomas. Rarely, they extend into the medullary space, which can

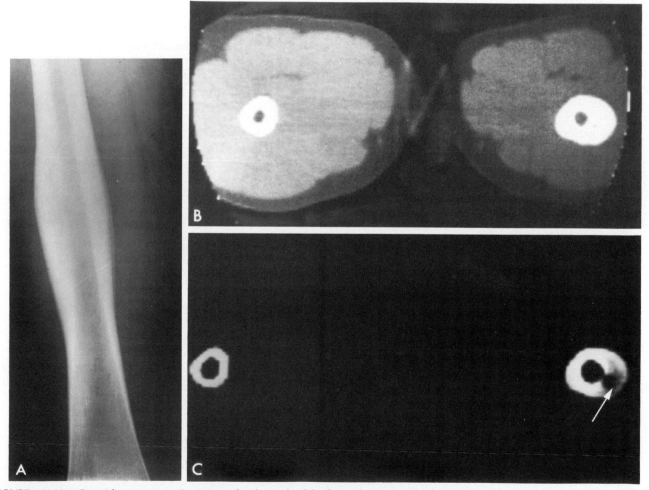

FIGURE 14–19 ■ Osteoid osteoma. *A*, Conventional radiograph of the femur demonstrates solid periosteal reaction circumscribing the femur. CT scans are shown at two different window settings, one optimal for soft tissues *(B)* and one optimal for skeletal structures *(C)*. The lucent nidus *(arrow)* surrounded by dense bone on CT is nearly diagnostic of an osteoid osteoma.

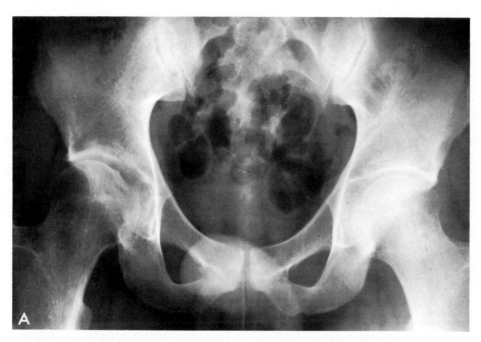

FIGURE 14–20 ■ Osteoid osteoma of the acetabulum. *A,* Conventional radiograph of the pelvis of a young man with right hip pain reveals periarticular demineralization.

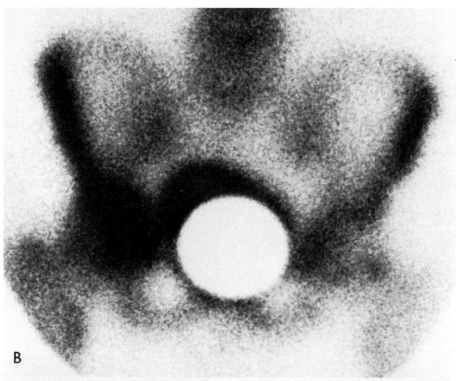

FIGURE 14–20 *Continued B,* Bone scan shows increased radionuclide uptake in the acetabulum. *C,* CT scan identified the nidus of an osteoid osteoma and defines its position in the acetabulum, facilitating surgical resection.

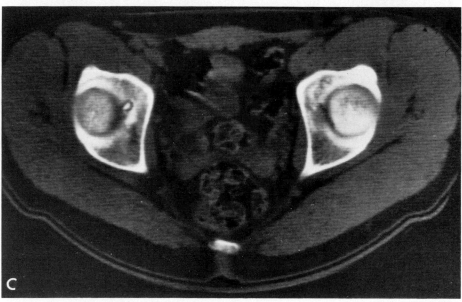

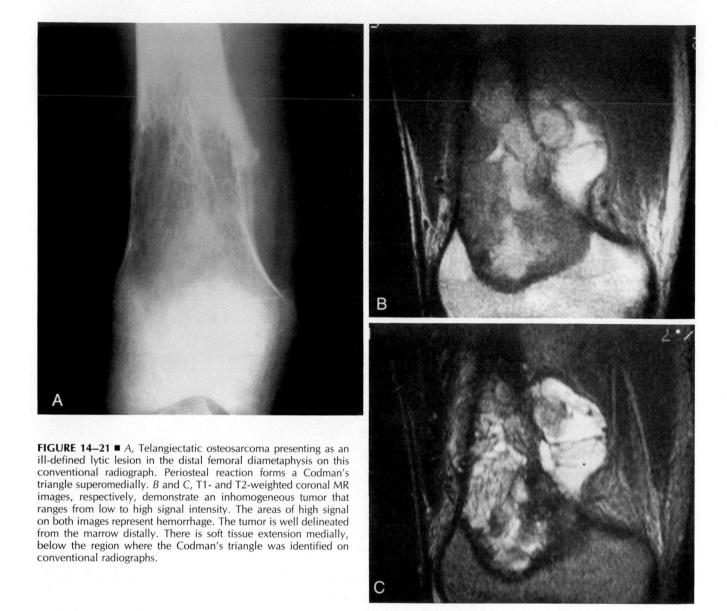

FIGURE 14–21 ■ *A*, Telangiectatic osteosarcoma presenting as an ill-defined lytic lesion in the distal femoral diametaphysis on this conventional radiograph. Periosteal reaction forms a Codman's triangle superomedially. *B* and *C*, T1- and T2-weighted coronal MR images, respectively, demonstrate an inhomogeneous tumor that ranges from low to high signal intensity. The areas of high signal on both images represent hemorrhage. The tumor is well delineated from the marrow distally. There is soft tissue extension medially, below the region where the Codman's triangle was identified on conventional radiographs.

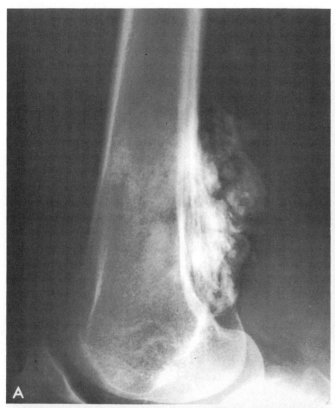

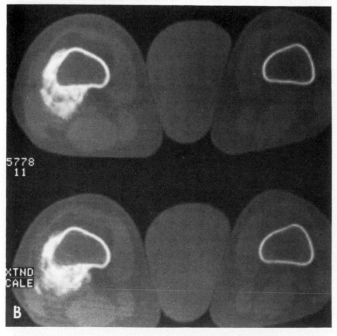

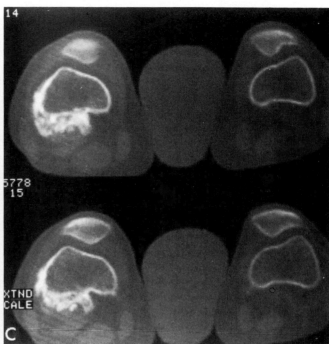

FIGURE 14–22 ■ Parosteal osteosarcoma. *A,* Lateral radiograph demonstrates a large ossifying mass encircling the posterior cortex of the distal femur. *B* and *C,* CT scans demonstrate the intimate relationship of the ossifying mass to the underlying cortex and sparing of the medullary space, supporting a diagnosis of parosteal sarcoma and bearing prognostic significance.

alter both prognosis and treatment. CT and MRI can be utilized to evaluate for medullary invasion (see Figs. 14–16 and 14–22).[55, 56]

Periosteal osteosarcomas are osteoid-containing spiculated lesions limited in extent to the cortex and periosteum. Unlike parosteal osteosarcomas, the tumor mass does not tend to outgrow the base of origin in length.[57]

Tumors with Chondroid Matrix

Calcifications are best seen by CT (Figs. 14–23 through 14–25). If there is a question regarding the presence of tumor calcification on a conventional radiograph, a CT scan should be obtained.

The unmineralized matrix of well-differentiated cartilaginous tumors is of moderate-to-high signal intensity on T1-weighted MR images and intermediate-to-high signal intensity on T2-weighted MR images (see Fig. 14–24C, D).[26] This is primarily because of the uniform composition, high water content, and low cellularity of chondroid matrix.[58] If there is heavy mineralization of cartilaginous tumors, they will be hypointense on both T1- and T2-weighted images as a result of the low proton density and short T2 relaxation time of calcium.[52, 59] Higher grade cartilaginous tumors, which have less mature chondroid matrices and high cellularity, may be isointense or hypointense with muscle on T2-weighted images. Chondroid tumors usually have well-defined lobulated margins.

Enchondromas are well-circumscribed benign tumors that contain hyaline cartilage and varying amounts of calcified cartilage that can be identified on CT and MRI scans (Fig. 14–26). Expansion or osseous scalloping of an enchondroma is suggestive of malignant degeneration.

Osteochondromas are exostoses continuous with the adjacent medullary marrow and surrounded by cortical bone. Overlying the cortical rim is a hyaline cartilaginous cap that contains varying degrees of calcification. CT and MRI demonstrate the attachment site of the tumor, particularly in complex joints, where conventional radiographs can be confusing. The absence of bone destruction and the thickness of the cartilaginous cap are important criteria for a benign osteochondroma (Fig. 14–27). A cartilaginous cap that contains dense, disorganized calcification or is larger than 1 cm increases the suspicion of chondrosarcoma.[59, 60] CT[61] and T2-weighted MR images[62] clearly delineate the cartilaginous cap.

Chondroblastomas are well-defined lytic epiphyseal lesions that often contain calcified matrix.[63] The calcifications are easily identified by CT, thereby increasing the certainty of diagnosis (see Figs. 14–23 and 14–24). The degree of calcification in the tumor influences the signal intensity on MR images. A heavily calcified tumor is predominantly low in signal intensity on T1- and T2-weighted images.[64] Chondroblastomas frequently produce a thick solid or layered periosteal response distant from the lesion, along the diametaphyseal shaft, associated with changes in the marrow that are consistent with edema.

Chondrosarcomas are destructive cartilaginous lesions that occur in patients in their fourth to sixth decades. On CT and MRI scans high-grade chondrosarcomas are frequently characterized by necrosis accompanied by faint, nonuniform, amorphous, eccentric calcification (see Fig. 14–25).

Text continued on page 579

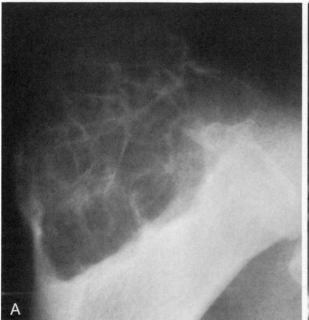 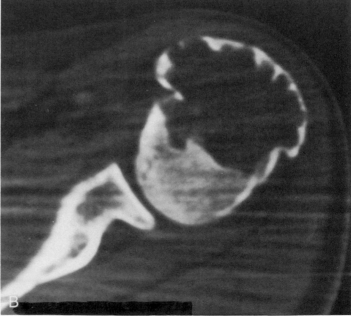

FIGURE 14–23 ■ *A,* Trabeculated lytic expansile tumor of the proximal humerus involving the greater tuberosity. *B,* CT scan demonstrates internal calcification with certainty, suggesting that this is a chondroblastoma, which was surgically proven.

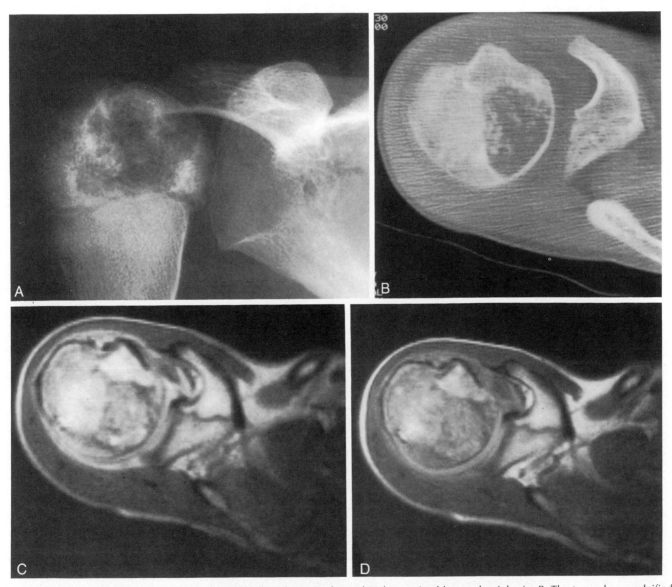

FIGURE 14–24 ■ *A,* Well-defined lytic lesion with scalloped margins located in the proximal humeral epiphysis. *B,* The tumor has a calcified matrix by CT, characteristic of a chondroblastoma. On T1- *(C)* and T2-weighted *(D)* axial MR images, the tumor contains areas of high and intermediate signal, respectively, representing chondroid matrix. The calcification has low signal intensity.

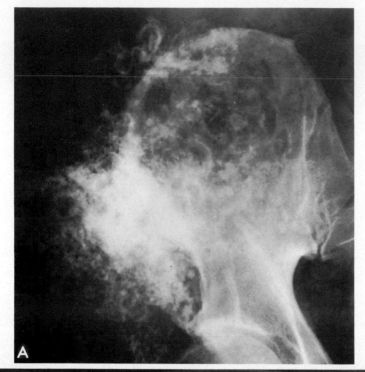

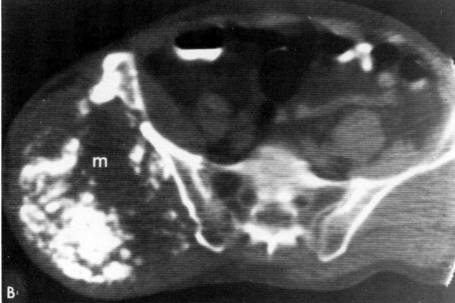

FIGURE 14–25 ■ Chondrosarcoma. *A*, Plain radiograph of the pelvis shows a densely calcified cartilaginous mass in the region of the right buttock. *B*, CT scan of the pelvis accurately defines the extent of the mass and reveals erosion of the ileum. A soft tissue mass (m) located beyond the calcified portion of the mass has invaded the inner pelvic wall. These findings indicate malignancy and help to determine an appropriate therapeutic approach. Chondrosarcoma was confirmed at surgery.

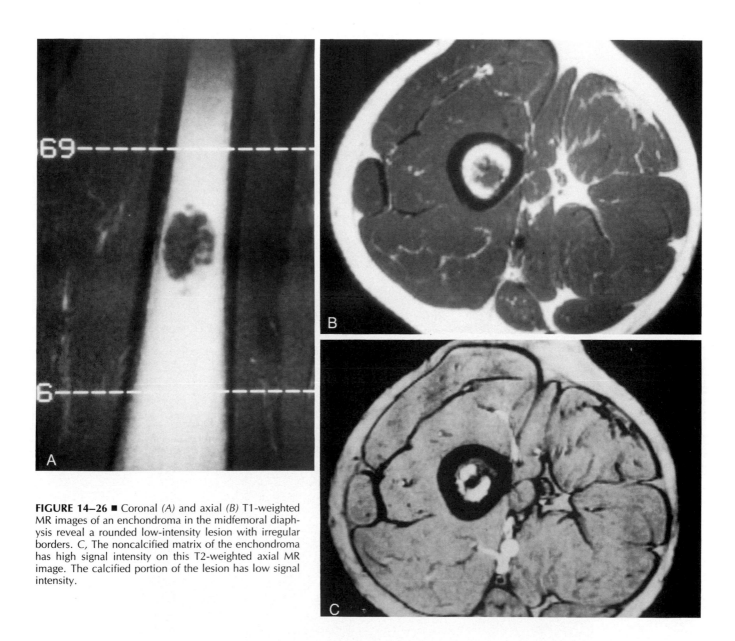

FIGURE 14–26 ■ Coronal *(A)* and axial *(B)* T1-weighted MR images of an enchondroma in the midfemoral diaphysis reveal a rounded low-intensity lesion with irregular borders. C, The noncalcified matrix of the enchondroma has high signal intensity on this T2-weighted axial MR image. The calcified portion of the lesion has low signal intensity.

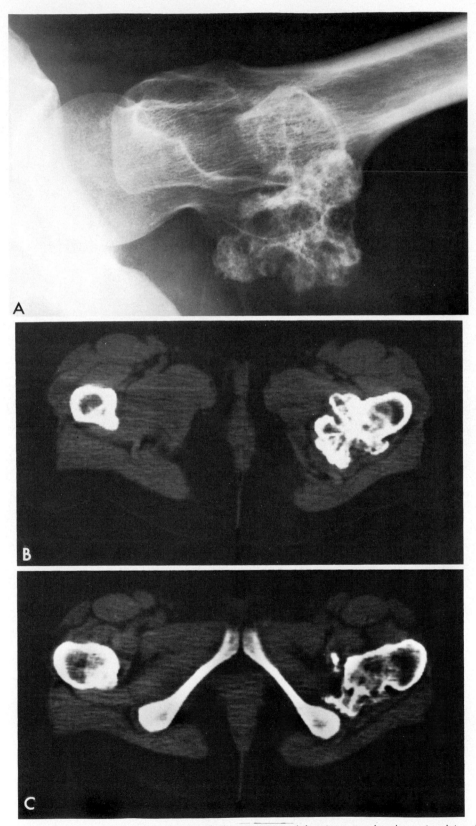

FIGURE 14–27 ■ Osteochondroma. *A,* Conventional radiograph demonstrates a deforming osteochondroma involving the proximal femur. *B* and *C,* CT scans demonstrate the exact relationship of the stalk of the osteochondroma to the shaft of the femur, the proximity of the calcified cap to the ischium, and the absence of a significant soft tissue mass, suggesting benignancy.

Miscellaneous Primary Osseous Tumors

Bone cysts are central, well-circumscribed lesions that are characterized by their fluid contents on CT and MRI scans. Proteinaceous material or hemorrhage may occasionally be seen within bone cysts, rendering them more dense or high in signal intensity on CT and T1-weighted MR scans, respectively. We have seen fluid-fluid levels in bone cysts on MRI. Lack of a sclerotic or low-signal rim often differentiates them from aneurysmal bone cysts.[65]

Aneurysmal bone cysts are benign, lytic, expansile lesions of unknown etiology. CT characteristically demonstrates a thin cortical shell or a well-defined soft tissue margin (Figs. 14–28 through 14–30). On MRI scans, aneurysmal bone cysts are characterized by an intact rim of low signal intensity and multiple internal septations.[66] These lesions may also extend into surrounding bone with diverticula-like projections.[66] Fluid-fluid levels have been demonstrated in aneurysmal bone cysts by CT and MRI (see Figs. 14–28 through 14–30). Fluid-fluid levels have also been described in giant cell tumors, telangiectatic osteosarcomas, and chondroblastomas[14, 26, 67–69] and represent layering of fluid of different composition. The fluid can be hemorrhagic or cystic in nature. Theoretically any tumor that contains fluid could contain a fluid-fluid level and the finding is nonspecific.[69a] To capture the fluid levels, it is best to have the patient motionless for at least 10 minutes prior to scanning.

Giant cell tumors are expansile, eccentric lesions that extend to the articular surface. They are often associated with a soft tissue mass and may occasionally extend through subchondral bone to enter the joint. CT and MRI can be used to determine whether the tumor has entered the joint (Fig. 14–31). Giant cell tumors may be inhomogeneous on CT and MRI scans and do not enhance on CT scans with intravenous contrast, despite their hypervascularity.[70] With MRI, they usually have low signal intensity on T1-weighted images and low-to-high signal intensity

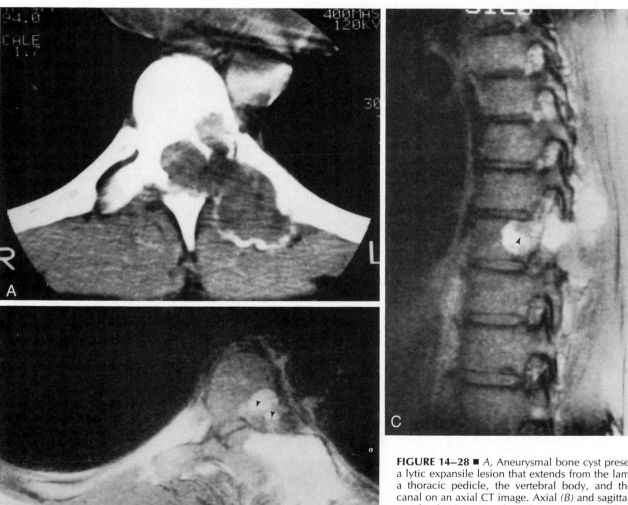

FIGURE 14–28 ■ *A,* Aneurysmal bone cyst presenting as a lytic expansile lesion that extends from the lamina into a thoracic pedicle, the vertebral body, and the spinal canal on an axial CT image. Axial *(B)* and sagittal *(C)* T2-weighted MR images show the tumor to have high signal intensity with some internal fluid-fluid levels *(arrowheads).*

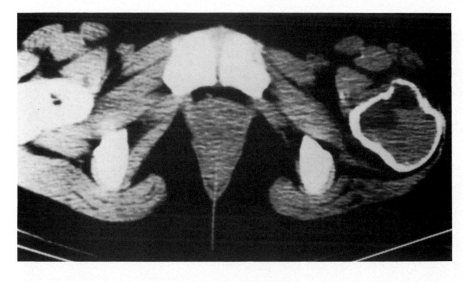

FIGURE 14–29 ■ Aneurysmal bone cyst of the left femur containing fluid-fluid levels on CT.

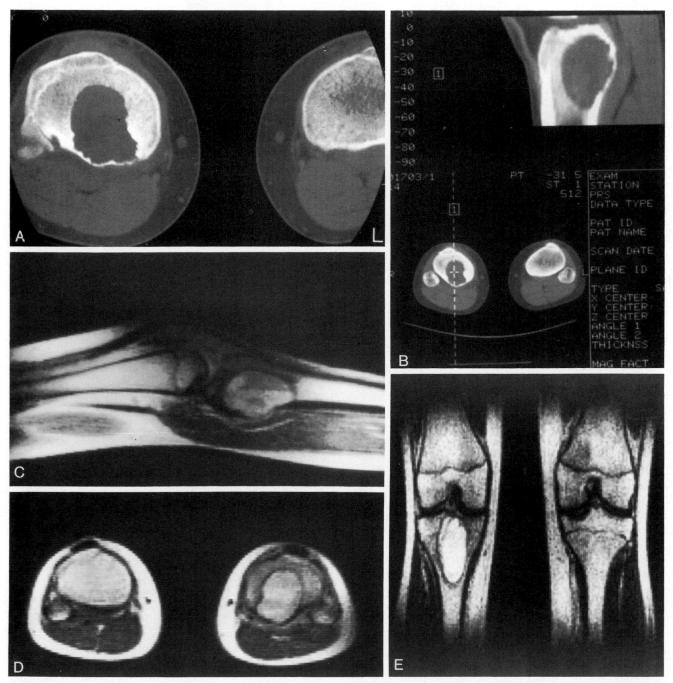

FIGURE 14–30. ■ *A,* Aneurysmal bone cyst in the proximal tibia is expansile and lytic, thinning the posterior cortical margin on this axial CT. *B,* The cyst is well delineated on a CT reformation in the sagittal plane. *C,* Fluid-fluid levels are apparent on a sagittal T1-weighted MR image obtained with the patient lying supine. The dependent blood cells have high signal intensity, whereas the supernatant plasma has intermediate signal intensity. *D,* Fluid-fluid levels are again demonstrated on an axial T2-weighted MR image. *E,* The tumor has homogeneous high signal intensity on a coronal T2-weighted MR image. A characteristic low–signal intensity rim surrounds this tumor.

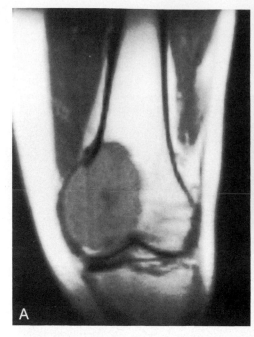 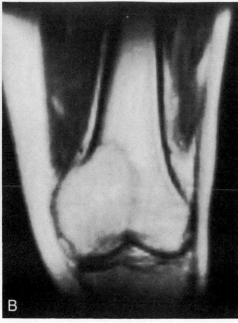

FIGURE 14–31 ■ *A,* Giant cell tumor extending to the distal medial femoral condylar surface. It is expansile and has homogeneous intermediate signal intensity on a T1-weighted coronal MR image. The overlying cortex is intact.

B, On a corresponding T2-weighted coronal MR image, the tumor has high signal intensity. There is no surrounding low-intensity rim, thus differentiating it from an aneurysmal bone cyst.

on T2-weighted images.[65] Unlike aneurysmal bone cysts, giant cell tumors lack a sclerotic or low-signal rim on CT and MRI, respectively. Giant cell tumors frequently recur and should be followed at 6-month intervals with either CT or MRI (Fig. 14–32).[71]

Chordomas are malignant tumors believed to arise from notochordal rests. They may contain calcium or residual bone. Approximately 50 per cent arise in the sacrum.[72] Sacral tumors are difficult to evaluate by conventional radiography. However, CT and MRI are useful for determining their extent, as well as any spread to surrounding vital structures (Fig. 14–33). Involvement of sacral foramina are easily identified in the direct coronal plane by CT and MRI.[73] Rectal invasion is difficult to assess by either CT or MRI.[73]

Round cell tumors such as Ewing's sarcoma and primary histiocytic lymphoma permeate the cortex and medullary cavity with little bone destruction. These tumors are relatively homogeneous unless there is necrosis, and they are often associated with large soft tissue masses.[74] CT and MRI are particularly helpful in defining the extent of such permeative tumors (Fig. 14–34).[75, 76]

Primary Soft Tissue Tumors

Lipomas are an exception to the general rule of nonspecificity. They are usually sharply marginated, have characteristic low attenuation coefficients by CT (-65 to -120 H), and lack significant contrast enhancement (Figs. 14–35 through 14–37). They have high signal on MR images obtained with a short TE but decrease in signal with increasing TE times, similar to subcutaneous fat (Figs. 14–35 through 14–38). Because of the specificity of the low attenuation coefficient of fat, CT is more specific than MRI in

diagnosing lipomas.[77–79] With MRI, lipomas can be confused with other processes that have high signal intensity on T1-weighted images (e.g., subacute hemorrhage), although a distinction might be made with heavily T2-weighted images; in this case fat is not as high in signal as is hemorrhage. On T1-weighted MR images, lipomas are usually homogeneously hyperintense, whereas hemorrhage in a tumor is usually inhomogeneous, presenting as high signal within a predominantly low-signal mass. Within lipomas there may be thin streaks of soft tissue, hemorrhage, or necrosis that may simulate a liposarcoma on CT and MRI scans.[80] Infiltrating lipomas are often poorly defined and very vascular, making them also difficult to distinguish from liposarcomas.[13] Atypical lipomas can simulate liposarcomas, as they have a variable composition of multinucleated cells, collagen bundles, and adipocytes with large hyperchromatic nuclei.[80] *Angiolipomas* (Fig. 14–39) may also show features (e.g., heterogeneity, ill-defined margins, and CT contrast enhancement) quite similar to those of liposarcoma.[81]

Liposarcomas are the most common soft tissue sarcoma.[13] There are five different histologic categories—differentiated, embryonal, myxoid, pleomorphic, and round cell—with varying amounts of fat and soft tissue components. With CT, the malignant forms are more opaque because of fibrous, myxomatous, and vascular elements that enhance with intravenous contrast (see Fig. 14–10).[13, 77] They often have areas of high signal intensity on T1-weighted MR images, attributable to fat, which may distinguish them from other soft tissue tumors.[80a] They generally have lower signal intensity with T1 weighting than do lipomas, particularly myxoid liposarcomas, which have a high water content.[80b] Liposarcomas are usually ill defined, inhomogene-

Text continued on page 591

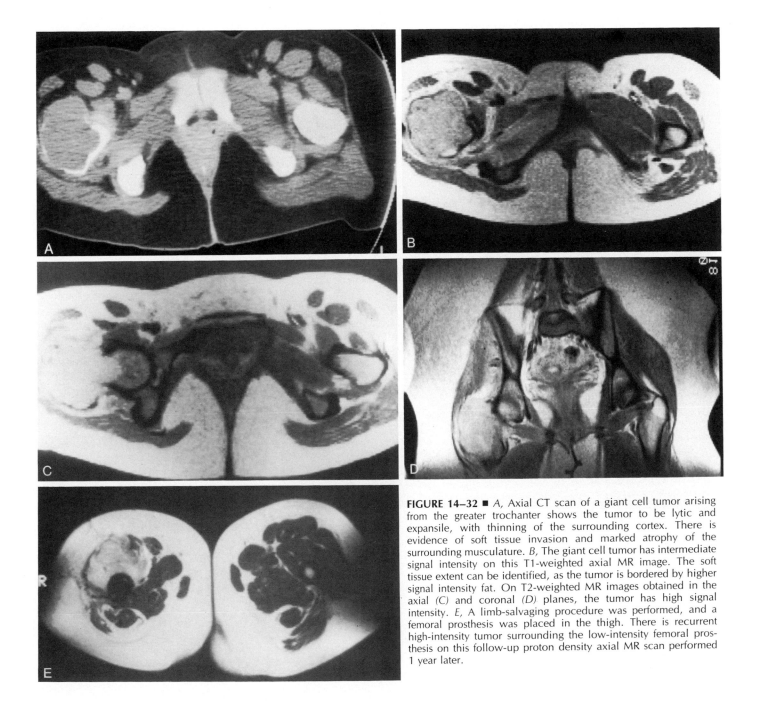

FIGURE 14–32 ■ *A,* Axial CT scan of a giant cell tumor arising from the greater trochanter shows the tumor to be lytic and expansile, with thinning of the surrounding cortex. There is evidence of soft tissue invasion and marked atrophy of the surrounding musculature. *B,* The giant cell tumor has intermediate signal intensity on this T1-weighted axial MR image. The soft tissue extent can be identified, as the tumor is bordered by higher signal intensity fat. On T2-weighted MR images obtained in the axial *(C)* and coronal *(D)* planes, the tumor has high signal intensity. *E,* A limb-salvaging procedure was performed, and a femoral prosthesis was placed in the thigh. There is recurrent high-intensity tumor surrounding the low-intensity femoral prosthesis on this follow-up proton density axial MR scan performed 1 year later.

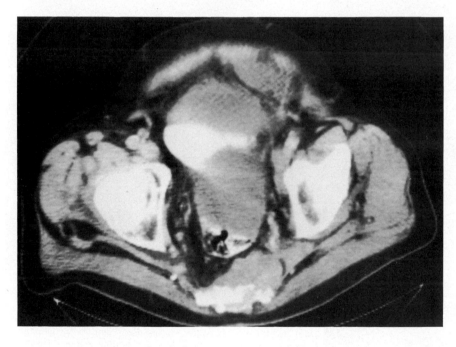

FIGURE 14–33 ■ A chordoma produces sacral destruction and a large soft tissue mass that extends into the presacral region, as demonstrated on this axial CT image. The presence of a fat plane between the chordoma and the rectum indicates rectal sparing.

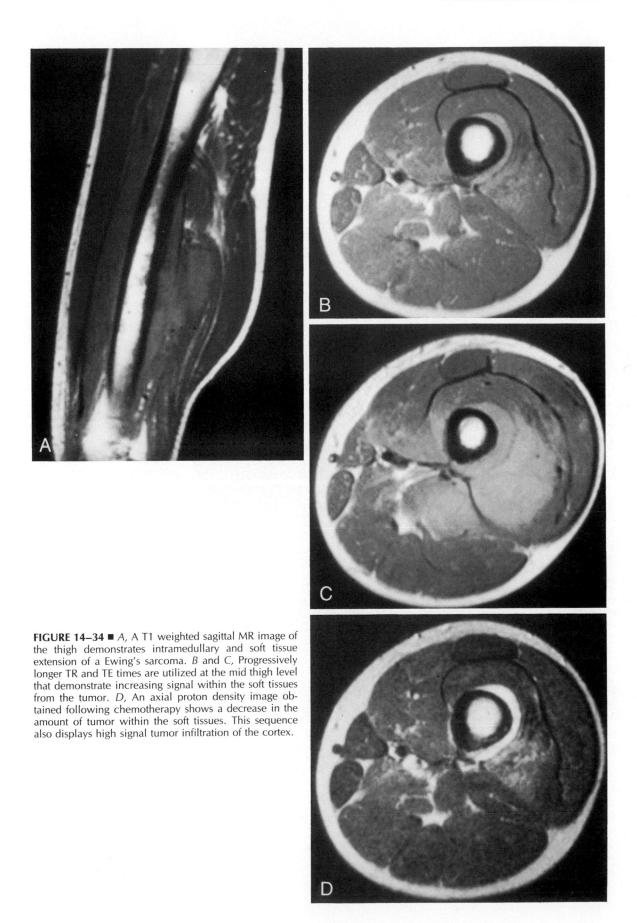

FIGURE 14–34 ■ *A,* A T1 weighted sagittal MR image of the thigh demonstrates intramedullary and soft tissue extension of a Ewing's sarcoma. *B* and *C,* Progressively longer TR and TE times are utilized at the mid thigh level that demonstrate increasing signal within the soft tissues from the tumor. *D,* An axial proton density image obtained following chemotherapy shows a decrease in the amount of tumor within the soft tissues. This sequence also displays high signal tumor infiltration of the cortex.

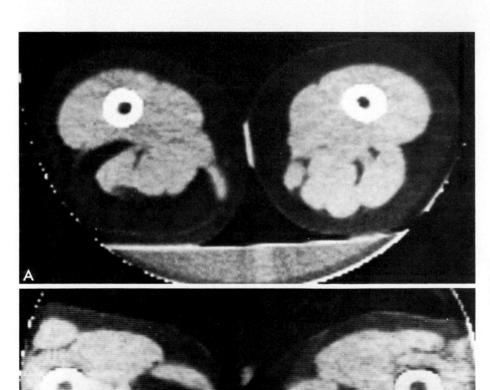

FIGURE 14–35 ■ Lipoma. CT scans of different cases reveal sharply marginated, homogeneous, low-density soft tissue masses diagnostic of lipomas.

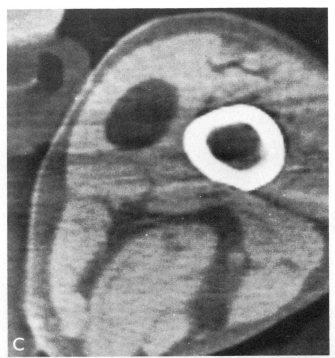

FIGURE 14-35 *Continued*

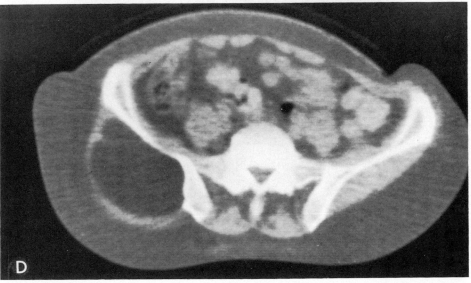

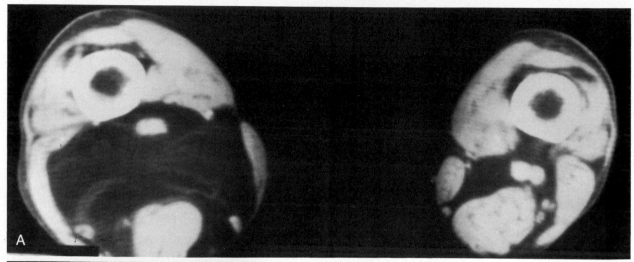

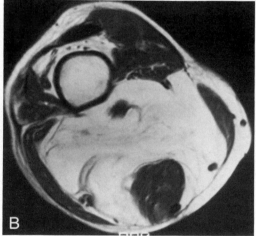

FIGURE 14–36 ■ *A,* Several high-density streaks are present within a lipoma of the thigh, characterized by its low attenuation on CT. *B,* T1-weighted axial MR image at the same level demonstrates the high-intensity lipoma (TR, 600; TE, 20). The lipoma has signal intensity equal to that of subcutaneous fat. The internal streaks are of low signal intensity.

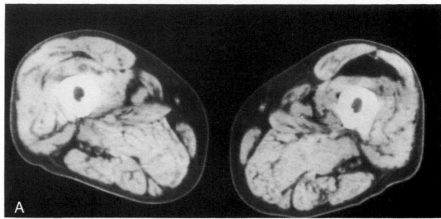

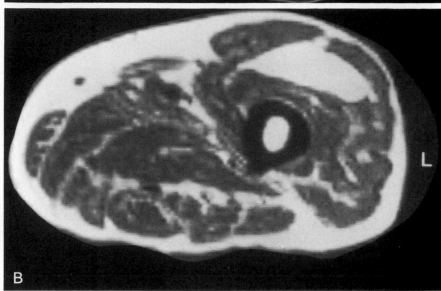

FIGURE 14–37 ■ *A*, A crescentic lipoma in the left thigh is well-delineated and of uniform low attenuation on this axial CT scan. *B*, The high-intensity lipoma is easily identified on the corresponding T1-weighted axial MR image (TR, 500; TE, 30).

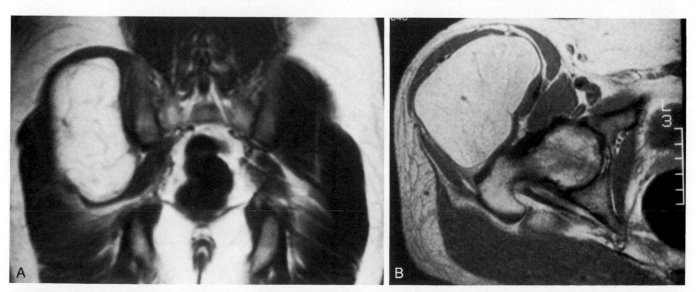

FIGURE 14–38 ■ *A*, Lipoma in the soft tissues lateral to the right ilium on a coronal T1-weighted MR image. *B*, The lipoma also lies anterior to the right hip, as demonstrated on this axial proton density image. It is well circumscribed and has a signal intensity consistent with fat. A few lower signal streaks run through it.

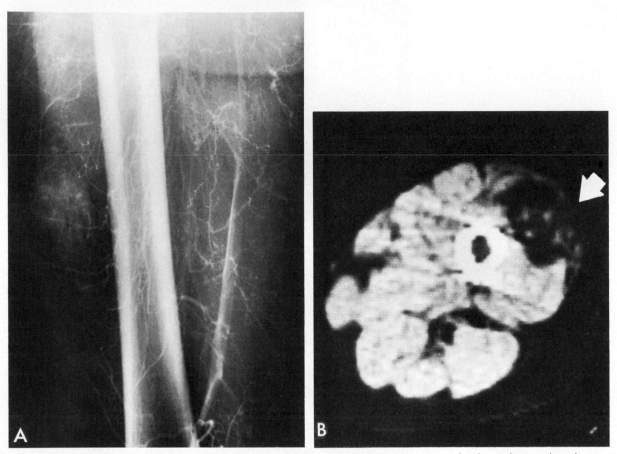

FIGURE 14–39 ■ *A,* Infiltrative angiolipoma in the right thigh. A right femoral angiogram shows a tangle of irregular vessels and a tumor stain. *B,* CT scan (without contrast) demonstrates the mass *(arrow)* to have poorly defined margins and to be a heterogeneous mixture of fat and water and calcific density elements.

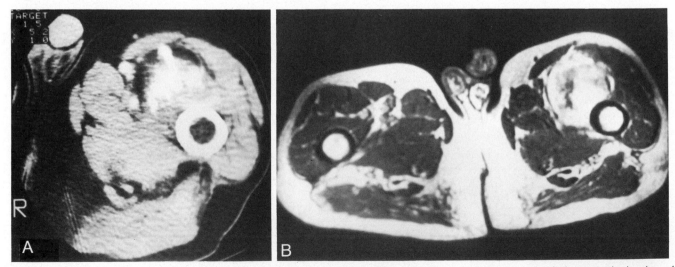

FIGURE 14–40 ■ *A,* CT scan of a liposarcoma of the thigh reveals fat density along the anterior rim and internal calcification. The borders of the tumor are not well seen. *B,* Calcification within the tumor is of low intensity on this axial proton density MR image (TR, 2000; TE, 35). The rest of the tumor is of high signal intensity. The tumor margins are easily identified.

ous, and may occasionally contain metaplastic bone or cartilage (Fig. 14–40).

In addition to tumors that contain fat or hemorrhage, *angiodysplasias* occasionally produce high signal on T1-weighted MR images. Angiodysplasias are the most common benign congenital anomaly and include *arteriovenous malformations* (high-flow lesions with arteriovenous shunting), *hemangiomas* (small-vessel malformations with little arteriovenous shunting), and *venous malformations* (enlarged, saccular veins with stagnant flow). These are usually well-defined and inhomogeneous tumors that frequently contain phleboliths. On CT scans, angiomatous tumors have values ranging between 30 and 40 H and they markedly enhance following rapid injection of contrast (Fig. 14–41).[13, 20, 82] Angiomatous lesions may be high or low in signal intensity on T1-weighted MR images but are very high in signal intensity with T2 weighting (Fig. 14–42).[83–86] Arteriovenous malformations contain rapidly flowing blood, producing serpiginous zones of low signal intensity on T1- and T2-weighted images secondary to high flow. There may be round foci of low signal intensity scattered throughout that represent rapidly flowing blood,

thrombosed or hyalinized vessels, or phleboliths. Fat may also contribute to the inhomogeneity of these lesions.[83–85] MRI is more helpful in defining the extent of angiomatous masses, which aids in planning for surgery or laser therapy, in evaluating the effectiveness of therapy, and in checking for recurrence. Venous or lymphatic occlusive disease can cause focal or generalized soft tissue enlargement (Fig. 14–43).

Neurogenic tumors such as *neurofibromas* and *schwannomas* (Figs. 14–44 through 14–46) are often homogeneous, smoothly marginated cylindrical lesions. Their morphology and location in the neurovascular bundle may strongly suggest the correct diagnosis.[4] On CT scans, they have a density lower than that of muscle. On MRI scans they usually have low to intermediate signal intensity with T1 weighting and intermediate to high signal intensity with T2 and T2* weighting (see Fig. 14–46). Multiple neurofibromas tend to form a grape cluster configuration.

Benign fibrous soft tissue tumors such as *desmoids* contain dense collagen and are relatively acellular. They range in density on CT and enhance with intravenous contrast.[87] These tumors often have low signal on T1- and variable signal on T2-weighted MR

Text continued on page 597

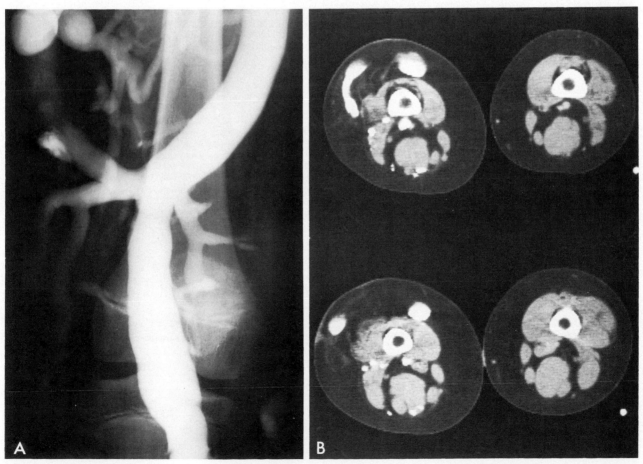

FIGURE 14–41 ■ Arteriovenous malformation. *A,* Angiogram demonstrates massive dilatation of venous channels in the left lower extremity as a result of extensive arteriovenous malformation. *B,* CT scans delineate the spatial relationship of the enlarged vascular channels following intravenous contrast but fail to demonstrate a significant vascular neoplasm.

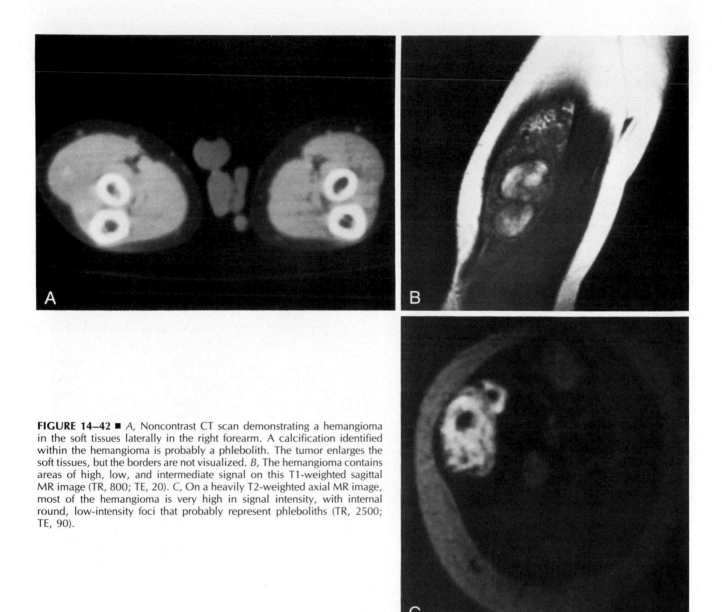

FIGURE 14–42 ■ *A,* Noncontrast CT scan demonstrating a hemangioma in the soft tissues laterally in the right forearm. A calcification identified within the hemangioma is probably a phlebolith. The tumor enlarges the soft tissues, but the borders are not visualized. *B,* The hemangioma contains areas of high, low, and intermediate signal on this T1-weighted sagittal MR image (TR, 800; TE, 20). *C,* On a heavily T2-weighted axial MR image, most of the hemangioma is very high in signal intensity, with internal round, low-intensity foci that probably represent phleboliths (TR, 2500; TE, 90).

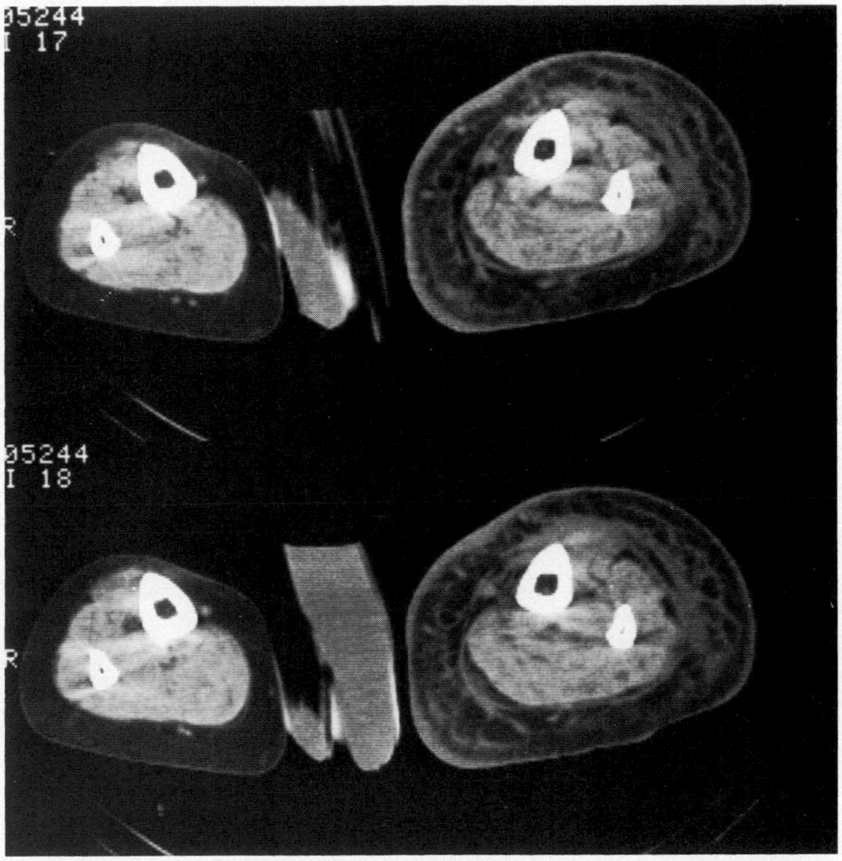

FIGURE 14–43 ■ Filariasis. CT scans through the legs demonstrate massive enlargement of the left lower extremity as a result of involvement with filariasis. The CT study shows tremendous engorgement of lymphatic and venous channels with collections of fluid deep in the subcutaneous fat and marked thickening of the skin.

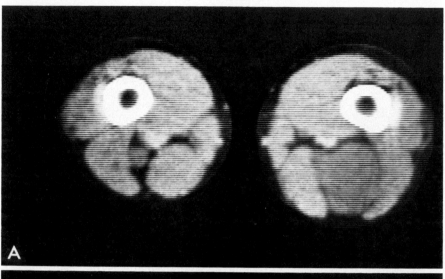

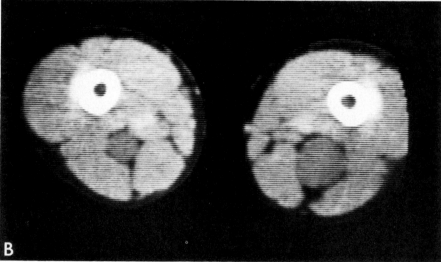

FIGURE 14–44 ■ Neurofibroma. CT scans in a patient with von Recklinghausen's disease and painful swelling of the left leg reveal a sharply marginated, low-density mass in the popliteal space. The mass extends, on contiguous sections, in a cylindrical fashion over many centimeters. Biopsy demonstrated the mass to be a neurofibroma. A second smaller neurofibroma was found incidentally in the right popliteal space.

FIGURE 14–45 ■ Schwannoma. CT scans demonstrate a relatively low density mass within the neurovascular bundle of the posterior thigh. This cylindrical mass was shown by CT to extend over 15 cm, suggesting the correct diagnosis of schwannoma.

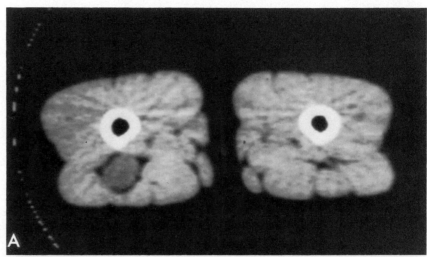

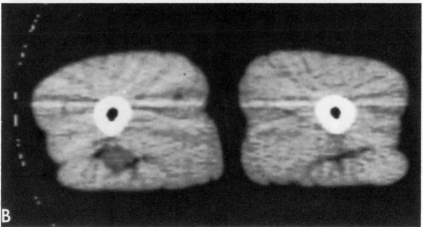

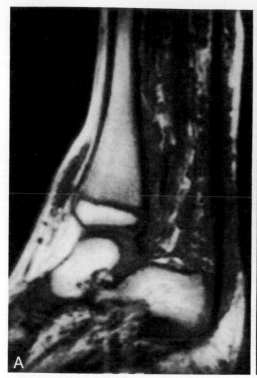
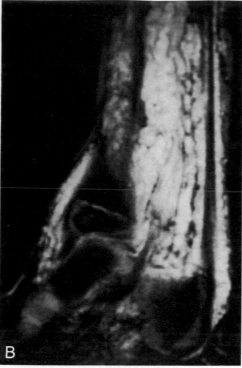

FIGURE 14–46 ■ *A*, T1-weighted sagittal MR image reveals extensive involvement of the soft tissues in the lower leg by low-intensity neurofibromatosis. The neurofibromas surround the Achilles tendon and extend into the subcutaneous fat posterior and anterior to the tibia. *B*, The area of involvement by neurofibromatosis has very high signal intensity on this sagittal gradient-echo MR image. There is high contrast between the tumor and low-intensity fat, marrow, tendon, and cortex.

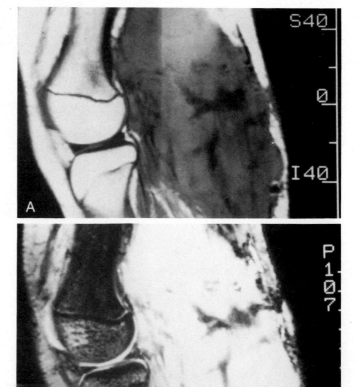

FIGURE 14–47 ■ A desmoid arising in the popliteal space is demonstrated on *(A)* T1- and *(B)* T2-weighted sagittal MR images. The desmoid has predominantly intermediate signal intensity on T1 weighting and high signal intensity on T2 weighting, with the exception of some low-intensity fibrous strands within it.

scans (Fig. 14–47). Underlying factors that contribute to occasional low signal intensity within fibrous tumors on T2-weighted images are the low mobile proton density and short T2 of fibrous tissue.[52, 88]

Malignant soft tissue tumors such as *malignant fibrous histiocytoma, rhabdomyosarcoma,* and *synovial sarcoma* are usually inhomogeneous with infiltrative margins on both CT and MRI scans. They have low-to-moderate signal intensity on T1-weighted MR images, whereas T2-weighted MR images often demonstrate central, high-intensity hemorrhage and necrosis with occasional low-signal hemosiderin or fibrosis. Edema may surround these tumors. Calcification may be seen within these soft tissue tumors.

Masses simulating tumors can result from intramuscular injections, hemorrhage into the soft tissues, abscess, myositis ossificans, and calcific tendinitis.[13, 89–92] Some of these pseudotumors can be distinguished from tumors by following them serially with CT or MRI to see if they decrease in size or undergo changes in density or signal intensity.

Biopsy

Prior to biopsy, one must have a thorough knowledge of the anatomic location of a tumor. Proper selection of biopsy sites is crucial to ensure that all existing surgical alternatives remain available to the patient after biopsy. Staging studies such as CT and MRI should be performed prior to biopsy; interpretation of images after biopsy is much less reliable because of local soft tissue alterations and possible complications such as hematoma or fascial tumor spread.[93, 94] Edema, hematoma, and inflammation can be confused with residual tumor.[25, 95]

If a biopsy has been performed prior to the imaging study, it is better that the staging imaging study be postponed until wound repair is mature, if feasible (generally 8 to 12 weeks following the biopsy). Hemorrhage following biopsy may lead to spread of tumor cells, increased surgical margins, and limitations on limb-salvaging procedures (Fig. 14–48).[96, 97]

Postoperative Follow-up

Imaging studies are indicated for postoperative follow-up of musculoskeletal tumors to obtain a baseline scan and check for recurrence. A baseline scan is particularly important if the tumor has not been completely resected or a local recurrence is likely.

Differentiation between recurrent tumor and postoperative change can be difficult, especially because there may be obliteration of soft tissue planes, scarring, hemorrhage, or infection.[21] When trying to differentiate scar and hematoma from recurrent tumor, MRI is more helpful than CT, provided that the study is obtained at least several months following surgery. Scar, hemorrhage, necrosis, inflammation, and tumor appear hypodense on CT and cannot be differentiated.[95] Chronic scarring is of low signal intensity on T1- and T2-weighted images and can be distinguished from most tumors and hematomas by

MRI.[98] Acute scarring may have an appearance similar to that of tumor and may not be distinguishable (Fig. 14–49). CT cannot differentiate tumor recurrence from chronic hemorrhage, although this distinction can usually be made by MRI. Subacute and chronic hemorrhage have high signal on T1 weighting, unlike most tumors. Only acute hemorrhage simulates the signal characteristics of tumor. To distinguish tumor from acute hemorrhage, follow-up scans are helpful. Active tumor cannot be reliably distinguished from inflammatory changes by CT or MRI.

Areas of necrosis and liquefaction within tumor have higher T2 values than the tumor and background tissues and may be distinguished from them on a T2-weighted image.[26, 37] Paramagnetic contrast agents such as gadolinium can aid in this distinction. On T1-weighted images obtained following gadolinium administration, tumor enhances relative to necrosis and edema.[45–48]

A postoperative abscess often has a thick, irregular capsule and may be seen on MRI scans without contrast. One problem with MRI is that air within the abscess may be missed, as the low signal produced by air is nonspecific. If an abscess is suspected, conventional radiographs or CT are suggested to evaluate for its presence.

High-risk areas for tumor recurrence include the track of the previous procedure, the previous resection site, and planes and tissues exposed by the previous procedure. If there has been prior radiation, recurrence usually occurs along the margins of the previous radiation field and extends proximally along the course of the major neurovascular bundle.

MRI is more helpful than CT in detecting recurrence of tumor in patients with nonferromagnetic prostheses, fixation devices, or surgical clips. These metallic objects have low signal intensity on MRI and cause minimal artifact when compared with CT. The surrounding tumor is usually easily identified as an area of high signal intensity on the T2-weighted image (Figs. 14–32 and 14–50).[21, 27, 32, 36]

Radiation and Chemotherapy

Radiation or chemotherapy may be utilized to decrease tumor bulk prior to surgery or following surgery, depending on the extent and histology of the tumor.[75, 94–98] Because MRI and CT allow for more precise evaluation of tumor extent, they enable the radiation dose to the tumor to be increased while minimizing radiation to the surrounding normal tissues.[31] Direct sagittal and coronal images provided by MRI are of particular use to the radiation therapist because of their similarity to lateral and anteroposterior simulator radiographs used to outline proposed therapy portals.[99]

Response of tumor to radiation or chemotherapy is indicated on CT or MRI scans by a decrease in size, as well as by a change in CT density and signal intensity within the tumor. On MRI scans, signal

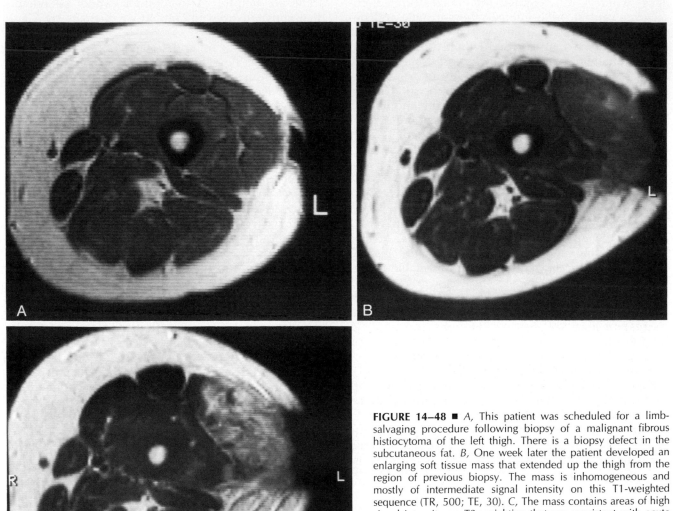

FIGURE 14–48 ■ *A*, This patient was scheduled for a limb-salvaging procedure following biopsy of a malignant fibrous histiocytoma of the left thigh. There is a biopsy defect in the subcutaneous fat. *B*, One week later the patient developed an enlarging soft tissue mass that extended up the thigh from the region of previous biopsy. The mass is inhomogeneous and mostly of intermediate signal intensity on this T1-weighted sequence (TR, 500; TE, 30). *C*, The mass contains areas of high signal intensity on T2 weighting that are consistent with acute hemorrhage from biopsy. Because of the possible spread of tumor within the hemorrhage, the left leg had to be amputated.

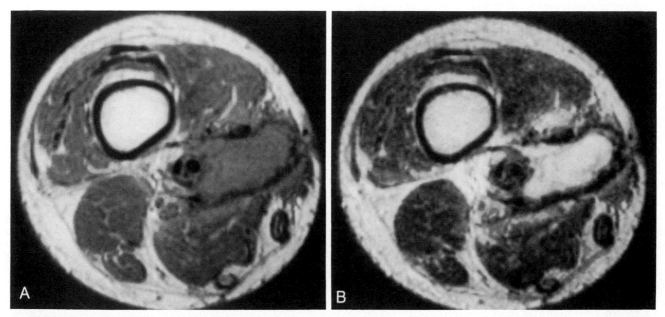

FIGURE 14–49 ■ *A*, Well-circumscribed mass of intermediate signal on an axial T1-weighted MR image obtained several months following resection of a liposarcoma. *B*, This region is of high signal intensity on a corresponding axial T2-weighted MR image. Both images reveal a low–signal intensity rim surrounding the mass consistent with fibrous tissue and/or hemosiderin. The mass represents an area of granulation tissue and scarring rather than recurrent tumor.

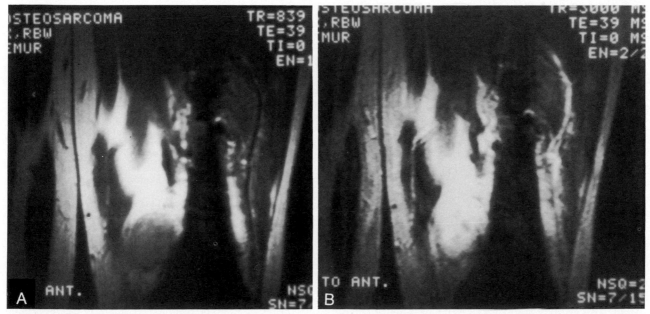

FIGURE 14–50 ■ *A*, Minimal artifact produced by a limb-salvaging prosthesis in the distal femur does not interfere with the significant finding of recurrent tumor, seen as an area of intermediate signal intensity in the soft tissues medial to the femur on this T1-weighted coronal MR image (TR, 839; TE, 39). *B*, The same region is high in signal intensity on a T2-weighted coronal MR image (TR, 3000; TE, 78). (Courtesy of Catherine Mills, MD, San Francisco, CA.)

intensity changes often precede changes in tumor volume.[26, 99a] A decrease in signal intensity on a T2-weighted image may be seen following radiation or chemotherapy as a result of a combination of factors, including dehydration, fibrosis, and calcification. Vanel et al.[100] observed that low signal intensity within the tumor on MR scans obtained following radiation had a 96 per cent sensitivity for indicating the absence of neoplasm. Residual tumor may be confused with necrosis, hemorrhage, or inflammation following radiation or chemotherapy. The ability of CT and MRI to distinguish among these was discussed in the previous section. Radiation also produces high signal intensity in normal bone marrow on T1-weighted sequences; this is thought to be caused by a radiation-induced increase in the lipid composition of the marrow.[101]

Conclusion

CT and MRI are important in the assessment and subsequent management of musculoskeletal tumors. We believe that MRI is the imaging procedure of choice with which to evaluate the extent of tumor; its advantages include direct multiplanar imaging capability and high soft tissue contrast between tumor and normal tissues. MRI is not as helpful as CT in identifying calcification, ossification, periosteal reaction, or gas formation. This information can usually be obtained from conventional radiographs. Neither CT nor MRI can distinguish benign from malignant tumors, and both are specific only in a few tumor types, primarily lipomas. MRI is more effective than CT in monitoring the effects of surgery, radiation, and chemotherapy on tumor viability.

References

1. Richardson ML, Kilcoyne RF, Gillespy T, et al: Magnetic resonance imaging of musculoskeletal neoplasms. Radiol Clin North Am 24:259, 1986.
2. Bloem JL, Taminlau AHM, Eulderink F, et al: Radiologic staging of primary bone sarcoma: MR imaging, scintigraphy, angiography, and CT correlated with pathologic examination. Radiology 169:805, 1988.
3. Gillespy T, Manfrini, Ruggieri P, et al: Staging of intraosseous extent of osteosarcoma: correlation of preoperative CT and MR imaging with pathologic macroslides. Radiology 167:765, 1988.
4. Genant HK, Cann CE, Chafetz NI, et al: Advances in computed tomography of the musculoskeletal system. Radiol Clin North Am 19:645, 1981.
5. Genant HK, Wilson JS, Bovill EG, et al: Computed tomography of the musculoskeletal system. J Bone Joint Surg 62A:1088, 1980.
6. Hardy DC, Murphy WA, Gilula LA: CT in planning percutaneous bone biopsy. Radiology 134:447, 1980.
7. Schreiman JS, Crass JR, Wick MR, et al: Osteosarcoma: role of CT in limb-sparing treatment. Radiology 161:485, 1986.
8. Enneking WF, Kagan A: Skip metastases in osteosarcoma. Cancer 36:2192, 1975.
9. Bohndorf K, Reiser M, Lochner B, et al: Magnetic resonance imaging of primary tumors and tumor-like lesions of bone. Skeletal Radiol 15:511, 1986.
10. Petterson H, Springfield DS, Enneking WF: Radiologic Management of Musculoskeletal Tumors. New York, Springer-Verlag, 1987.
11. Thrall JH, Geslein GE, Corcoran RJ, et al: Abnormal radionuclide deposition patterns adjacent to focal skeletal lesions. Radiology 115:659, 1975.
12. Chew FS, Hudson TM: Radionuclide bone scanning of osteosarcoma: falsely extended uptake patterns. AJR 139:49, 1982.
13. Scott WW, Magid D, Fishman EK: Computed Tomography of the Musculoskeletal System. New York, Churchill Livingstone, 1987.
14. Hudson TM, Hamlin DJ, Enneking WF, et al: Magnetic resonance imaging of bone and soft tissue tumors: early experience in 31 patients compared with computed tomography. Skeletal Radiol 13:134, 1985.
15. Coffre C, Vanel D, Contesso G, et al: Problems and pitfalls in the use of computed tomography for the local evaluation of long bone osteosarcoma: report on 30 cases. Skeletal Radiol 13:147, 1985.
16. Hudson TM, Schiebler M, Springfield DS, et al: Radiologic imaging of osteosarcoma. Role in planning surgical treatment. 10:137, 1983.
17. Simon MA, Kirchner PT: Scintigraphic evaluation of primary bone tumors. J Bone Joint Surg 62A:758, 1980.
18. Boyko OB, Cory DA, Cohen MD, et al: MR imaging of osteogenic and Ewing's sarcoma. AJR 148:317, 1987.
19. Sundaram M, McGuire MH, Herbold DR: Magnetic resonance imaging of osteosarcoma. Skeletal Radiol 16:23, 1987.
20. Weekes RG, McLeod RA, Reiman HM, et al: CT of soft-tissue neoplasms. AJR 144:355, 1985.
21. Sundaram M, McGuire MH, Herbold DR: Magnetic resonance imaging of soft tissue masses: an evaluation of fifty-three histologically proven tumors. Magn Reson Imaging 6:237, 1988.
22. Demas BE, Heelan RT, Lane J, et al: Soft-tissue sarcomas of the extremities: comparison of MR and CT in determining the extent of disease. AJR 150:615, 1988.
23. Chang AE, Matory YL, Dwyer AJ, et al: Magnetic resonance imaging versus computed tomography in the evaluation of soft tissue tumors of the extremities. Ann Surg 205:340, 1987.
24. Petasnick JP, Turner DA, Charters JR, et al: Soft-tissue masses of the locomotor system: comparison of MR imaging with CT. Radiology 160:125, 1986.
25. Pettersson H, Gillespy T, Hamlin DJ, et al: Primary musculoskeletal tumors: examination with MR imaging compared with conventional modalities. Radiology 164:237, 1987.
26. Bloem JL, Bleumm RG, Taminiau AHM, et al: Magnetic resonance imaging of primary malignant bone tumors. Radiographics 7:425, 1987.
27. Schumacker TM, Genant HK, Korobkin MT, et al: Computed tomography: its use in space-occupying lesions of the musculoskeletal system. J Bone Joint Surg 60A:600, 1978.
28. Wilson JS, Korobkin M, Genant HK, et al: CT of musculoskeletal disorders. AJR 131:55, 1978.
29. Weinberfer G, Levinsohn EM: Computed tomography in the evaluation of sarcomatous tumors of the thigh. AJR 130:115, 1978.
30. Kanal E, Burk L, Brunberg JA, et al: Pediatric musculoskeletal magnetic resonance imaging. Radiol Clin North Am 26:211, 1988.
31. deSantos LA, Bernardino ME, Murray JA: Computed tomography in the evaluation of osteosarcoma: experience with 25 cases. AJR 132:535, 1979.
32. Weekes RG, Berquist TH, McLeod RA, et al: Magnetic resonance imaging of soft-tissue tumors: comparison with computed tomography. Magn Reson Imaging 3:345, 1985.
33. Reiser M, Rupp N, Biehl RH, et al: MR in diagnosis of bone tumors. Eur J Radiol 5:1, 1985.
34. Totty WG, Murphy WA, Ganz WY, et al: Magnetic resonance imaging of the normal and ischemic femoral head. AJR 143:1273, 1984.
35. Wetzel LH, Levine E, Murphey MD: A comparison of MR imaging and CT in the evaluation of musculoskeletal masses. Radiographics 7:851, 1987.
36. Zimmer WD, Berquist TH, McLeod RA, et al: Bone tumors:

magnetic resonance imaging versus computed tomography. Radiology 155:709, 1985.

37. Petterson H, Hamlin DJ, Scott KN: Magnetic resonance imaging of primary musculoskeletal tumors. CRC Crit Rev Diagn Imaging 241, 1987.

38. Soye I, Levine E, DeSmet AA, et al: Computed tomography in the preoperative evaluation of masses arising in or near the joints of the extremities. Radiology 143:727, 1982.

39. Campanacci M, Costa P: Total resection of distal femur or proximal tibia for bone tumors. J Bone Joint Surg [BR] 61B:455, 1979.

40. Watts HG: Introduction to resection of musculoskeletal sarcomas. Clin Orthop 153:31, 1980.

41. Totty WG, Murphy WA, Lee JKT: Soft-tissue tumors: MR imaging. Radiology 160:135, 1986.

42. Wehrli FW. Fast-scan imaging: principles and contrast phenomenology. In (eds): Higgins CB, Hricak H, Magnetic Resonance Imaging of the Body. New York, Raven Press, 1987.

43. Shuman WP, Baron RL, Conrad EU, et al: High-field multisection MR STIR imaging versus spin-echo imaging of extremity tumors: lesion conspicuity and extent. Radiology 169P:23, 1988.

44. Dwyer AJ, Frank JA, Sank VJ, et al: Short-Ti inversion-recovery pulse sequence: analysis and initial experience in cancer imaging. Radiology 168:827, 1988.

45. Erlemann R, Reiser M, Stoeber U, et al: MR imaging with static and dynamic Gd-DTPA studies in neoplasms of the musculoskeletal system. Radiology 169(P):135, 1988.

46. Imhof H, Hajek PC, Kramer J, et al: Gd-DTPA: Help in diagnosis of malignant bone lesions? Radiology 169(P):136, 1988.

47. Yousry T, Tilling R, Hahn D, et al: MR imaging in bone tumors: gradient-echo sequences and Gd-DTPA compared with CT. Radiology 169(P:):136, 1988.

48. Von Schulthess GK, Kuoni W, Wuthrich R, et al: Soft-tissue and bone lesions examined with 1.5 T MR imaging and Gd-DTPA. Radiology 169(P):136, 1988.

49. Bloem JL, Doornbos J, Taminiau AH, et al: Gd-DTPA-enhanced MR imaging of bone tumors. Presented at the 74th Annual Meeting of the Radiologic Society of North America, Chicago, IL, 1988.

50. Pettersson H, Eliasson J, Egund N, et al: Gadolinium-DTPA enhancement of soft tissue tumors in magnetic resonance imaging—preliminary clinical experience in five patients. Skeletal Radiol 17:319, 1988.

51. Pettersson H, Slone RM, Spanier S, et al: Musculoskeletal tumors: T1 and T2 relaxation times. Radiology 167:783, 1988.

52. Aisen AM, Martel W, Braunstein EM, et al: MRI and CT evaluation of primary bone and soft-tissue tumors. AJR 146:749, 1986.

53. Yeager BA, Schiebler ML, Wertheim SB, et al: MR imaging of osteoid osteoma of the talus. J Comput Assist Tomogr 11:916, 1987.

54. Bloem JL, Fulke THM, Taminlau AHM, et al: Magnetic resonance imaging of primary malignant bone tumors. Radiographics 5:853, 1985.

55. Lindell MM, Shirkhoda A, Raymond AK, et al: Parosteal osteosarcoma: radiologic-pathologic correlation with emphasis on CT. AJR 148:323, 1987.

56. Picci P, Campanacci M, Bacci G, et al: Medullary involvement in parosteal osteosarcoma. J Bone Joint Surg [Am] 69A:131, 1987.

57. de Santos LA, Murray JA, Finklestein JB, et al: The radiographic spectrum of periosteal osteosarcoma. Radiology 127:123, 1978.

58. Cohen EK, Kressel HY, Frank TS, et al: Hyaline cartilage-origin bone and soft-tissue neoplasms: MR appearance and histologic correlation. Radiology 167:477, 1988.

59. Lichtenstein L: Bone Tumors, Ed 4. St Louis, CV Mosby, 1972, p 21.

60. Kenney PJ, Gilula LA, Murphy WA: The use of CT to distinguish osteochondroma and chondrosarcoma. Radiology 139:129, 1981.

61. Goldberg RR, Genant HK, Johnston WA: Case report: a case

of differentiated chondrosarcoma of the scapula demonstrated on CT. Skeletal Radiol 3:179, 1978.

62. Nurenber P, Harms SE: Magnetic resonance imaging of musculoskeletal tumors. CRC Crit Rev Diagn Imaging 28:331, 1988.

63. Bloem JL, Mulder JD: Chondroblastoma: a clinical and radiologic study of 104 cases. Skeletal Radiol 14:1, 1985.

64. Fobben ES, Dalinka MK, Schiebler ML: The magnetic resonance imaging appearance at 1.5 Tesla of cartilaginous tumors involving the epiphysis. Skeletal Radiol 16:647, 1987.

64a. Brower AC, Moser KP, Kransdorf MJ: The frequency and diagnostic significance of periostitis in chondroblastoma. AJR 154:309–314, 1990.

65. Herman SD, Mesgarzadeh M, Bonakdarpour A, et al: The role of magnetic resonance imaging in giant cell tumor of bone. Skeletal Radiol 16:635, 1987.

66. Beltran J, Simon DC, Levy M, et al: Aneurysmal bone cysts: MR imaging at 1.5T. Radiology 158:689, 1986.

67. Kaplan PA, Murphey M, Greenway G, et al: Fluid-fluid levels in giant cell tumors of bone: report of two cases. J Comput Tomogr 11:151, 1987.

68. Hertzanu Y, Mendelsohn DS, Gottschalk F: Aneurysmal bone cyst of the calcaneus. Radiology 151:51, 1984.

69. Hudson TM: Fluid levels in aneurysmal bone cysts: a CT feature. AJR 141:1001, 1984.

69a. Tsai JC, Dalinka MK, Fallon MD, Zlatkin MB, Kressel HY: Fluid-fluid level—a nonspecific finding in tumors of bone and soft tissue. Radiology 175:779, 1990.

70. De Santos LA, Goldstein HM, Murray JA, et al: Computed tomography in the evaluation of musculoskeletal neoplasms. Radiology 128:89, 1978.

71. Eckardt JJ, Grogan TJ: Giant cell tumor of bone. Clin Orthop 204:45, 1986.

72. Sundaresan N: Chordomas. Clin Orthop 204:135, 1986.

73. Rosenthal DI, Scott JA, Mankin HJ, et al: Sacrococcygeal chordoma: magnetic resonance imaging and computed tomography. AJR 145:143, 1985.

74. Levin E, Levin C: Ewing tumor of rib: radiologic findings and computed tomography contribution. Skeletal Radiol 9:227, 1983.

75. Vanel D, Contesso G, Couanet D, et al: Computed tomography in the evaluation of 41 cases of Ewing's sarcoma. Skeletal Radiol 9:8, 1982.

76. Ginaldi S, de Santos LA: Computed tomography in the evaluation of small round cell tumors of bone. Radiology 134:441, 1980.

77. Hatldorsdottir A, Ekelund L, Rydholm A: CT-diagnosis of lipomatous tumors of the soft tissues. Arch Orthop Trauma Surg 100:211, 1982.

78. Dooms GC, Hricak H, Sollitto RA, et al: Lipomatous tumors and tumors with fatty component: MR imaging potential and comparison of MR and CT results. Radiology 157:479, 1985.

79. Sundaram M, McGuire MH, Herbold DR, et al: High signal intensity soft tissue masses on T1 weighted pulsing sequences. Skeletal Radiol 6:30, 1987.

80. Bush CH, Spanier SS, Gillespy T: Imaging of atypical lipomas of the extremities: report of three cases. Skeletal Radiol 17:472, 1988.

80a. London J, Kim EE, Wallace S, Shirkoda A, Coan J, et al: MR imaging of liposarcomas: correlation of MR features and histology. J Comput Tomogr 13:832, 1989.

80b. Sundaram M, Baran G, Merenda G, McDonald DJ: Myxoid liposarcoma: magnetic resonance imaging appearance with clinical and histological correlation. Skeletal Radiol 19:359, 1990.

81. Hunter JC, Johnston WH, Genant HK: Computed tomography evaluation of fatty tumors of the somatic soft-tissues: clinical utility and radiographic pathologic correlation. Skeletal Radiol 4:79, 1979.

82. Hill JH, Mafee MF, Chow JM, et al: Dynamic computerized tomography in the assessment of hemangioma. Am J Otolaryngol 6:23, 1985.

83. Yuh WTC, Kathol MH, Sein MA, et al: Hemangiomas of skeletal muscle: MR findings in five patients. AJR 149:765, 1987.

84. Kaplan PA, Williams SM: Mucocutaneous and peripheral soft-tissue hemangiomas: MR imaging. Radiology 163:163, 1987.

85. Ross JS, Masaryk TJ, Modic MT, et al: Vertebral hemangiomas: MR imaging. Radiology 165:165, 1987.

86. Cohen JM, Weinreb JC, Redman HC: Arteriovenous malformations of the extremities: MR imaging. Radiology 158:475, 1986.

87. Rubenstein WA, Gray G, Auh YH, et al: CT of fibrous tissues and tumors with sonographic correlation. AJR 147:1067, 1986.

88. Sundaram M, McGuire MH, Schajowicz F: Soft-tissue histologic bases for decreased signal (short T2) on T2-weighted MR images. AJR 148:1247, 1987.

89. Huber DJ, Sumers E, Klein M: Soft tissue pseudotumor following intramuscular injection of "DPT": a pitfall in magnetic resonance imaging. Skeletal Radiol 16:469, 1987.

90. Swensen SJ, Keller PL, Berquist TH, et al: Magnetic resonance imaging of hemorrhage. AJR 145:921, 1985.

91. Wilson DA, Prince JR: MR imaging of hemophilic pseudotumors. AJR 150:349, 1988.

92. Beltran J, Simon DC, Katz W, et al: Increased MR signal intensity in skeletal muscle adjacent to malignant tumors: pathologic correlation and clinical relevance. Radiology 162:251, 1987.

93. Simon MA: Biopsy of musculoskeletal tumors: current concepts review. J Bone Joint Surg 64A:1253, 1982.

94. Schubiner JM, Simon MA: Primary bone tumors in children. Orthop Clin North Am 18:577, 1987.

95. Hudson TM, Schakel M, Springfield DS: Limitations of computed tomography following excisional biopsy of soft tissue sarcomas. Skeletal Radiol 13:49, 1985.

96. Springfield DS, Enneking WF, Neff JR, et al: Principles of tumor management. In Murray JA (ed): AAOS Instructional Course Lectures. St Louis, CV Mosby, 1984.

97. Murray JA: Biopsy in musculoskeletal tumors. In Evarts CM (ed): Surgery of the Musculoskeletal System. Vol 4. New York, Churchill Livingstone, 1983, pp 11–39.

98. Glazer HS, Lee JKT, Levitt RG, et al: Differentiation of radiation fibrosis from recurrent tumor by MRI. Radiology 156:721, 1985.

99. Shuman WP, Griffin BR, Haynor DR, et al: MR imaging in radiation therapy planning. Radiology 156:143, 1985.

99a. Holscher HC, Bloem JL, Nooy MA, Taminian AHM, Eulderink F, et al: Monitoring the effect of chemotherapy on bone sarcomas. AJR 154:763, 1990.

100. Vanel D, Lacombe MJ, Couanet D, et al: Musculoskeletal tumors: follow-up with MR imaging after treatment with surgery and radiation therapy. Radiology 164:243, 1987.

101. Ramsey RG, Zacharias CE: MR imaging of the spine after radiation therapy: easily recognizable effects. AJNR 6:247, 1985.

CHAPTER 15

MARROW-INFILTRATING DISORDERS

BRUCE A. PORTER

Until relatively recently the radiographic diagnosis of marrow-infiltrating diseases has relied heavily on detection of cortical or trabecular bone destruction, which is a rather specific but insensitive diagnostic finding. Many marrow-infiltrating malignant processes, such as leukemia, lymphoma, myeloma, and even metastatic disease, are often rather extensive before radiographic evidence of bone destruction can be detected.[1-4]

The radionuclide bone scan,[5-8] although generally considered the "gold standard" for marrow tumor, often fails to detect diffuse marrow infiltration by primary hematologic malignancies,[9] especially myeloma.[10] Some very aggressive metastatic lesions, such as lung carcinoma, may also not be detected in the context of rapid lytic destruction.[2] The bone scan also has poor spatial resolution and frequently cannot discriminate between benign and malignant causes of increased uptake.[2] As a result of the limitations of conventional imaging methods and the infrequent utilization of guided bone biopsy, diagnostic imaging of marrow disorders remains quite undeveloped when compared with that of other organ systems.

Computed tomography (CT), because of its high spatial resolution, soft tissue contrast, and tomographic image display, has improved the assessment of both benign and malignant bone and marrow lesions[2, 7, 11-16] and allowed the detection of more subtle abnormalities than was previously possible. As with plain radiography, the CT findings of neoplasms involving or arising from the bone marrow, although of limited diagnostic sensitivity, may be quite diagnostically specific and are therefore complementary to the bone scan. Additionally, CT is excellent for detection of soft tissue extension of marrow-based lesions.

Magnetic resonance (MR) imaging, unlike other imaging methods, visualizes bone marrow and marrow disorders directly[10, 14, 17-24] and has extremely high soft tissue contrast, excellent anatomic detail, and direct multiplanar imaging capabilities. As a result, utilization of MR for musculoskeletal and bone diseases is increasing rapidly.[23, 24]

The purposes of this chapter are to discuss techniques, advantages, limitations, and the complementary nature of MR and CT as they apply to marrow diseases and to present examples of MR and CT images of malignant and benign disorders involving the bone marrow. Magnetic resonance will be emphasized, as it is becoming the preferred method for marrow imaging.

This work was supported in part by Grant CA-18029 from the National Cancer Institute and the Medical Research Service of the Department of Veterans Affairs.

Technique

Magnetic Resonance Imaging

GENERAL CONSIDERATIONS

Because normal adult marrow (Fig. 15–1A) is composed predominantly of fat with an admixture of water-containing hematopoietic cells,[1, 25] its MR characteristics are determined primarily by the short T1 and moderately long T2 times of fat. Most benign and malignant disorders that involve marrow have long T1 and long T2 times and high proton density, with the exception of fibrotic or densely blastic lesions, hemangiomas, bone islands, or hematomas. Hence there is intrinsically high MR contrast available for imaging pathologic processes that infiltrate or replace the normal marrow fat, especially with T1-weighted imaging sequences. MR of marrow disorders[1, 17–20] relies heavily on T1 contrast, more so than the intrinsically lower contrast of T2-weighted spin-echo (T2 SE) images. Short TR, short TE, T1-weighted spin-echo (T1 SE) images (see Fig. 15–1B) have high contrast resolution for most marrow abnormalities and also have a high signal-to-noise ratio, good anatomic detail, and relatively short image acquisition times. Therefore these are the primary imaging sequences for most marrow-based diseases.

At our field strengths (0.15 T and 0.5 T), we utilize a combination of short TR, short TE spin-echo and short TI inversion recovery (STIR) sequences (see Fig. 15–1C) for marrow imaging and have discontinued T2 SE sequences in favor of the STIR technique. The clinical applications of STIR for CNS and body imaging were originally described by Bydder, Young, Steiner, and colleagues[26–29]; technical details of the inversion recovery sequence have also been reported by Droege and colleagues[30–32] and others.[33, 34] We utilize this method extensively for body and oncologic MR,[18, 19, 21, 35–43] but marrow applications are perhaps where it is most valuable. The following attributes make STIR images particularly useful for marrow and body MR imaging:

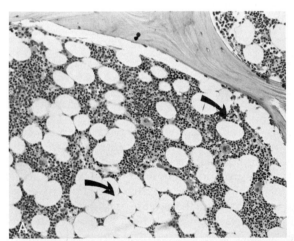

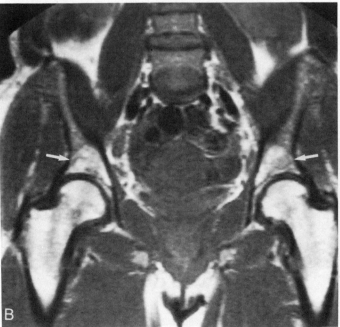

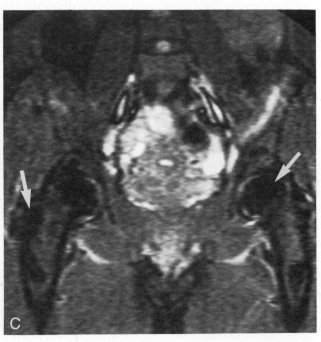

FIGURE 15–1 ■ *A,* Photomicrograph of bone marrow biopsy specimen. Normal marrow is composed of globules of fat *(arrows)* interspersed between water-containing hematopoietic (red) marrow. Bone spicules contribute to low signal intensity within the marrow as well, depending on the degree of weight bearing of the bone. *B,* Coronal T1-weighted spin-echo (T1 SE) image of the pelvis in a 50-year-old female. The signal intensity of normal adult marrow is slightly lower than that of subcutaneous or peritoneal fat. Mild heterogeneity of the marrow, particularly in the iliac bones *(arrows),* is representative of the normal distribution of red versus yellow marrow in an adult (TR, 500; TE, 26; 0.5 T). *C,* Corresponding coronal STIR image portrays subcutaneous and peritoneal fat as dark black; red marrow is slightly higher in signal intensity and more heterogeneous. Yellow marrow areas of the greater trochanter and the femoral epiphysis *(arrows)* are dark black. Normal long-T1 materials such as urine in the bladder, as well as slow-flowing blood in pelvic vessels, are portrayed as high signal intensity. (*A* courtesy of A. Shields, MD, PhD; Seattle, WA.)

1. Marked suppression of the high signal intensity from fat. This "background subtraction" displays fat as black, and most pathologic tissues are intensely white (Fig. 15–2A). This markedly increases lesion contrast. Highly T2-weighted, reduced flip angle, gradient-echo sequences may be similarly used if STIR is not available or in the extremities where motion is not a problem.

2. Because STIR is an inversion spin-echo sequence, it is *additive* of both T1 and T2 contrast,[26] unlike conventional spin-echo sequences, which are either predominantly T1- or T2-weighted or often contain variable degrees of T1 and T2 effects (see Fig. 15–2B). Also, twice the magnetization range is available with STIR, compared with conventional SE images.[26] The result is very high signal from long T1, long T2 pathologic tissues. Somewhat longer TI times are required at higher field strengths for comparable degrees of fat signal suppression.[26]

The images produced by the STIR sequence are intrinsically noisy and have very high contrast and less anatomic detail and spatial resolution than SE images. STIR images are initially difficult to interpret without a matching set of T1 SE images, and acceptance of these images by both clinicians and radiologists has been limited by their unusual appearance. With time and experience, however, the very high diagnostic yield of the STIR technique and its complementarity to T1 SE for detection of pathologic processes in the bone marrow and elsewhere become obvious.

Imaging marrow pathology with T2-weighted spin-echo sequences is less reliable with more variable contrast,[1, 44] unless very long TR and TE times are utilized. Large, lytic, water-containing lesions from bladder, kidney, or thyroid carcinomas or myeloma may be detected with T2 SE sequences (see Fig. 15–2C). However, many diffuse or mixed lytic-blastic

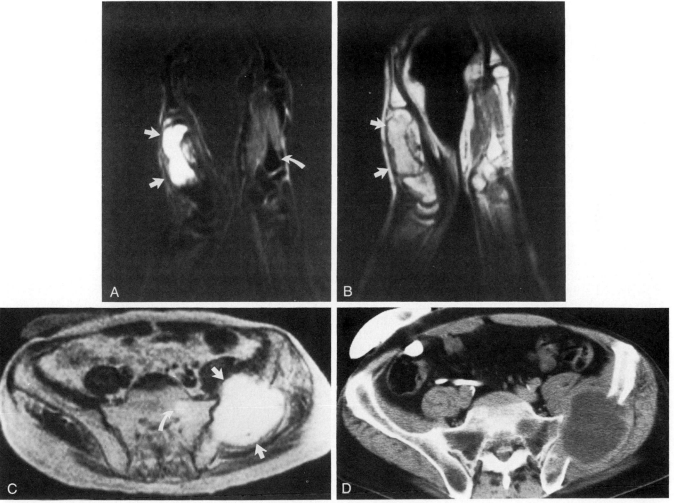

FIGURE 15–2 ■ *A,* Coronal STIR image of the hands with a Ewing's sarcoma of the second metacarpal depicted as marked hyperintensity on STIR *(arrows).* Normal marrow fat, particularly in the extremities, is dark black *(curved arrow)* (TR, 1600; TE, 40; TI, 125; 0.15 T). *B,* Corresponding intermediate spin-echo sequence (TR, 1000; TE, 40; 0.15 T) detects the abnormal marrow signal intensity in the metacarpal. However, the improper choice of pulse parameters, with resulting low T1 contrast, yields low lesion contrast. *C,* Transverse T2 spin-echo (TR, 2000; TE, 60; 0.15 T) image reveals high signal intensity of this large bladder metastasis *(arrows).* A second, smaller lesion is faintly seen more medially *(curved arrow)* but was easily identified on a T1 SE image. *D,* The lytic nature of this lesion, as well as its centrally necrotic core, is confirmed on the corresponding CT image. The smaller lesion cannot be detected except in retrospect. (*C* and *D* from Porter BA, Shields AF, Olson DO: Radiol Clin North Am 24:269–289, 1986.)

tumors may be virtually isointense with normal marrow on T2 SE sequences,[17, 35, 40, 42] and as a result we have discontinued the use of T2 SE sequences for marrow tumors in favor of the higher contrast and shorter imaging times with STIR. On the other hand, the extraosseous component of bone tumors may have a signal intensity similar to that of surrounding muscle[45] and hence may be poorly delineated on the anatomically oriented T1 SE sequences.

MR evaluations of suspected diffuse marrow disorders usually begin with coronal imaging of the pelvis and proximal femurs, which, along with the spine, are the areas most likely to contain hematogenous metastases, as they are the predominant red marrow areas in adults.[25, 46, 47] When a sufficiently large field of view (40 to 45 cm) is used, these images include substantial portions of the lumbar spine as well. If localized symptoms indicate pathologic abnormalities elsewhere, the examination is begun there, as the area of greatest probable yield should be imaged first, particularly in patients who are in pain or claustrophobic. Combining coronal T1 spin-echo images with STIR images of matching slice thickness and registration provides the anatomic detail of the T1 SE with the sensitivity to marrow disorders of STIR and allows assessment of the relative cellularity or osteoblastic component of an abnormality. If marrow tumor is present and is predominantly blastic (i.e., dark on both T1 SE and STIR), then the remainder of the examination is done with T1 SE images. This occurs frequently with metastatic prostate or breast cancer. However, for leukemia, myeloma, lymphoma, and diffuse marrow disorders, STIR produces images with substantially greater lesion conspicuity, and therefore it is used subsequently. An additional benefit of this combined approach is markedly better detection of lymphadenopathy and pulmonary, hepatic, or abdominal metastases by STIR than is possible with T1 SE either alone or in combination with T2 SE sequences.

Suspected spinal malignancies are imaged initially in the sagittal plane.[17, 21, 35, 42, 48, 49] If a lesion is detected adjacent to the spinal canal or radiculopathy or myelopathy is present, axial images improve delineation of the relationship of the marrow or epidural tumor to the spinal cord (see Figs. 15–13B and 15–18C). Sagittal images are usually sufficient if radiation therapy is planned, although coronal images may further facilitate treatment planning.

MR Pulse Sequences

Attention to imaging technique is important for MR in general and particularly for evaluation of marrow abnormalities.[1, 3, 17, 49–51] T1-weighted spin-echo images should generally utilize the shortest TE available on the machine; TE times of 10 to 30 ms are preferred. The TR time selected depends on the number of slices necessary to cover the pathologic area but should be as short as feasible; TR values should range from 350 to not more than 700 ms. If longer TR and intermediate TE images are utilized

(e.g., TR, 1000; TE, 40–60), many lesions will be either isointense with marrow or have low lesion contrast (see Fig. 15–2B). Conventional inversion recovery sequences using intermediate TI times of 400 to 500 ms have excellent T1 contrast,[26] although they require longer imaging times than T1 SE.

Slice thicknesses of 7 to 10 mm are adequate unless smaller lesions require thinner sections, in which case 5-mm slices are helpful. Thinner sections (3 mm) of large bones (particularly the spine) produce noisier and more heterogeneous-appearing marrow images, which are harder to interpret. Two or four signal averages with the T1 spin-echo images produce excellent signal-to-noise ratio and spatial resolution. Typically a 256 × 256 or 256 × 192 imaging matrix is used, depending on field of view. We recommend vertical phase encoding on spinal studies, with large fields of view (>40 cm) to decrease the severity of pulsation, peristalsis, and respiratory motion artifact over the spine.[52] If T2-weighted sequences are used for marrow imaging, they often require TR times of 2000 to 2500 ms or more, and TE times of 80 to 100 ms or greater are necessary. In the spine and pelvis (normal red marrow areas in adults), these sequences may not have adequate contrast to definitively detect marrow abnormality, especially with diffuse or minimal disease.

Our STIR acquisitions on the 0.15-T system use a TR of 1200 to 1600 ms with interleaved slices, whereas the 0.5-T system images require a TR of 1600 to 2100 ms for comparable numbers of slices and contrast. For most marrow STIR evaluations, 7-mm or 10-mm sections, either contiguously or with 1- or 2-mm gaps, are used with large (40- to 45-cm) fields of view. This allows rapid, high-contrast screening of large volumes of marrow. Typically 128 × 256 imaging matrices are used with one or two signal averages on the 0.15-T system and one or two signal averages on the 0.5-T unit. For small bones or knees, thin slices of 5 mm with smaller fields of view and surface coils are useful, although the extreme contrast of STIR substantially reduces the need for both high spatial resolution and thin slices. Phase-sensitive (real) image reconstruction[26, 34] is favored because of its optimal contrast, although it is quite artifact prone; a practical alternative is magnitude reconstruction, which is more reliable but substantially lower in contrast. Flowing blood may be very bright with STIR, especially when motion artifact suppression techniques (MAST) are used.[53]

Gradient-echo techniques[54, 55] use echoes refocused by changes in the magnetic gradients for image production (see Fig. 15–9). They have variable degrees of T1 or T2 contrast depending on TR, TE, and the flip angle[56] used; these sequences are increasingly available, although marrow imaging experience with them is limited. Gradient-echo images with flip angles of 10 to 30° and TR times of 150 to 450 ms and TE times of 20 ms or more have substantial T2* contrast.[54] The resulting images are rather similar in appearance to STIR images (see Fig. 15–9B,C). Gradient-echo techniques are artifact prone because of high motion sensitivity, image distortion at interfaces of tissues of markedly different magnetic susceptibility, and oversensitivity to normal variations in marrow susceptibility that may simulate marrow tumor. However, gradient-echo sequences are rapid and complement T1 spin-echo imaging for marrow imaging, as long as the physician is aware of their limitations. These sequences also improve MR detection of soft tissue calcium, hemosiderin, and blood flow—all important diagnostic observations.

Chemical shift imaging[57-61] relies on the temporal separation of the returning MR signal of water and fat to produce images displaying predominantly the water or fat components of the marrow. Although theoretically well suited to marrow imaging and quantitative assessment of marrow fat and water, the lesion contrast and clinical use of chemical shift methods have so far been limited.

Computed Tomography

The usefulness of CT for evaluation of marrow-infiltrating disorders is primarily a result of its ability to sensitively detect changes in local bone density[1, 7, 62] caused by lytic or blastic lesions (Fig. 15–3A; see also Fig. 15–16D). However, CT is generally not as sensitive as the bone scan for marrow-based tumors.[63, 64] CT examinations, of necessity, are usually done in the axial plane; however, sagittal or coronal images (see Fig. 15–3B,C) can be produced by computer reformation of serial thin-section CT images.

Slice thickness, field of view, and display algorithm are determined by the site of the suspected abnormality, as well as by individual CT machine parameters and capabilities. Slice thickness for initial lesion-localizing scans are 5 to 10 mm, with 1- to 3-mm sections and smaller fields of view used as necessary for high bone detail. Detection of subtle abnormalities, as in differentiating stress fractures from tumor,

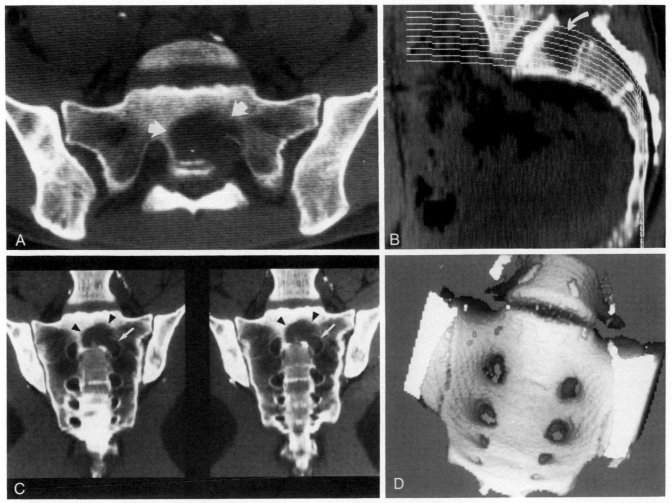

FIGURE 15–3 ■ *A,* Axial CT image through a lytic lesion in S2 caused by marrow lymphoma *(arrows). B,* Reformatted sagittal CT image clearly defines the destructive process in the S2 vertebral body *(arrow).* The curvilinear lines represent the planes of section of the reformatted images in *C. C,* Curved coronal reformatted images (Dimensional Medicine, Inc.) display particularly well the lytic process *(arrowheads)* with soft tissue extending into the left S1 neural foramen *(arrow).* Reformatted images improve assessment of the relationship of tumor to normal structures. *D,* Three-dimensional CT image shows the absence of anterior cortical penetration by the marrow tumor. The S1 foramen is intact caudally.

requires 1- to 2-mm sections with magnification. Intravenous contrast may improve detection and delineation of the margins of both benign and malignant, marrow-based lesions. Both bone and soft tissue algorithms may be necessary for maximal utilization of the CT data, as a wide range of densities may be present in cortical bone, medullary cavity, and adjacent soft tissues. Filming at bone and soft tissue window width and levels optimizes display of diagnostic information. In selected cases, three-dimensional or nonorthagonal two-dimensional reformatted images (see Fig. 15–3) may improve display of the spatial relationships of lytic bone lesions to important structures.

Processes that do not destroy bone are much more difficult to detect with CT. Asymmetry or increases in medullary density can be measured with CT[62, 65] because of replacement of low-density marrow fat by higher density tumor infiltrate or infection; however, this technique is nonspecific and not suited to general diagnostic studies. Patients with leukemia, lymphoma, or myeloma may have extensive marrow tumor that is not detectable by conventional methods, including CT.[9, 10] Computed tomography is not suited as a marrow-screening method because of its limited lesion sensitivity and the fact that the axial imaging plane confines evaluation to relatively small areas. The primary advantage of marrow CT is added diagnostic specificity[7] when bone scans, plain films, or MR (examinations more suitable to screening of large areas) indicate sites of probable abnormality, and further lesion characterization is necessary. CT displays the extent of bone destruction well and, in combination with its very sensitive detection of osteoid or chondroid matrix or soft tissue calcification, often yields critically important differential diagnostic information.

MR detects calcification rather poorly and is therefore intrinsically more limited in diagnostic specificity when compared with CT and plain films for many primary bone and soft tissue tumors. CT-guided biopsy of bone (Fig. 15–4) is a valuable tool for definitive diagnosis of bone or marrow lesions,[63] and although not a common procedure, it has high diagnostic yield with substantially lower morbidity than the surgical alternative. Its value is greatest when bony metastases are solitary, which occurs in 10 per cent of cases.[66] As MR detection of marrow disorders increases, the importance of CT-guided bone biopsies should also increase.

Clinical Applications

MR Appearance of Normal Marrow

The signal intensity of normal adult marrow on T1 spin-echo images is moderate to high[1, 17] and is similar to that of adjacent subcutaneous or peritoneal fat (Fig. 15–5A; see also Fig. 15–1B). Subtly lower signal intensity is seen in areas of red (hematopoietic) versus yellow (nonhematopoietic) marrow in the

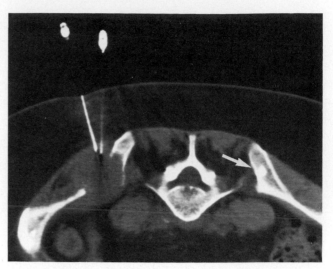

FIGURE 15–4 ■ CT-guided bone biopsy for identification of a lytic metastasis of the left iliac bone. The patient had two primary tumors, and histologic identification of the origin of the metastatic disease was crucial for therapy planning. An additional smaller and more blastic lesion that was dark centrally and hyperintense peripherally on STIR is identified in the opposite iliac bone (arrow). Biopsy indicated breast carcinoma.

proximal femurs, pelvis, and lumbar spine on T1 SE images. The fat suppression of STIR images (Fig. 15–5B; see also Fig. 15–1C) more capably demonstrates the distinction between normal red and yellow marrow. Long T1 materials such as urine, cerebrospinal fluid (CSF), kidney, and spleen also have high signal intensity on STIR. Areas of dense weight-bearing trabecular bone in the femoral head and neck have low signal intensity on both sequences as a result of low proton density. In adults the primary areas of hematopoiesis are the central skeleton, particularly the spine, pelvis, and proximal one third of the femurs.[1, 25, 47] The peripheral appendicular skeleton contains mostly yellow marrow, although irregular areas of somewhat lower signal intensity on T1 SE images are occasionally visualized incidentally elsewhere[67] (i.e., in the distal femurs on MR knee examinations, particularly in premenopausal women; for example, see Fig. 15–29) and should not be mistaken for leukemia, marrow infarction, or other infiltrating processes. This observation is more frequent and pronounced at higher field strengths and probably reflects normal variability in hematopoietic marrow distribution, as well as differences in magnetic susceptibility of hemoglobin of varying degrees of oxygenation. It is also seen in patients with benign hyperproliferative anemias.[17, 68]

Normal sagittal spine images with T1 spin-echo images (see Fig. 15–5A) demonstrate marrow signal intensity that is higher than that of the adjacent intervertebral disks. Diffuse homogeneous marrow infiltration may be difficult to detect on T1 SE sequences alone, unless the relative intensities of vertebral bodies and intervertebral disks are carefully compared. STIR imaging of the spine[21, 35] produces low signal intensity in the marrow (see Fig. 15–5B)

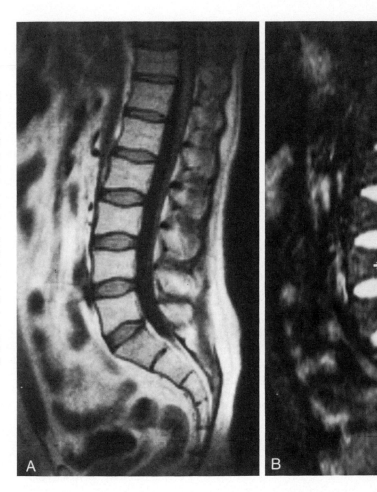

FIGURE 15–5 ■ *A,* Normal spinal marrow shown in a T1 SE image of a 47-year-old male. The signal intensity of the normal spinal marrow is slightly lower than that of retroperitoneal fat but higher than that of the intervertebral disks. The T1 SE images provide excellent anatomic detail of the spinal canal, cord, and paraspinous tissues (TR, 500; TE, 22; 0.15 T). *B,* The vertebral signal intensity on the corresponding STIR image is slightly higher than that of retroperitoneal fat because of hematopoietic material. High intensity of the basivertebral veins is seen dorsally *(arrows).* Normal intervertebral disks also have high signal. CSF is somewhat less intense with this relatively short TR image (TR, 1400; TE 36; TI, 100; 0.15 T), which improves delineation of lesions that abut the thecal sac.

and very high signal intensity in nondegenerated intervertebral disks, as well as in the basivertebral veins and CSF. Prolongation of the TR with STIR, as with T2 spin-echo sequences, results in progressively increasing CSF signal and decreased ability to delineate margins of tumors that are in apposition to the thecal sac. Keeping the TR short decreases the relative hyperintensity of the CSF.[26, 35] There is marked suppression of abdominal, peritoneal, and marrow fat on STIR images.

In children, hematopoietic marrow extends much further into the appendicular skeleton,[25, 47] producing lower signal intensity on T1 spin-echo images (Fig. 15–6) than in adults and with distribution and signal characteristics that may simulate neoplastic infiltration if the physician is not familiar with this age-related finding. The physeal plates are particularly hypointense on T1 spin-echo sequences; MR can diagnose focal tumor that may be very difficult to discern adjacent to these areas on radionuclide bone scans.

Marrow Malignancies

LEUKEMIA

Leukemic marrow infiltration,[17, 19, 20, 60, 69, 70] whether on initial presentation or when advanced, is usually diffuse, symmetric, and rather homogeneously dis-

tributed throughout the marrow in both adults and children. A marrow biopsy of a patient with chronic myelogenous leukemia (Fig. 15–7*A*) reflects the marked change in marrow composition. When compared with normal marrow (see Fig. 15–1*A*), the marrow fat has been almost entirely replaced by water-containing, long T1, leukemic cellular infiltrate. As expected, leukemic marrow on T1 spin-echo images has low signal intensity (see Fig. 15–7*B*) as a result of the replacement of the high-signal fat. Marrow hypercellularity is depicted on STIR (see Fig. 15–7*C*) as high intensity instead of the usual dark marrow of normal individuals. Although diffuse marrow tumors typically appear substantially more intense on STIR images than do benign marrow proliferative or replacement disorders, this cannot be relied on to definitively indicate or exclude malignancy.[48]

Most subacute or chronic forms of leukemia involve primarily the red marrow areas, with relative sparing of the normal yellow marrow areas,[20] as shown in Figure 15–7*B,C.* Acute-phase leukemias, leukemics in blast phase, or aggressive lymphomas[43] frequently have complete to near complete replacement of both red and yellow marrow areas.[19] In such cases the signal intensity of epiphyseal yellow marrow areas is also abnormal on both sequences—a finding very suggestive of malignancy. The inherent nonspecificity of MR must be remembered whenever

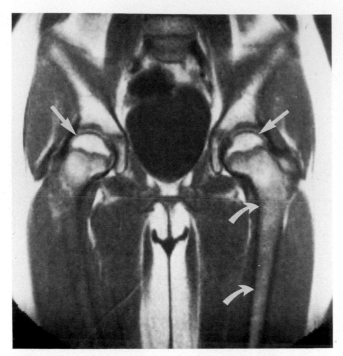

FIGURE 15–6 ■ T1 spin-echo coronal pelvic image of normal marrow of an 8-year-old female. The signal intensity in the femoral epiphyses *(straight arrows)* is relatively higher at this age, because it contains more fat than the hematopoietic red marrow *(curved arrows)* in the femoral shaft. This appearance in an adult can simulate leukemia or hyperproliferative change such as that caused by anemia. In a child it is a normal finding.

diffuse marrow signal abnormality is identified, as various benign disorders may have a similar appearance,[18, 48] as will be demonstrated later.

Leukemic infiltration of marrow is more difficult to detect by MR in children than in adults, because the appearance of the normally very cellular, hematopoietic marrow of children is very similar to that of the hypercellular, neoplastic marrow of leukemia. Quantitative measurement of marrow relaxation times has been proposed to aid in this assessment,[69] but the reliability of this method has not been established for the great variety of diseases that may occur in the marrow. Spectroscopic techniques for marrow malignancies[71] are investigational only. In clinical practice, assessment of leukemia in children is done reliably with posterior iliac crest aspiration or biopsies and monitoring of peripheral blood smears. Therefore MR has a limited role in childhood leukemias.

An exception to the usually very homogeneous tumor distribution in leukemia has been identified in hairy cell leukemia,[72] which has a propensity for somewhat more irregular and patchy marrow involvement (Fig. 15–8). Hairy cell leukemia is poorly detected and monitored by peripheral blood smears, and marrow aspiration is often nonproductive because of marrow fibrosis; large marrow biopsies are necessary for diagnosis and for serial monitoring of therapy. In a patient with vague systemic symptoms, splenomegaly, and this MR appearance, hairy cell leukemia is a diagnostic consideration, although this

combination may also be seen with Gaucher's disease.[73]

Clinical staging and monitoring of irregularly distributed tumors such as hairy cell leukemia, lymphoma, and metastatic disease is improved with MR,[19, 20, 72] as marrow biopsies are likely to understage focal marrow neoplasms as a result of sampling error. MR may obviate the need for serial marrow biopsies and in focal marrow malignancies seems to correlate better with clinical course than the more variable marrow biopsies.[72]

Tumor relapse in acute leukemias may be irregularly distributed, with patchy areas of dense tumor replacement interspersed with normal-appearing marrow (Fig. 15–9). This is logical, as relapse presumably occurs from focal "rests" of tumor cells that have survived therapy. The appearance simulates metastatic disease, although it is more patchy and irregularly marginated than is typical with metastatic tumor.

The great sensitivity of magnetic resonance imaging may allow preclinical detection of marrow disease, as was the case with the patient in Figure 15–9 who was believed to be in remission at the time of imaging but was subsequently confirmed to be in leukemic relapse. Figure 15–9 also illustrates the complementarity of T1 spin-echo and STIR imaging for assessing cellularity (water content) of marrow neoplasms and the potential for reduced flip angle gradient-echo imaging (see Fig. 15–9C) to complement T1 SE images in the assessment of marrow cellularity. However, in our experience, gradient-echo images appear to have less lesion conspicuity and contrast than the STIR images.[42] They additionally may introduce confusion by indicating abnormality that is actually the result of normal or posttherapeutic variations in marrow magnetic susceptibility (see Fig. 15–9D), implying that tumor is present when or where it is not. Caution is therefore necessary in interpreting both T1- and T2-weighted gradient-echo images of marrow.

Further experience with various TR/TE times and flip angles should improve the utility of gradient-echo techniques, which are rapid and increasingly available.

MR imaging soon after effective chemotherapy or radiotherapy may initially result in a worse MR appearance as a result of marrow edema, tumor debris, necrotic material, or inflammatory or osteoblastic cells. These findings may persist for several months or more, and T1 SE images may remain at least somewhat abnormal for an indeterminate time. However, by 3 to 12 months the marrow should no longer be hyperintense on STIR or heavily T2-weighted sequences, unless focal necrosis and cyst formation have occurred. The MR findings must therefore be carefully interpreted within the appropriate clinical context, and a follow-up examination or biopsy should be considered if clinical suspicion for residual tumor or relapse is high. A similar finding of paradoxically apparent worsening on bone scans has also been described.[74] The latter probably

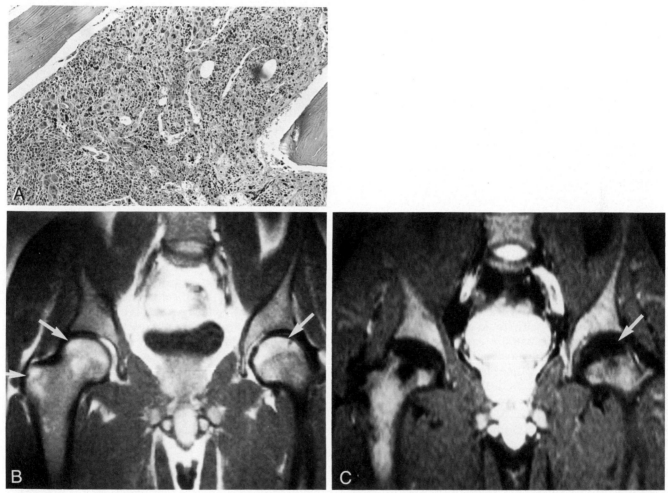

FIGURE 15–7 ■ *A*, Photomicrograph of a bone marrow biopsy specimen from a patient with chronic myelogenous leukemia. Hypercellularity of the marrow caused by leukemic infiltration and displacement of normal marrow fat is evident when compared with Figure 15–1. The higher water content of such marrow is portrayed as low signal intensity on T1 spin-echo images and as high signal intensity on STIR. *B*, MR appearance of leukemia. Coronal TR 600/TE 40 spin-echo image of a 30-year-old male with chronic myelogenous leukemia. The decreased signal intensity in the iliac bones and proximal femurs is caused by leukemic infiltration. Most chronic or subacute forms of leukemia, as seen here, do not involve the normal yellow marrow areas *(arrows)*, but more advanced disease does. When abnormal marrow signal in the epiphyses of long bones is identified, malignancy should be strongly suspected. *C*, The corresponding STIR image with the same slice registration portrays the hyperintense cellular infiltrate readily differentiated from the very low signal intensity of normal yellow marrow *(arrow)*. (*A* courtesy of A. Shields, MD, PhD; Seattle, WA.)

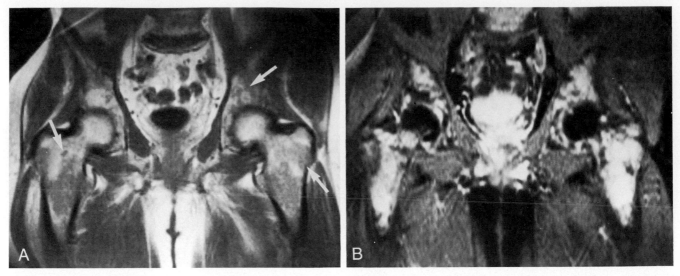

FIGURE 15–8 ■ *A,* T1 SE image of hairy cell leukemia. This form of leukemia is typically somewhat more heterogeneous, patchy, and asymmetric than seen here. Islands of tumor cells (*arrows*) interspersed throughout normal-appearing or fibrotic marrow are common. *B,* STIR image. The marrow hypercellularity is clearly defined by the very high contrast of the STIR technique. Sampling errors caused by random posterior crest iliac biopsies are common with hairy cell leukemia because of its irregular distribution. Marrow tumor is more extensive in this case than usual.

represents repair processes in the bone adjacent to successfully treated tumor. Newer bone scan techniques, such as three-phase scanning, may improve the diagnostic accuracy of the radionuclide study in marrow malignancy.

When CT- or plain film–detectable bone abnormalities are present with leukemic marrow infiltration, the findings are usually irregular lytic destruction within the metaphyseal portions of long bones, cortical erosions, or diffuse areas of punctate medullary osteolysis. Increased thickness of the bone trabecula is readily detected by CT, and areas of dense osteosclerosis may also be visualized. These findings are intrinsically nonspecific; however, when they are detected in children, the likelihood of leukemia is high. The CT findings of leukemia may be nearly identical to those of diffuse metastatic neuroblastoma, another marrow malignancy common in children. However, the latter is more likely to produce focal sclerotic marrow lesions on MR and CT.

The distribution of leukemia is different in children than in adults. Because leukemia arises from red marrow, the abnormalities are more likely to be identified in the central skeleton, pelvis, and proximal femurs in adults but may be more peripherally located in children. Again, widespread areas of lytic abnormality, cortical erosions, or disruption in the spine, pelvis, or metaphyseal portion of long bones are seen. CT and plain films accurately demonstrate periosteal reaction or elevation when cortical disruption has occurred, a diagnostically useful and specific finding indicating the malignant nature of the lesion. Similar findings can be detected with MR when appropriate imaging sequences and planes are utilized.

MYELOMA

Multiple myeloma is the most common primary marrow malignancy in adults.[75] Myelomatous marrow involvement is typically, though not invariably, multifocal and is more sensitively detected by MR than by bone scan, CT, or skeletal radiographs. The distribution of myeloma ranges from complete marrow replacement simulating leukemia to patchy asymmetric or focal deposits indistinguishable from multiple metastases (Fig. 15–10A). Solitary lesions (plasmocytomas) in young or middle-aged adults (see Fig. 15–10B) may present with back pain and cord compression symptoms as the initial manifestation of disease.

Myeloma may be a difficult clinical diagnosis, as bone pain, vertebral collapse, and osteopenia are common in the elderly. Plain films and radionuclide bone scans are clearly inadequate for detection and determination of the extent of myeloma[10] and may soon be replaced by magnetic resonance imaging. Analysis of urinary protein or serum protein electrophoresis determinations may confirm the diagnosis. MR appears well suited to evaluate the extent of myelomatous disease, particularly when epidural tumor or involvement of areas with potentially serious clinical consequences is suspected.[10, 21] Magnetic resonance is particularly indicated when routine evaluation with standard modalities has supplied information discordant with the clinical impression. In such situations, MR frequently detects much more extensive disease than was suspected on conventional scans[10, 21, 76] and substantially improves clinical staging and detection of spinal cord–threatening lesions.

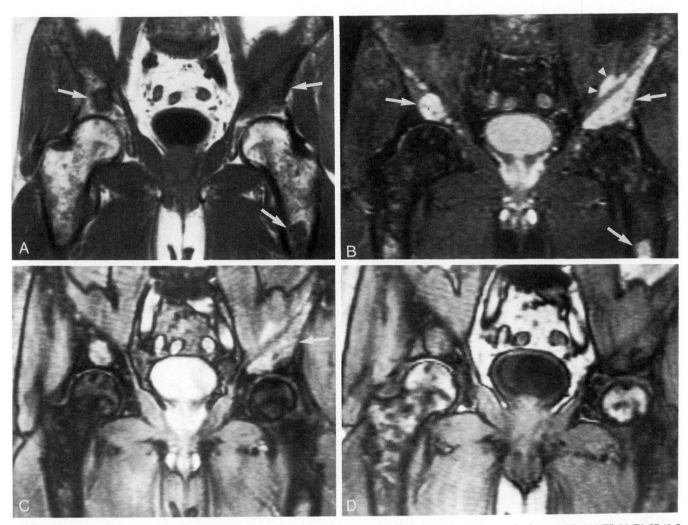

FIGURE 15–9 ■ *A,* Preclinical detection of marrow relapse in a 50-year-old male with acute myelogenous leukemia. TR 600/TE 20 T1 SE (0.5 T) coronal image of the pelvis shows multiple patchy marrow signal abnormalities, particularly in the supraacetabular left iliac bone *(arrows).* *B,* STIR image (TR, 2200; TE, 30; TI, 100) has much higher contrast and lesion conspicuity than the T1 spin-echo sequence. Hyperintense peritumoral edema of the left iliacus muscle is seen on the left *(arrowheads).* *C,* T2*-weighted gradient-echo image in the same plane as *B* (TR, 450; 20° flip angle; TE, 20; 0.5 T) confirms the fluidlike nature of the largest lesions in the supraacetabular bone but has lower lesion contrast than STIR. Some of the marrow heterogeneity in this patient is residual from prior therapy but may also be seen in normal individuals. This probably reflects variability in marrow magnetic susceptibility, as well as in T1 and T2. *D,* T1-weighted gradient-echo image (TR, 450; 90° flip angle; TE, 20) primarily portrays variations in the marrow magnetic susceptibility.

The extremely high contrast of the STIR sequence is particularly helpful in diagnosing diffuse myeloma, particularly in the spine. T2-weighted spin-echo sequences in these patients may distinguish normal from focally abnormal marrow; however, diffuse marrow involvement is much more difficult to identify with T2 SE than with STIR, as the latter displays marked marrow hyperintensity that is usually not subtle (see Fig. 15–10C). Small focal lesions are also substantially more conspicuous. It is not currently known whether MR can distinguish between myeloma-associated marrow amyloid and active myeloma; correlation with clinical history, quantitative serum protein electrophoresis, biopsy, or follow-up examination may be necessary for this determination. It must be remembered that not all marrow lesions appearing on MR scans are necessarily malignant, even in oncology patients.

CT findings in myeloma (see Fig. 15–10D) are typically multifocal areas of discretely marginated lysis that may be punctate or contiguously involve large volumes of medullary bone. Pathologic compression of thoracic and lumbar spine vertebral bodies, which is frequent, may mask the underlying malignant involvement on CT, plain x-ray, and MR films. When the sternum or ribs are involved, the lesions are frequently expansile and painful, although this finding is not specific to myeloma; lymphoma may behave similarly, for example. Of particular importance in CT of the spine in patients with myeloma, as well as those with other spinal malignancies, is detection of disruption of the posterior cortical margin of a vertebra adjacent to the spinal canal.[15] This is a reliable indicator of epidural tumor extension, a serious clinical problem. Posterior cortical disruption has been considered a definitive

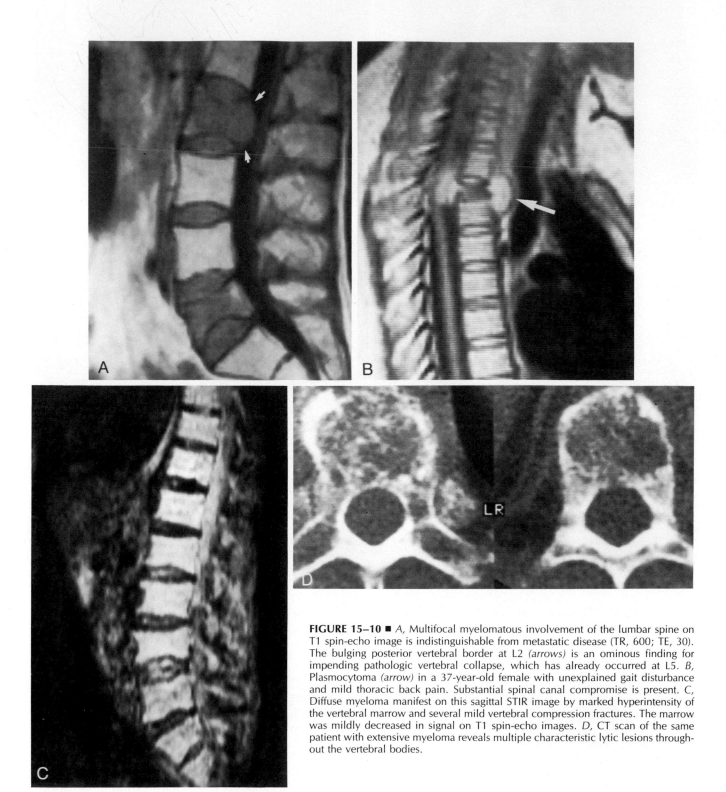

FIGURE 15–10 ■ *A,* Multifocal myelomatous involvement of the lumbar spine on T1 spin-echo image is indistinguishable from metastatic disease (TR, 600; TE, 30). The bulging posterior vertebral border at L2 *(arrows)* is an ominous finding for impending pathologic vertebral collapse, which has already occurred at L5. *B,* Plasmocytoma *(arrow)* in a 37-year-old female with unexplained gait disturbance and mild thoracic back pain. Substantial spinal canal compromise is present. *C,* Diffuse myeloma manifest on this sagittal STIR image by marked hyperintensity of the vertebral marrow and several mild vertebral compression fractures. The marrow was mildly decreased in signal on T1 spin-echo images. *D,* CT scan of the same patient with extensive myeloma reveals multiple characteristic lytic lesions throughout the vertebral bodies.

indication for myelography;[15] however, myelography is currently being supplanted by MR in this situation.[21] MR is less time consuming, is noninvasive, and gives a better overall assessment of the extent of spinal and extraspinal tumor.[21] Detection of imminent vertebral collapse and spinal cord compression may be improved with MR[10, 17, 21, 42, 76] in patients with myeloma, as well as in those with primary and metastatic marrow disease. Hopefully, early MR diagnosis of threatened cord compression can improve the therapy and patient prognosis for this serious complication of spinal malignancy.

LYMPHOMA

During our early experience with imaging of marrow malignancies,[19, 20] it became evident that a frequent feature of lymphoma was focal infiltration (Fig. 15–11) of red marrow areas and that MR imaging would become an important method for staging and monitoring lymphoma. Although the marrow involvement may be minimal, detection of and relative quantitative assessment of the amount of marrow tumor is important for staging, treatment, and monitoring of therapy (Fig. 15–12). Marrow biopsies are inherently limited by sampling error in focal disorders, and considering that approximately 50 per cent of patients have lymphomatous marrow involvement at autopsy, routine biopsies probably underestimate tumor extent in many cases. MR is capable of "sampling" large volumes of marrow and detecting early

marrow infiltration and is more sensitive than the bone scan in this situation.[9] Bone scan abnormalities in lymphoma are relatively infrequent and often subtle.[77] The frequency of marrow tumor as determined by bone scan abnormality is probably substantially underestimated.

In some cases, marrow lymphoma may be distributed as diffusely as leukemia or myeloma, although patchy areas of relatively normal marrow are still commonly seen.[19] Radionuclide bone scans,[9] even in patients with rather extensive disease, frequently appear normal or equivocal (see Fig. 15–12A).

Experience indicates that staging and overall evaluation of lymphoma patients can be substantially improved with MR,[19, 43, 78, 79] which can detect focal marrow tumor deposits, chest wall or lymph node tumor, or other abnormalities, such as avascular necrosis, not detected by bone scan, CT, plain films, marrow biopsy, or other methods (Fig. 15–13). As a result, STIR marrow imaging of lymphoma patients has become a major part of our body MR practice. Solitary marrow lesions in any patient population are always problematic and may require biopsy, but follow-up studies after tumor-specific therapy are quite confirmatory when the lesion resolves (see Fig. 15–12). Sensitive detection of numerous lesions generally increases the likelihood that MR-detected marrow abnormalities are neoplastic,[10] as does typically malignant behavior such as that seen in Figure 15–13. An additional advantage of MR over CT and bone

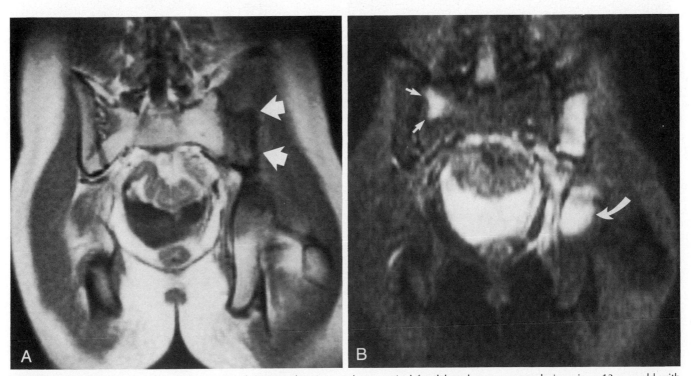

FIGURE 15–11 ■ *A,* Marrow lymphoma. Coronal T1 SE pelvic image shows typical focal lymphoma marrow lesions in a 13-year-old with Hodgkin's disease. Low signal in the left posterior iliac crest *(arrows)* is caused by tumor, whereas the right posterior iliac crest is normal. Low signal in the midleft iliac bone is either tumor or partial volume averaging of cortex and soft tissues. *B,* Corresponding high-contrast STIR image improves detection of tumor infiltration in the lateral right sacrum *(small arrows)* and confirms that the suspected abnormality in the left iliac bone *(curved arrow)* is tumor.

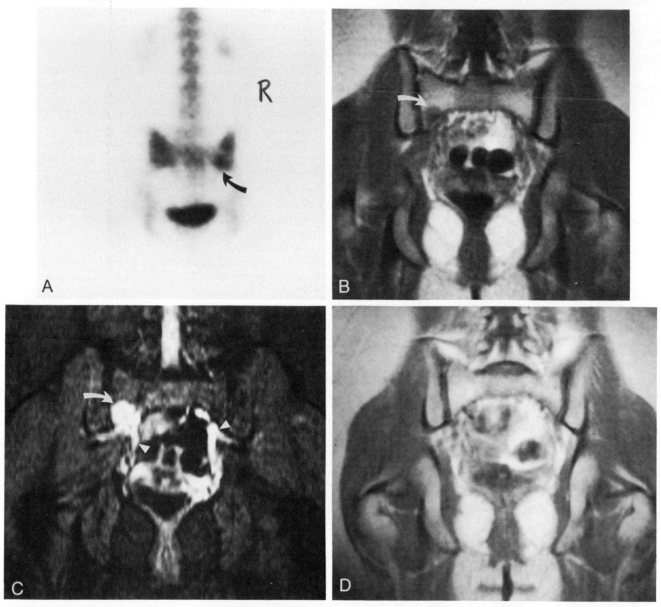

FIGURE 15–12 ■ *A,* Focal marrow lymphoma in the right sacrum with resolution after successful therapy. Bone scan in this patient with Hodgkin's lymphoma appeared normal but in retrospect may have detected rounded area of increased uptake in the right sacrum *(arrow). B,* Coronal T1 spin-echo image of the same patient detected a focal signal abnormality in the inferior lateral margin of the right sacrum *(arrow).* C, This lesion was hyperintense on STIR, a very typical feature of lymphoma, whether in the marrow or elsewhere. Slow-flowing venous blood in pelvic veins is also very bright on this sequence *(arrowheads). D,* After successful chemotherapy, the sacral lesion resolved completely on both this T1 spin-echo and STIR images. (Reprinted with permission from Hoane BR, Shields DF, Porter BA, Shulman HM, et al: Detection of lymphomatous bone marrow involvement with magnetic resonance imaging. Blood 78:728–738, 1991.)

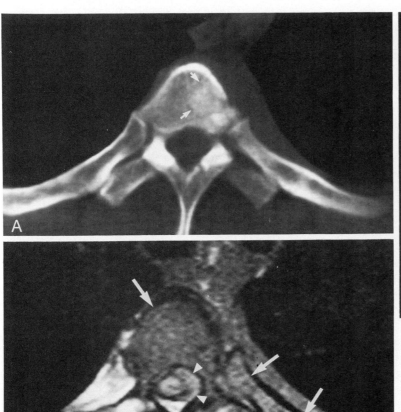

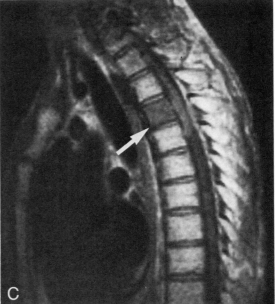

FIGURE 15–13 ■ *A*, CT versus MR for marrow lymphoma. CT scan of T4 vertebral body detected the paravertebral soft tissue mass, but the slight increase in density of the left lateral vertebral body *(arrows)* was only detectable in retrospect. Marrow tumor was not suspected in this patient, who had a negative marrow biopsy result and no symptoms of marrow or spinal tumor. *B*, Corresponding oblique axial T1 SE (TR, 500; TE, 26; 0.5 T) image more sensitively detected both the extensive marrow lymphoma in the vertebral body and adjacent rib *(arrows)* and the foraminal and epidural tumor *(arrowheads)*. The spinal cord is displaced to the right. The presence of unsuspected marrow and spinal canal tumor had first been detected on a coronal marrow screening STIR sequence done at 0.15 T and was confirmed with a sagittal T1 SE image *(C)*.

scan in lymphoma is the ability to simultaneously detect lymphadenopathy and marrow tumor involvement.[38, 43]

A negative result on MR marrow study does not exclude diffuse microscopic marrow tumor.[40, 42] Therefore marrow biopsies and MR are complementary. When T1 SE and STIR imaging of the marrow in a lymphoma patient are negative or only minimally heterogeneous or hyperintense on STIR, a posterior iliac crest marrow biopsy can be considered to be representative of the marrow elsewhere; this can provide very useful clinical information.

A negative result on MR scan helps exclude clinically significant macroscopic marrow tumor. If MR is focally abnormal, CT-guided or operative biopsy can be performed, unless the MR appearance, clinical situation, and multiplicity of marrow lesions indicate a high probability of marrow disease.

Computed tomography scans of both Hodgkin's and non-Hodgkin's lymphoma in patients with bone pain and marrow tumor may initially be normal. However, with more advanced disease, osteolytic or osteoblastic changes within adult red marrow areas may be seen, as previously illustrated. Other radiographic patterns of lymphomatous bone involvement

are diffuse sclerosis or mixed areas of either variably decreased or increased x-ray absorption within the axial skeleton (see Fig. 15–13*A*). The distribution of Hodgkin's versus non-Hodgkin's lymphoma is substantially different; Hodgkin's involves the proximal bones almost three times as often as non-Hodgkin's lymphoma.[77]

Dense sclerosis of trabecular and cortical bone with advanced lymphoma ("ivory vertebra") is readily recognized on plain radiographs or CT scans, but early changes are often subtle (see Fig. 15–13*A*). However, MR readily detects the marrow abnormality when bone scan,[9] plain films, or CT scans are negative or equivocal (see Fig. 15–13*B*). Lymphomatous involvement of the chest wall and spine is quite common[78, 79] and is usually associated with an osteolytic, often expansile destructive process of either a rib or the sternum, with an associated soft tissue or pleural-based mass. Neural foraminal encroachment by tumor with erosion of vertebral bodies and invasion into the spinal canal (see Fig. 15–13*B*) is another not infrequent finding.

Oncology patients, particularly lymphoma and leukemia patients treated with steroids and radiation, are at risk for developing avascular necrosis of the hip,[79a, 80] which may be detected in its advanced stages by CT and earlier with MR. Underlying, clinically unsuspected osteonecrosis may be difficult to detect by bone scan, CT, and radiography and even by MR when marrow tumor is also present (Fig. 15–14). Persistent hip pain in patients with leukemia or lymphoma[43, 137] should suggest osteonecrosis, as well as marrow tumor.

METASTATIC MARROW DISEASE

The most common focal pathologic abnormality in the bone marrow of oncology patients is metastatic disease (Fig. 15–15), which spreads hematogeneously and hence involves predominantly red marrow areas, with the frequency and location of lesions depending on tumor type and patient population.[5, 6, 66, 81] Most skeletal metastases in women arise from breast tumors; in men the prostate is the most common origin.[66] MR appears to be the most sensitive method for detection of secondary tumor deposits in the marrow,[48] but it is not yet as feasible for routine whole body screening as the bone scan because of greater cost and a more limited field of view. Because most marrow metastases occur in the red marrow areas of the axial spine, pelvis, and proximal long bones, many are detected by MR studies done for other reasons. Additionally, whole-body MR screening for marrow metastases is possible, with reasonable imaging time, with high-contrast sequences such as STIR. Because marrow metastases, like primary marrow malignancies, are characterized by long T1 and long T2, they are detected readily by MR, because they displace the marrow fat.

With predominantly blastic metastatic disease, such as prostate cancer, the metastatic lesions are often discrete and better delineated on T1 spin-echo images than on T2 spin-echo or STIR (Fig. 15–16). The bone blastic activity often far exceeds the amount of tumor present with prostate metastases.[82] As illustrated, in a patient with metastatic prostate carci-

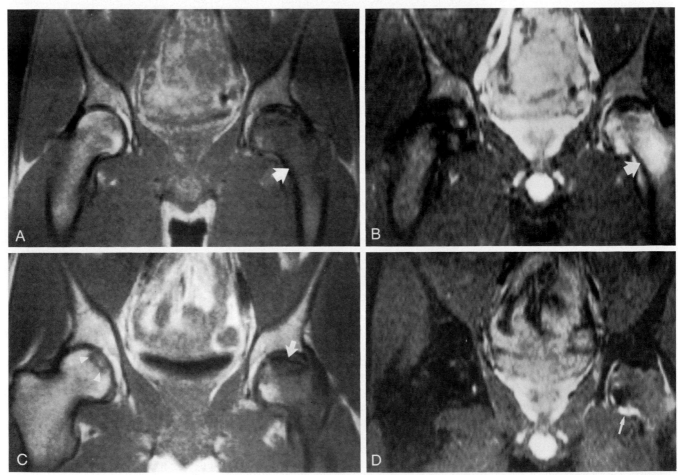

FIGURE 15–14 ■ *A,* Occult avascular necrosis. Diffusely decreased marrow signal with focally asymmetric involvement of the painful proximal left femur *(arrow)* was attributed clinically and by MR scan to tumor infiltration. *B,* STIR image detects the diffuse mild marrow hypercellularity (positive marrow biopsy result), as well as a more focally intense signal in the left intertrochanteric region *(arrow),* probably caused by superimposed edema. In retrospect this abnormality is more poorly marginated than is usually seen with focal marrow lymphoma. *C,* Coronal T1 spin-echo image after therapy reveals circular areas of decreased signal in the subchondral portion of the left femoral head *(arrow)*—typical findings of avascular necrosis. Similar early findings are visible on the right *(arrowheads)* as well. Both lesions were probably present on the initial examination (see *A*) but not recognized. Left hip pain persisted after a successful bone marrow transplant. *D,* The generalized decrease in marrow tumor is well depicted on STIR as lower signal in the iliac bones. Osteonecrotic (dead) bone in the cranial portion of the left femoral head has very low signal intensity on both T1 spin-echo and STIR images. A small effusion is present in the left hip joint *(arrow).*

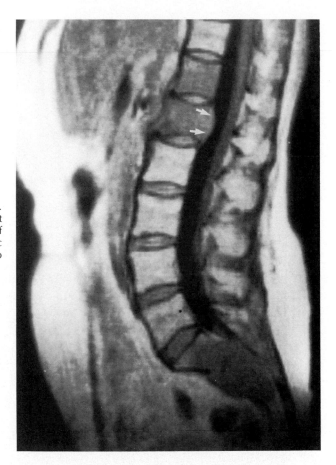

FIGURE 15–15 ■ Metastatic breast carcinoma to T12, L1, and the sacrum. Low signal intensity on this T1 spin-echo image was the result of replacement of the normal short-T1 marrow fat by long-T1 tumor. The posterior bulge of the L1 vertebral body *(arrows)* is worrisome for impending pathologic collapse and nerve root compression. Notice the similarity in appearance to marrow myeloma (see Fig. 15–10A).

noma, an abnormal bone scan, and degenerative intervertebral disk disease, MR can discriminate among benign focal end plate abnormalities of reactive discogenic sclerosis, areas of blastic metastatic tumor, and radiation-induced marrow changes. Successful hormonal therapy may not change the CT appearance of prostate metastases (see Fig. 15–16D) or some bone scan findings in lymphoma,[77] but the decreased cellularity can be documented with STIR (see Fig. 15–16E,F), in both marrow and extraskeletal masses,[43, 136] as marked decrease or absence of abnormal signal on STIR images in follow-up MR studies. The bone scan may revert to a negative result, despite persistence of blastic deposits of bone.[150]

Follow-up studies indicating such substantial decreases in lesion signal intensity and extent on STIR or T2 SE sequences appear to correlate well with clinical response,[43, 60, 136, 151] although these observations need further investigation to determine their reliability.

The greater specificity and spatial resolution of MR is a clear advantage over the bone scan, even with newer bone scan techniques. In addition, the greatly superior soft tissue resolution of MR allows assessment of nerve root– or cord-threatening tumors (see Fig. 15–15) and delineation of the spinal cord–compressing metastatic lesions (Fig. 15–17). With advanced and cord-threatening metastatic disease, most of the vertebral body is involved, and morphologic changes in the vertebral contour are identifiable,

implying impending pathologic fracture and cord compression.[21] CT detection of penetration of posterior cortical bone is an ominous finding compatible with epidural tumor[15] and can also be visualized on T1 spin-echo or STIR images (Fig. 15–18) when sufficient epidural soft tissue mass, cortical interruption, or obliteration of the spinal canal is present. However, MR has the advantages of direct sagittal imaging and much greater sensitivity to marrow tumor.

Axial images (see Fig. 15–18C) depict the relationships of the spinal cord and marrow tumor well when cord compression is present. Gadolinium-enhanced T1 SE or STIR images can improve the depiction of epidural and paraspinous soft tissue involvement,[35] as addressed later in this chapter. Acute angulation of vertebral end plate fractures further increases diagnostic confidence that a visualized marrow abnormality is neoplastic; smooth concave end plate depression is more likely benign.[83]

Attention to the relative signal intensity of the intervertebral disks and to the vertebral marrow may be necessary to detect diffuse spinal involvement (Fig. 15–19A) when lesser degrees of blastic activity are present. The complementary nature of STIR (see Fig. 15–19B) for detection of diffuse marrow tumor, as well as extraspinous disease, is evident. The detection of pulmonary, hepatic, or nodal metastases by STIR[42] can decrease the need for other diagnostic studies, thus decreasing the time and cost of diagnosis and staging.

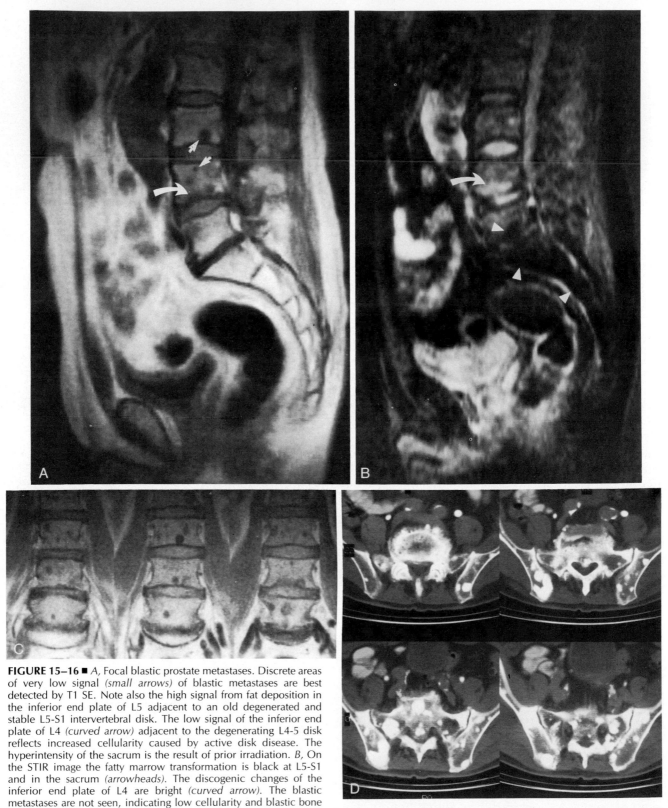

FIGURE 15–16 ■ *A,* Focal blastic prostate metastases. Discrete areas of very low signal *(small arrows)* of blastic metastases are best detected by T1 SE. Note also the high signal from fat deposition in the inferior end plate of L5 adjacent to an old degenerated and stable L5-S1 intervertebral disk. The low signal of the inferior end plate of L4 *(curved arrow)* adjacent to the degenerating L4-5 disk reflects increased cellularity caused by active disk disease. The hyperintensity of the sacrum is the result of prior irradiation. *B,* On the STIR image the fatty marrow transformation is black at L5-S1 and in the sacrum *(arrowheads)*. The discogenic changes of the inferior end plate of L4 are bright *(curved arrow)*. The blastic metastases are not seen, indicating low cellularity and blastic bone with little, if any, residual tumor after successful hormonal therapy. *C,* Multiple images from a coronal T1 SE acquisition of the pelvis and lumbosacral spine in the same patient showing the extensive distribution and sharply demarcated margins of blastic prostate metastases. *D,* CT of another patient after successful hormonal therapy for prostate carcinoma. Densely blastic lesions remain.

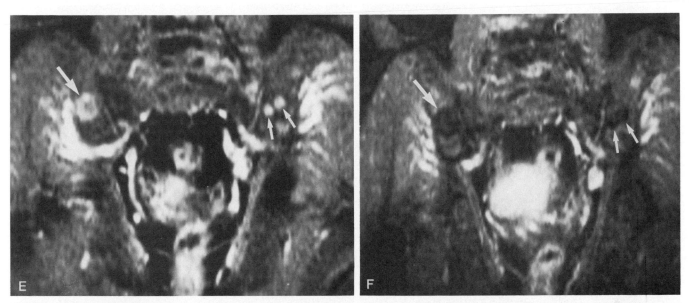

FIGURE 15–16 *Continued* ■ *E,* STIR coronal pelvic image of the patient in *D* 1 year earlier indicates hypercellularity of the posterior iliac crest metastases *(arrows). F,* Lesions that were bright at the time of the CT scan in *D* are now dark *(arrows),* corresponding to the clinical response of this tumor. The bone scan remained abnormal.

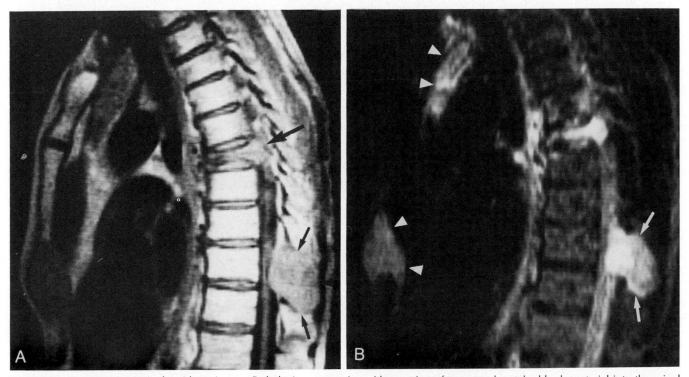

FIGURE 15–17 ■ *A,* Metastatic thyroid carcinoma. Pathologic compression with extrusion of tumor and vertebral body material into the spinal canal is present at T6 *(large arrow)* on this T1 SE image. An additional soft tissue mass arising from the lamina of T9 *(small arrows)* and extending into the spinal canal is also seen. *B,* The substantially higher contrast of the STIR image improves tumor conspicuity and margin delineation at T9 *(arrows)* and confirming metastases in the retromanubrial space and sternum *(arrowheads).* Tumor invasion of the spinal canal is rather well seen on this short-TR (1400 ms) STIR image at 0.15 T.

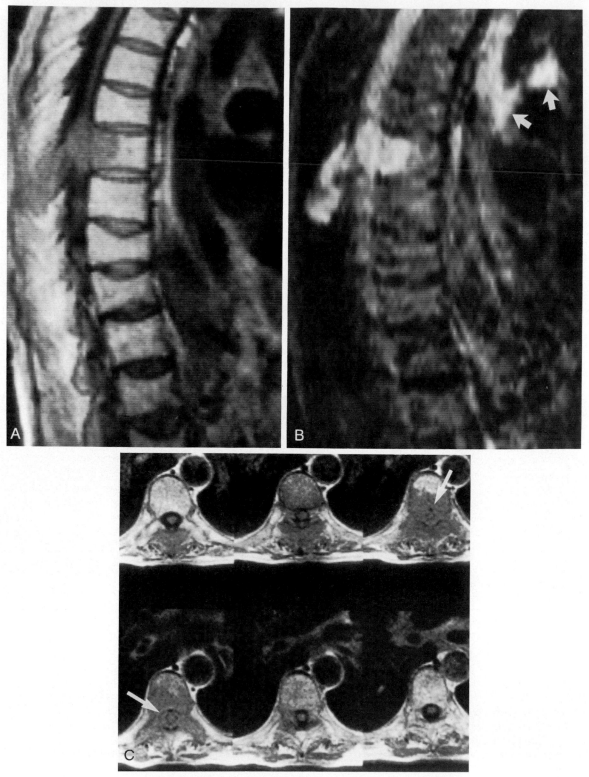

FIGURE 15–18 ■ *A,* Sagittal T1 SE image of metastatic lung carcinoma demonstrates a cord-compressing epidural tumor, as well as benign appearance of lower thoracic and upper lumbar vertebrae compression fractures. *B,* Corresponding STIR images illustrate the normal signal of old, benign compression fractures, hyperintense marrow tumor at T8, and mediastinal lymphadenopathy *(arrows). C,* Axial T1 SE images of metastatic lung carcinoma. At the level of a midthoracic near-complete block of the spinal canal, the CSF space is occupied by tumor, and the cord is circumferentially compressed *(arrows).*

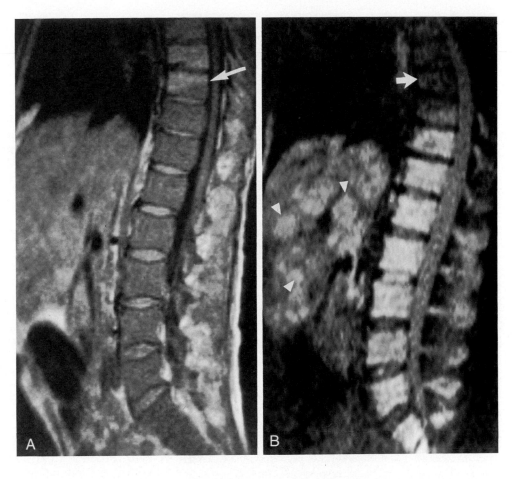

FIGURE 15–19 ■ *A*, T1 SE image of diffuse marrow metastatic disease after previous radiation therapy for lung carcinoma. There is a sharp demarcation of signal intensity *(arrow)* with relative tumor sparing of marrow in the cranial thoracic spine in areas of prior irradiation. Signal intensity of the tumor-involved lower thoracic and lumbar marrow is diffusely abnormal and substantially lower than that of the intervertebral disks. *B*, Marked hyperintensity of the tumor-involved spine with more normal (low) signal in areas of prior irradiation *(arrow)* is seen on STIR image. Extensive hepatic edema and multifocal liver metastatic disease is also present *(arrowheads)* (TR, 1400; TE, 36; TI, 100; 0.15T).

Clinically advanced marrow metastatic disease, particularly from breast, prostate, or lung carcinoma, may cause anemia as a result of extensive tumor replacement of hematopoietic marrow. T1 spin-echo images on these patients show markedly low signal intensity (Fig. 15–20). Similarly, dark marrow may also be seen with hemosiderosis as a result of marked T2 shortening by excess marrow iron.[84] Characteristic MR changes in bone marrow are seen after radiation therapy[1, 60, 85] for malignancy. On T1 spin-echo images, previously irradiated marrow is hyperintense (see Fig. 15–16A), reflecting the decreased cellular component of the marrow. Irradiated marrow on STIR is often deep black (see Fig. 15–16B) as a result of the very fatty nature of this nonhematopoietic marrow. Acutely, irradiated marrow may have increased signal on STIR images, probably reflecting increased marrow water caused by edema or vascular congestion.[60] Care should be exercised in diagnosing recurrent, primary, or metastatic disease in heavily irradiated marrow, as tumor necrosis, edema, marrow infarction, fractures,[149] or nonviable debris may simulate persistent or recurrent tumor.[86] Detection of recurrent malignancy in irradiated marrow has also occasionally been a problem with radionuclide bone scans[2, 134] as a result of the absence of osteoblastic cells within irradiated bone. Although more sensitive than the bone scan for detecting recurrent tumor in

irradiated marrow, MR suffers from potentially false-positive results, whereas the bone scan may miss recurrent disease or mistake bone repair or hyperemia for tumor. The margins of radiation fields with extensive metastatic disease may be strikingly portrayed by MR (see Fig. 15–19), and the therapeutic effect of the prior marrow irradiation is evident.

Differentiation of benign from malignant compression fractures may be difficult by CT and MR.[132] Findings that favor a malignant process include extensive marrow signal abnormality with pedicle involvement, sharply angled end plate fractures,[83] malignant-appearing or invasive characteristics, and the presence of multiple lesions elsewhere with similar signal characteristics (see Fig. 15–23). Benign vertebral collapse is usually wedge-shaped or has smoothly rounded end plate depression[83] and normal signal on T1 and STIR images (see Fig. 15–18), unless the collapse is very recent and marrow edema, particularly near the end plates, is detectable. Focal depressions at the site of Schmorl's nodes may occur with either benign or malignant disease. STIR hyperintensity at the end plates only (low signal on T1 SE) helps indicate a benign fracture. Gadolinium enhancement of vertebral tumors[35] versus lack of enhancement with benign fractures has been reported to improve differentiation of malignant from benign lesions.[87] Acute benign fractures may espe-

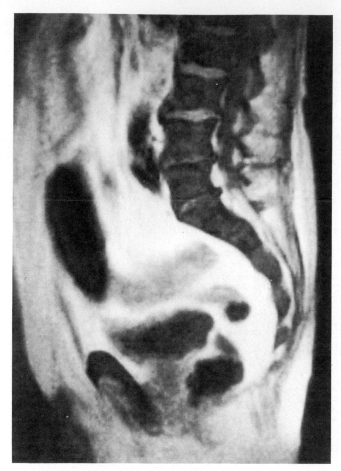

FIGURE 15–20 ■ Sagittal TR 600/TE 40 SE image of markedly blastic, extensive prostate metastatic disease. The signal intensity of the marrow is extremely low because of replacement of normal marrow fat and hematopoietic material by dense bone.

cially simulate tumor because of marrow edema, but after 1 to 3 months the marrow signal usually returns to normal or near normal.

MR and the Bone Scan ■ The radionuclide bone scan has been the standard of diagnosis for metastatic marrow disease for many years,[133] yet it may miss clinically significant marrow tumor.[10] The potential advantages of MR over bone scans for detection and clinical assessment of marrow malignancies are well illustrated in Figure 15–21. This young woman with metastatic Ewing's sarcoma to the lungs and pleura was imaged for suspected abdominal lymphadenopathy. A coronal large-field-of-view STIR image (see Fig. 15–21A) detected high signal intensity in the body of S2. The bone scan, done 2 days earlier (Fig. 15–21B), was negative. Sagittal T1 spin-echo and STIR images indicated focal abnormality with erosion of the posterior cortex of S2. This area underwent biopsy, and metastatic Ewing's sarcoma was confirmed; detection of such lesions substantially affects staging, therapy, and patient prognosis.

There is perhaps no more urgent and clinically useful application of magnetic resonance imaging in oncology than in the early detection of spinal cord–

threatening tumors,[21, 15, 76] as illustrated in the preceding examples. MR is a noninvasive, rapid, and accurate technique for this very important evaluation, yet some patients with clinically probable spinal tumor have negative results on conventional MR studies.

Improved detection and delineation of both intradural[88] and extradural[35] abnormalities (Fig. 15–22) can be obtained by T1 spin-echo images after administration of intravenous MR contrast agents such as gadopentetate dimeglumine; yet T2-weighted spin-echo images, obtained either before or after contrast, rarely add additional information.[35] On the other hand, unlike with contrast MR of the brain, enhancement with T1-shortening paramagnetic agents may actually decrease conspicuity of pathologic processes within the marrow.[35] Contrast-induced T1 shortening produces higher signal intensity on T1 SE images, and hence tumor enhancement may produce nearly normal-appearing bone marrow, even in the presence of extensive marrow tumor (Fig. 15–23). Therefore noncontrast T1 spin-echo images are routinely necessary.[35] Combined use of unenhanced T1 spin-echo, contrast-enhanced T1 spin-echo, and STIR sensitively detects marrow and intradural tumor and can provide better delineation of tumor margins, improved demarcation of the edges of tumor from adjacent CSF, and improved detection of intradural and intramedullary metastases when compared with conventional MR techniques. However, because in the majority of cases symptomatic spinal metastatic lesions arise from the vertebral bodies or pedicles,[21] contrast agents are of most use when the noncontrast study is normal and intradural or leptomeningeal tumor[88] is suspected. When spinal MR is negative for marrow or spinal canal tumor, a coronal STIR series may detect paraspinal or distal soft tissue lesions responsible for the patient's symptoms.

CT findings in marrow metastatic disease[7, 62, 89–91] depend on whether the tumor is predominantly lytic or blastic. Heavily blastic tumor such as prostate carcinoma (see Fig. 15–16) is usually discrete and focal but may be confluent and homogeneous with markedly increased density. This dense bone persists long after successful therapy. Focal areas of discretely marginated osteolytic metastatic disease, which are most commonly the result of breast or lung carcinoma, are clearly delineated by CT (Fig. 15–24), and although these lesions are diagnostically quite specific for malignant disease, neither CT nor MR can definitively indicate the origin of solitary lesions without bone biopsy, which is best guided by fluoroscopy or CT.[138] Variable amounts of reactive soft tissue edema adjacent to marrow tumor are detectable with CT, but are better seen with MR, which may lead the physician to the underlying abnormality. A negative CT scan does not exclude marrow tumor, because substantial bone destruction must occur for detection. MR may become the preferred method of simultaneous screening for visceral and

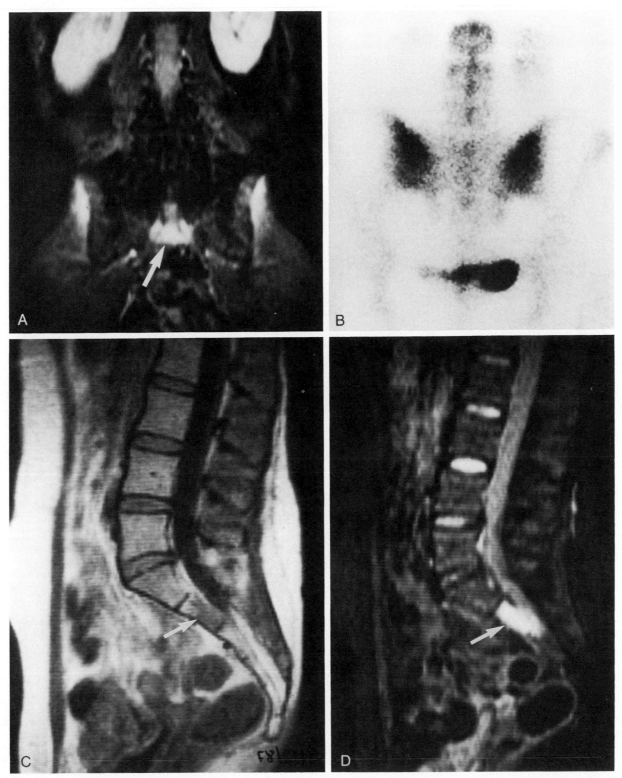

FIGURE 15–21 ■ Metastatic Ewing's sarcoma; MR versus bone scan. The sensitivity of STIR-MR for marrow tumor detection is illustrated by images of this 24-year-old female with thoracic Ewing's sarcoma. *A,* Coronal abdominal-pelvic STIR image detected high signal abnormality in S2 *(arrow).* The high signal intensity adjacent to the posterior iliac crests is muscle edema caused by recent iliac bone biopsy. *B,* Radionuclide bone scan done 2 days earlier does not indicate marrow abnormality in this region, even in retrospect. *C,* Sagittal T1 spin-echo image. *D,* STIR images confirm the marrow metastasis in S2.

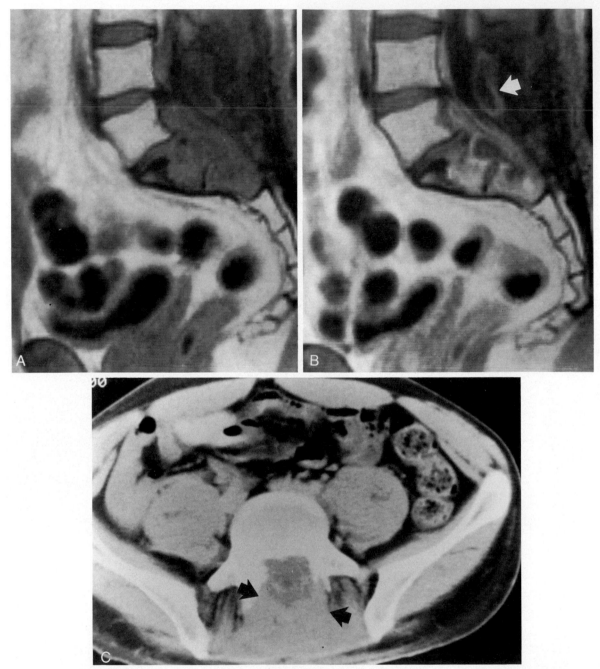

FIGURE 15–22 ■ *A*, Previously resected and irradiated giant cell tumor of the sacrum is rather well seen on unenhanced T1 SE image. *B*, The marrow component of this lesion was detected with very high contrast with STIR, although the interval architecture and CSF interface were best seen on this T1 SE after contrast enhancement with intravenous gadolinium, which also delineates the margin of a lesion dorsal to the thecal sac *(arrow)*. Because both scar tissue and tumor enhance, this is a nonspecific finding. *C*, The CT scan does not match the soft tissue contrast of MR imaging, which also has the advantage of direct sagittal imaging. Dense postoperative scar tissue is present dorsal to L5-S1 *(arrows)*. (*A* and *B* Reprinted with permission from Stimac GK, et al: Gadolinium-DPTA–enhanced imaging of spinal neoplasms. AJR 151:1185–1192, 1988. © American Roentgen Ray Society.)

FIGURE 15–23 ■ *A,* Gadolinium imaging of myeloma. An unenhanced T1-weighted spin-echo image of the lumbosacral spine in a patient with extensive myeloma, particularly involving L4. There is marked heterogeneity of the marrow from diffuse tumor infiltration. Acutely angulated collapse of the upper end plate of L4 (arrow) indicates a pathologic compression fracture. *B,* A moderately T2-weighted (TR, 2000; TE, 60; 0.15T) spin-echo image detects mild heterogeneity and higher signal in L4 but is of lower contrast and could be considered normal except for the pathologic compression fracture of L4, which is well seen. *C,* STIR image (TR, 1400; TE, 36; TI, 100) indicates almost complete involvement of L4 with patchy hyperintense foci in other vertebral bodies. *D,* T1 spin-echo image (TR, 600; TE, 22) after injection of gadopentetate dimeglumine. The contrast enhancement of the tumor results in a normal appearance of the marrow. If this examination was done without unenhanced T1 SE or STIR, the marrow tumor would be missed. (*D* Reprinted with permission from Stimac GK, et al: Gadolinium-DPTA–enhanced imaging of spinal neoplasms. AJNR 151:1185–1192, 1988. © American Roentgen Ray Society.)

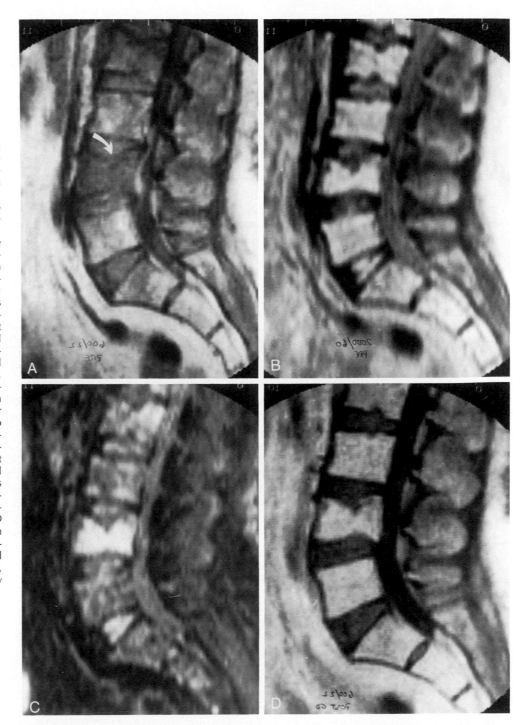

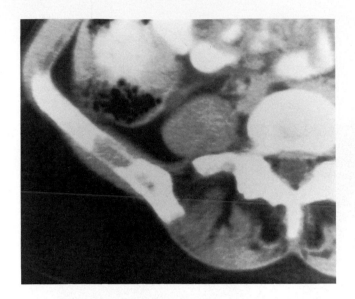

FIGURE 15–24 ■ Pelvic CT scan done for abdominal or pelvic adenopathy in a 54-year-old woman with breast carcinoma. The scan detected a discrete lytic lesion in the right iliac crest, which was asymptomatic but typical for metastatic breast carcinoma.

marrow metastatic disease as it becomes more rapid and as highly sensitive sequences like STIR become more prevalent.

Marrow Infiltration by Primary Bone Neoplasms ■ Clinical staging, treatment, and determination of prognosis in primary bone malignancies are affected by knowledge of the intramedullary and soft tissue extent of the tumor. Magnetic resonance is rapidly becoming the preferred method for imaging primary bone tumors, and one of its greatest contributions is in determination of the extent of infiltration within the medullary cavity.[1, 14, 92–97] The high contrast of MR allows not only delineation of the extent of contiguous intra- and extramedullary spread of tumor (Fig. 15–25), but also accurate detection of skip metastases (Fig. 15–26) from tumors such as osteogenic sarcoma or Ewing's sarcoma.[93, 98] The extreme clinical importance of detecting the limits of tumor extension, as well as metastatic skip lesions, warrants the use of MR for optimal evaluation. The fat suppression capability of STIR, together with the additive T1 and T2 contrast, is capable of detecting even microscopic marrow invasion. In Figure 15–25, gross examination of the pathologic specimen did not reveal any visible subcortical tumor extension. However, serial biopsies of the areas of high signal intensity on the preoperative STIR image confirmed the presence of subcortical microscopic tumor invasion. The penetration of the cortical bone, as well as the extent of extraosseous soft tissue mass, was also readily identified by MR.

Peritumoral soft tissue and marrow edema can extend a substantial distance from the margins of a tumor and to adjacent muscles.[99] This may result in overestimation of tumor volume (Fig. 15–27). However, it is very unlikely that tumor infiltration extends beyond the outer limits of STIR signal abnormality.

Detection of invasion of neural or vascular structures and soft tissue compartments in the extremities requires axial imaging and is very well done by MR.[95] If the lesion contrast is sufficient on T1 spin-echo images, the delineation of anatomy is superior with these sequences. If the lesion contrast is low, however, matching T1 spin-echo and STIR images will provide both the high anatomic resolution necessary, as well as the high soft tissue contrast for delineation of tumor margins. Primary tumors of bone are the subject of another chapter in this book and will not be covered in further detail here.

Benign Marrow Disorders Causing Tumorlike MR Appearance

An intrinsic feature of magnetic resonance imaging, whether in the bone marrow or elsewhere, is high sensitivity but limited specificity. This must be remembered whenever abnormal marrow signal intensity is identified.[131] Diffuse marrow hyperproliferation resulting from benign disease (as in sickle cell anemia,[68] polycythemia,[17, 143] hemolytic anemias, and thalassemia[17]) may be indistinguishable on MR from extensive marrow tumor (Fig. 15–28). Heterogeneous marrow signal in the distal femurs is frequently seen in young females and athletes (Fig. 15–29) and should not be confused with neoplastic conditions.[67]

Diffusely low signal in the bone marrow simulating tumor may be seen with Gaucher's disease[65, 73, 100, 101] and other lipid storage diseases as a result of intracellular deposition of long T1 materials within the reticuloendothelial cells of the bone marrow. In Gaucher's disease (Fig. 15–30), the low signal on T1 SE (and low signal on T2 SE as well)[73] results from the pathologic intracellular deposition of kerasin. Gaucher's disease involves the entire marrow space, with expansion of the distal femurs causing the characteristic Erlenmeyer flask configuration, which can be recognized on coronal MR images. Marrow infarction is rather common in Gaucher's disease and may be superimposed on the abnormal background signal of the involved marrow. Interpretive difficulty will be encountered in these patients when other

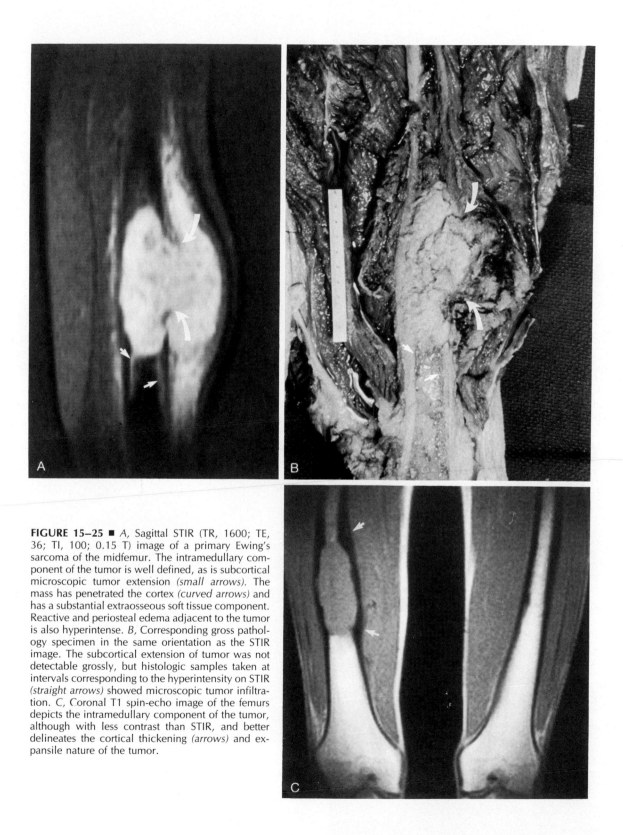

FIGURE 15–25 ■ *A,* Sagittal STIR (TR, 1600; TE, 36; TI, 100; 0.15 T) image of a primary Ewing's sarcoma of the midfemur. The intramedullary component of the tumor is well defined, as is subcortical microscopic tumor extension *(small arrows)*. The mass has penetrated the cortex *(curved arrows)* and has a substantial extraosseous soft tissue component. Reactive and periosteal edema adjacent to the tumor is also hyperintense. *B,* Corresponding gross pathology specimen in the same orientation as the STIR image. The subcortical extension of tumor was not detectable grossly, but histologic samples taken at intervals corresponding to the hyperintensity on STIR *(straight arrows)* showed microscopic tumor infiltration. *C,* Coronal T1 spin-echo image of the femurs depicts the intramedullary component of the tumor, although with less contrast than STIR, and better delineates the cortical thickening *(arrows)* and expansile nature of the tumor.

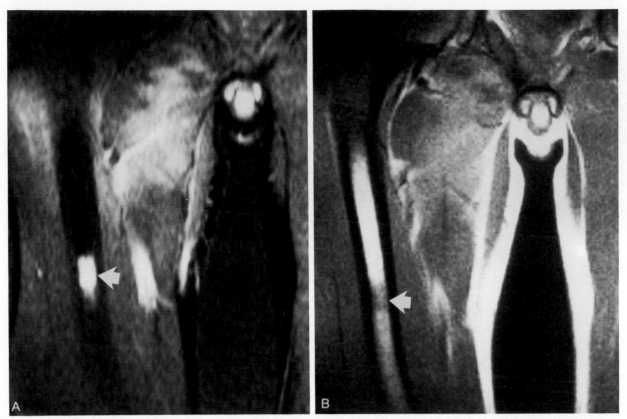

FIGURE 15–26 ■ *A,* Metastases from Ewing's sarcoma. A focal area of hyperintensity in the right midfemur is identified. Hyperintensity from prior radiation therapy to the more proximal tumor is seen in the adductor muscles. *B,* The corresponding T1 spin-echo image shows substantially lower contrast than the STIR image. Bone scan was positive in this area.

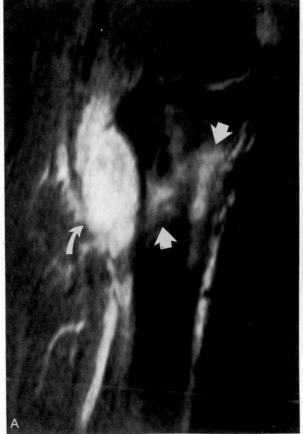

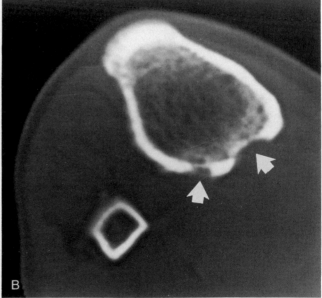

FIGURE 15–27 ■ *A,* Sagittal STIR image of metastatic melanoma to the soft tissues dorsal to the tibia *(curved arrow).* Reactive marrow edema is shown as hyperintensity in the proximal tibia *(straight arrows). B,* CT scan at the level of the soft tissue mass in *A* detects superficial cortical erosion *(arrows)* without gross penetration into the marrow space. The trabecular bone is not disrupted.

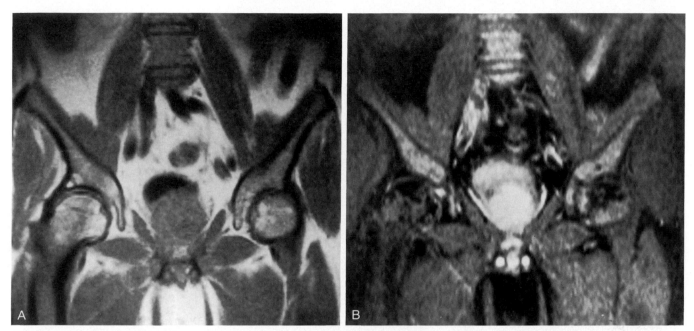

FIGURE 15–28 ■ Benign marrow hypercellularity. *A*, Coronal T1 spin-echo image of the pelvis in a 57-year-old male with polycythemia rubra vera reveals diffusely low signal intensity throughout the visualized marrow. The linear decrease in signal intensity in the capital femoral epiphyses is a result of the increased density of weight-bearing trabecular bone in this area. *B*, Corresponding STIR image detects mild diffuse hypercellularity of the red marrow areas, particularly those of the lumbosacral spine and pelvis. Signal intensity is not as bright as that seen with malignancies such as leukemia, diffuse metastatic disease, or lymphoma, but it cannot be reliably determined from this study alone.

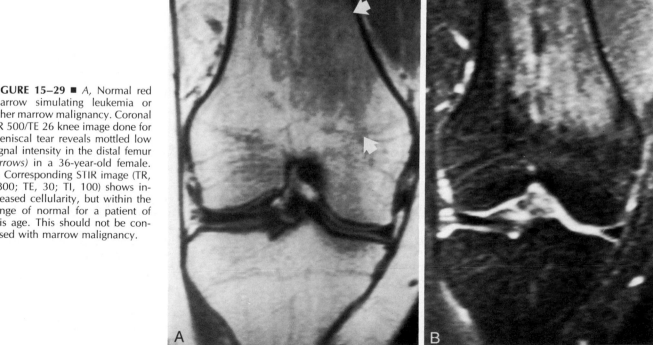

FIGURE 15–29 ■ *A,* Normal red marrow simulating leukemia or other marrow malignancy. Coronal TR 500/TE 26 knee image done for meniscal tear reveals mottled low signal intensity in the distal femur *(arrows)* in a 36-year-old female. *B,* Corresponding STIR image (TR, 1800; TE, 30; TI, 100) shows increased cellularity, but within the range of normal for a patient of this age. This should not be confused with marrow malignancy.

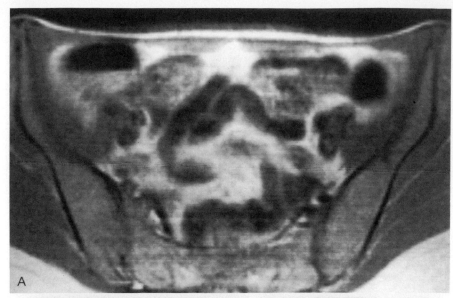

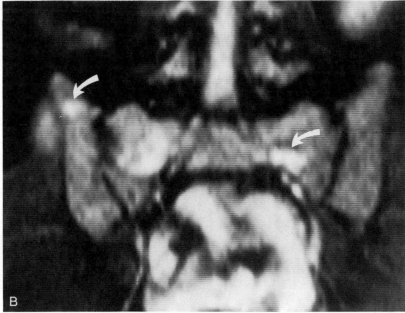

FIGURE 15–30 ■ *A,* MR appearance of Gaucher's disease. In Gaucher's disease, as with other replacement disorders, marrow fat is replaced by longer T1 infiltrative material and is diffusely and homogeneously darker than normal on this transverse T1 spin-echo image of the pelvis. *B,* Marrow abnormalities appeared diffuse and homogeneous on T1 SE, but on STIR, focal areas of further increased signal *(arrows)* were also detected. At subsequent posterior crest biopsy, 70% Gaucher's cells were present, but no tumor cells were seen. The nature of these focal areas of hyperintensity remains unclear.

disorders are also present, as demonstrated in Figure 15–30, which shows images from a patient with both Gaucher's and lymphoma. Focal areas of marrow STIR hyperintensity may be caused by tumor, infarction, or infection and require clinical correlation and possibly guided biopsy confirmation.

The histiocytoses, disorders caused by proliferative changes in the reticuloendothelial cells of the marrow, include eosinophilic granuloma, Hand-Schüller-Christian disease, and Letterer-Siwe disease. These disorders occur in children or young adults, and the diagnosis has usually been established before the patient is studied by MR. However, when diffuse marrow abnormality is identified on MR, histiocytosis should be considered in the differential diagnosis.

Osteochondritis and osteonecrosis are commonly associated with trauma or steroid therapy or may be idiopathic.[79a, 102, 103, 105, 116] Osteonecrosis is usually first

suspected and detected in the femoral heads (Fig. 15–31), although the shoulders, knees, and ankles may also be affected. MR is currently the most sensitive method for making this diagnosis,[22, 102, 104, 106] and the MR appearance may be quite complex,[107–110, 139, 140] depending on whether necrotic bone, marrow edema, or cellular debris is present. Careful attention to the MR patterns can affect and hopefully improve therapy. CT[149] and plain films add diagnostic specificity. Marrow edema is an early finding[39] and often has a background of abnormally fatty marrow.[103] Marrow edema and joint effusions are almost invariably detectable by MR when symptoms are present.

Transient edema of the femoral head not caused by osteonecrosis has been described both in the orthopedic and MR literature[111, 112] and can be differentiated from osteonecrosis by clinical and imaging

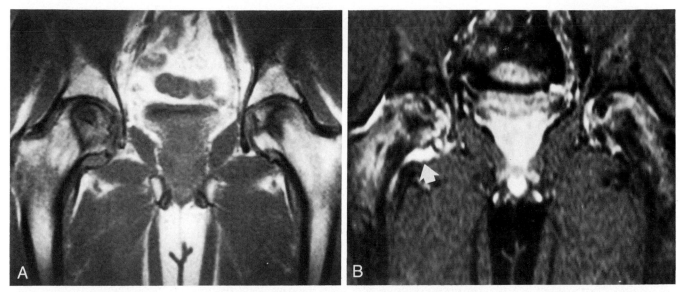

FIGURE 15–31 ■ *A,* Idiopathic bilateral avascular necrosis (osteonecrosis) of the femurs. Complex areas of variable signal intensity in the femoral heads on this T1-weighted spin-echo sequence (TR, 500; TE, 22; 0.15 T) image are characteristic of this disorder. *B,* Corresponding STIR image indicates diffuse mild marrow edema throughout the femoral head, neck, and proximal shaft, as well as areas of necrotic bone (indicated by low signal intensity on both T1 spin-echo and STIR images) and areas of persistent marrow fat. The moderate-sized right hip effusion *(arrow)* is better seen on STIR than T1 spin-echo images.

information. These patients have hip pain, and the femur demonstrates abnormally low signal intensity on T1 spin-echo images and high signal intensity on T2 spin-echo (or STIR) images, as well as increased (rather than decreased) radionuclide uptake on bone scans. The absence of predisposing factors and the abnormally high uptake on bone scan are differential diagnostic features that help distinguish this entity from osteonecrosis.

Marrow infarction typically occurs in the diaphyseal portions of the long bones (Fig. 15–32). In the early stages, marrow infarcts are associated with reactive marrow edema, which is well depicted on

STIR or heavily T2-weighted sequences. In later stages, characteristic serpiginous areas of low signal intensity are seen within the diametaphyseal portions of the femurs. Differentiation of marrow infarction and osteomyelitis can be difficult, as superinfection of marrow infarcts occurs fairly often, particularly in patients with sickle cell disease[68] or Gaucher's disease.[73] These entities may be very difficult to differentiate by CT, MR, and plain radiography, although clinical features and history may clarify the diagnosis.

Aplastic anemia[20, 113] appears on MR as either rather normal or diffuse, very fatty marrow (high signal on T1 SE), with patchy islands of hematopoietic material

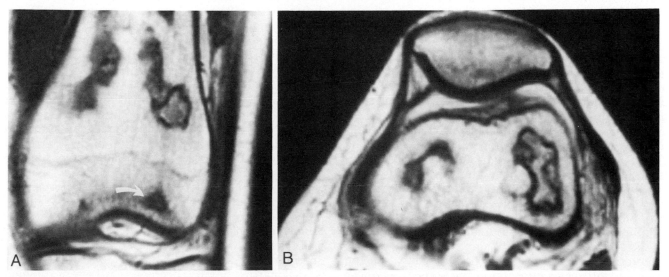

FIGURE 15–32 ■ Marrow infarcts in a patient on steroids. Characteristic serpiginous areas of well-demarcated signal abnormality in the distal long bone are well seen on coronal *(A)* and axial *(B)* views. Epiphyseal lesions *(curved arrow)* may also be seen and are probably an indication of impending osteochondritis dissecans or avascular necrosis. (Courtesy of Christopher Eckel, MD; Reno, NV.)

against a background of high-signal fatty marrow, primarily in the vertebral column. Aplastic anemia may be very difficult to discriminate visually from normal marrow by MR. Chemical shift imaging methods may improve the diagnosis and monitoring of these patients.[60]

Marrow Edema

With increasing experience with MR, it has become clear that the bone marrow is very reactive to a variety of insults to both the marrow and cortical or trabecular bone. These changes are reflected by increased marrow water (edema), which can be readily detected by MR, particularly with sequences that suppress signal from marrow fat.[39] This is a sensitive but nonspecific finding. STIR, T1 SE, heavily T2-weighted SE, or gradient-echo images all detect edema associated with stress fractures.[114, 115] On T1 SE images, both edema and compressed bone are dark (Fig. 15–33A), but the more T2-weighted sequences are very helpful and complementary for confirmation of the acuteness of the lesion. Subchondral marrow edema in knees after trauma (see Fig. 15–33B,C) is very sensitively detected by the more T2- and water-sensitive sequences. Detection of subchondral marrow changes may prove to be one of the more clinically unique and important observations on MR knee imaging done for internal derangement. Reflex sympathetic dystrophy[1] is another cause of marrow signal abnormality caused by edema and, unlike most benign disorders, may also involve the epiphysis of long bones.

Infection

MR is becoming the preferred method for evaluation of suspected spinal osteomyelitis,[37, 117, 145, 146, 148] as well as osteomyelitis occurring elsewhere.[118, 119] Typical spinal MR findings involve the vertebral body, adjacent end plates, and disks, as expected from observations with other imaging modalities. Low signal intensity on T1 SE and high signal on T2 SE or STIR images (Fig. 15–34A,B) are seen, as is extension to adjacent soft tissues; focal abscesses have intensely high signal on STIR, which may also improve detection of epidural infections.[37] MR contrast agents are very valuable for improved detection of epidural infection.

Occult osteomyelitis in oncology patients may simulate spinal tumor on MR (see Fig. 15–34C,D). The clinical features in these immunosuppressed patients, many of whom have chronically indwelling venous catheters, are often atypical for infection; a high level of suspicion is necessary, or the infection may not be recognized. Diminished capability for inflammation and abscess formation may result in an atypical appearance. High signal intensity in the intervertebral disk and adjacent end plates are the cardinal features of infection of the spine, regardless of the presence or absence of a focal soft tissue mass.

CT[120] or plain films may add important diagnostic specificity in this clinical setting. Pyogenic infections are characterized by soft tissue involvement, gas, diffuse osteolysis, and an intervertebral disk origin.[120] Tumors are more likely to arise posteriorly, have less adjacent soft tissue mass, and be osteoblastic.

Paget's disease of the bone is typically seen in the fifth or sixth decade of life and involves the skull or flat bones primarily. A characteristic radiographic feature is marked cortical thickening. Osteolytic as well as reparative and quiescent phases are best characterized by radiographic modalities, although marrow and periosteal changes may be striking on MR (Fig. 15–35). Quiescent, old disease is of low signal on all MR sequences. Characteristic V-shaped margination of the anterior edge of the bone involvement in long bones is seen radiographically; whether the MR-visible counterpart can be defined within the marrow is uncertain, although probable. Detection of sarcomatous degeneration of Paget's disease may require serial studies, as with conventional methods to detect focal enlargement and aggressive behavior. The propensity of Paget's disease to involve vertebral bodies should be remembered when isolated vertebral abnormalities are detected in patients of the appropriate age imaged for spinal metastatic disease.

Vertebral hemangiomas[121, 122] have rather pathognomonic findings on MR. These common, benign, focal marrow hamartomas are the exception to the rule that most marrow lesions are characterized by long T1 (dark on T1 spin-echo images) and long T2. Hemangiomas (Fig. 15–36A) are moderate to very high in intensity on both T1- and T2-weighted images (see Fig. 15–36B). The increased signal on T1 spin-echo images results from a T1 that is relatively shorter than normal marrow. A study with chemical shift imaging[122] indicates that the high signal in vertebral hemangiomas is caused by adipose tissue rather than blood products. In our experience, vertebral hemangiomas are variably dark on STIR, which agrees with these observations. CT findings are coarse trabeculation with relative vertebral body lucency.[121] The most common site of occurrence is the thoracic spine.

As would be expected, bone islands are readily detected with MR and are dark on all sequences. Focal areas of fatty marrow within the central vertebral bodies[123] are also frequently seen in the spine of older individuals but are not as intense on T1 SE images as are hemangiomas. These focal deposits tend to occur near the basivertebral veins and are different from the fatty conversion of the marrow in vertebral end plates adjacent to old, stable degenerative disk disease (see Fig. 15–16A,B).[135] Neither should be confused with pathologic processes. Successfully fused vertebral bodies also undergo diffuse fatty transformation when the mechanical stress is removed from the vertebra;[123] this MR finding can be used as an indicator of the success or failure of intervertebral fusions. Diffuse fatty conversion of spinal marrow has also been reported after prolonged bed rest,[124] which appears to support the hypothesis

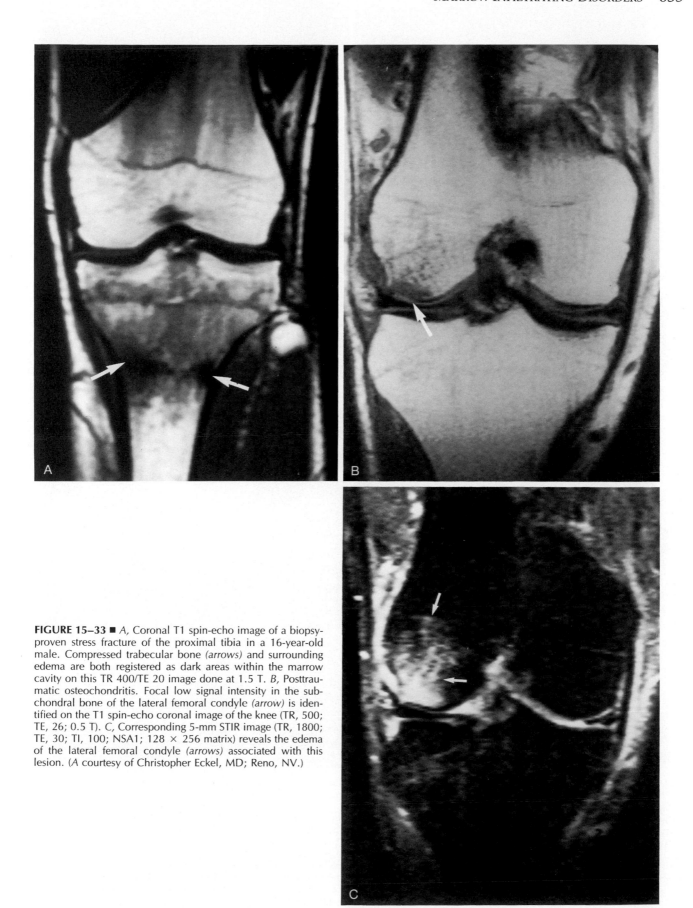

FIGURE 15–33 ■ *A,* Coronal T1 spin-echo image of a biopsy-proven stress fracture of the proximal tibia in a 16-year-old male. Compressed trabecular bone *(arrows)* and surrounding edema are both registered as dark areas within the marrow cavity on this TR 400/TE 20 image done at 1.5 T. *B,* Posttraumatic osteochondritis. Focal low signal intensity in the subchondral bone of the lateral femoral condyle *(arrow)* is identified on the T1 spin-echo coronal image of the knee (TR, 500; TE, 26; 0.5 T). *C,* Corresponding 5-mm STIR image (TR, 1800; TE, 30; TI, 100; NSA1; 128 × 256 matrix) reveals the edema of the lateral femoral condyle *(arrows)* associated with this lesion. *(A* courtesy of Christopher Eckel, MD; Reno, NV.)

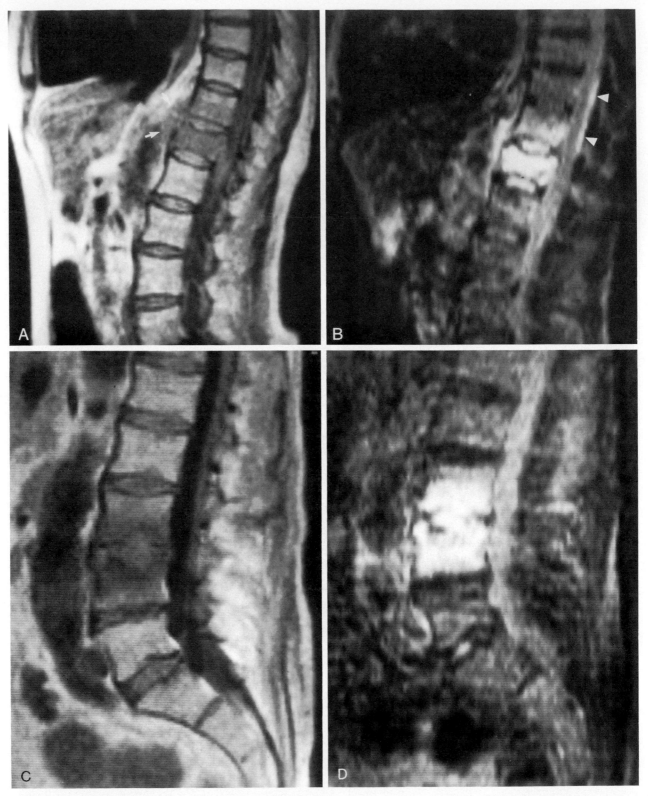

FIGURE 15–34 ■ *A*, Spinal osteomyelitis. Sagittal T1 spin-echo image of the lumbosacral spine indicates abnormal contour and signal intensity of T12 and T11 and of the intervertebral disk. There is a typical associated soft tissue mass anteriorly *(arrow)*, and compression of the conus medullaris has occurred. The appearance somewhat simulates metastatic disease. *B*, The higher contrast of the water-sensitive STIR sequence better reveals the anterior paraspinous abscess, as well as a linear area of high signal intensity dorsal to the thecal sac *(arrowheads)*. An epidural abscess was confirmed in this region by CT metrizamide myelography and surgery. *C*, Occult spinal osteomyelitis in an oncology patient with back pain. Abnormal signal intensity centered on the L3-4 intervertebral disk is a clue to the fact that this is osteomyelitis, not a tumor. Additionally, no other lesions were seen elsewhere. Notice that there is no paraspinous soft tissue mass or edema in this patient. *D*, Corresponding STIR image shows the focal hyperintensity of the intervertebral disk and adjacent vertebral bodies; this finding is typical for infection and very unusual for tumor. Biopsy revealed *Staphylococcus aureus* osteomyelitis arising from an indwelling venous catheter. (*A* and *B* Reprinted with permission from Bertino RE, Porter BA, Stimac GK, Tepper SJ: Imaging spinal osteomyelitis and epidural abscess with short TI inversion recovery (STIR). AJNR 9:563–564, 1988, © American Society of Neuroradiology.)

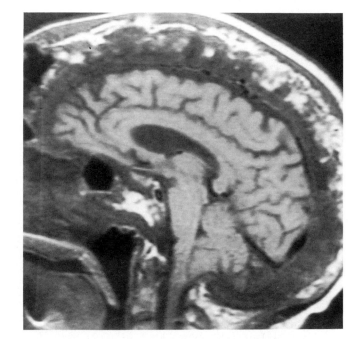

FIGURE 15–35 ■ Paget's disease of the skull. Marked thickening of the calvarium together with coarse trabecular bone and increased medullary fat are seen on this coronal T1 spin-echo image of the brain done at 1.5 T in a 65-year-old female. The marked thickening of cortex is a characteristic feature. (Courtesy of Christopher Eckel, MD, Reno, NV.)

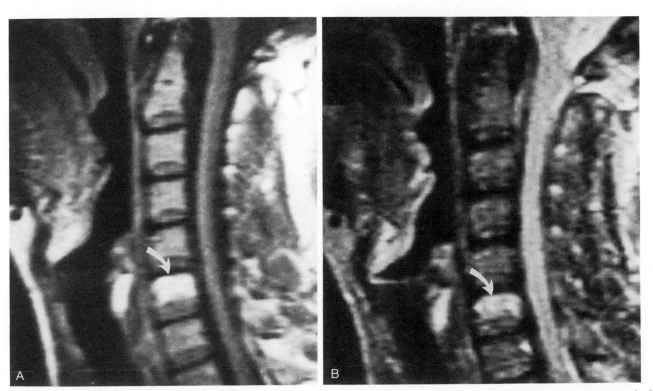

FIGURE 15–36 ■ *A,* Vertebral hemangioma. The high signal intensity in the body of C6 (*arrow*) on a TR 550/TE 26 sequence is typical of a benign vertebral hemangioma. *B,* On a corresponding T2 spin-echo (TR, 2000; TE, 80; 0.5 T) and STIR sequence, the behavior of the material within the vertebral body (*arrow*) was partially that of fat.

that hematopoietic activity in marrow is stimulated by mechanical stress.

A great variety of congenital, acquired, and metabolic abnormalities of the bones and marrow and benign bone lesions[1, 14, 17, 125–130, 131, 141, 144, 147, 152] can mimic tumors on MR and are beyond the scope of this chapter. When unexpected or unusual marrow lesions are detected by MR, the next logical diagnostic step, after a complete clinical history, is plain film radiography, which is unsurpassed for diagnostic specificity in a great variety of bone diseases. Additional experience with MR will certainly improve the differential diagnosis of the diverse entities that occur within the marrow. The MR findings of both benign and malignant marrow disorders can often be rather well predicted, based on the known plain film or CT manifestations of the individual disorder.

References

1. Vogler JB, Murphy WA: Bone marrow imaging. Radiology 168:679–693, 1988.
2. Thrall JH, Ellis BI: Skeletal metastases. Radiol Clin North Am 25:1155–1170, 1987.
3. Richardson ML, Kilcoyne RF, Gillespy T, et al: Magnetic resonance imaging of musculoskeletal neoplasms. Radiol Clin North Am 24:259–267, 1986.
4. Edelstyn GA, Gillespie PJ, Grebbel FS: The radiological demonstration of osseous metastases: experimental observations. Clin Radiol 18:185–162, 1967.
5. McNeil BJ: Rationale for the use of bone scans in selected metastatic and primary bone tumors. Semin Nucl Med 8:336–345, 1978.
6. McNeil BJ: Value of bone scanning in neoplastic disease. Semin Nucl Med 14:277–286, 1984.
7. Harbin WP: Metastatic disease and the non-specific bone scan: value of spinal computed tomography. Radiology 145:105–107, 1982.
8. Nelp WB, Larson SM, Lewis RJ: Distribution of the erythron and the RES in the bone marrow organ. J Nucl Med 8:430–436, 1967.
9. Weaver GR, Sandler MR: Increased sensitivity of magnetic resonance imaging compared to radionuclide bone scintigraphy in the detection of lymphoma of the spine. Clin Nucl Med 12:333–334, 1987.
10. Ludwig H, Tscholakoff D, Neuhold A, et al: Magnetic resonance imaging of the spine in multiple myeloma. Lancet 15:364–366, 1987.
11. Muindi J, Coombes RC, Golding S, et al: The role of computed tomography in the detection of bone metastases in breast cancer patients. Br J Radiol 56:233–236, 1983.
12. O'Rourke T, George CB, Redmond J, et al: Spinal computed tomography and computed tomography metrizamide myelography in the early diagnosis of metastatic disease. J Clin Oncol 4(4):576–583, 1986.
13. Durning P, Best JJ, Sellwood RA: Recognition of metastatic bone disease in cancer of the breast by computed tomography. Clin Oncol 9(4):343–346, 1983.
14. Hudson TM, Hamlin DJ, Enneking WF, et al: Magnetic resonance imaging of bone and soft tissue tumors: early experience in 31 patients compared with computed tomography. Skeletal Radiol 13:134–146, 1985.
15. Redmond J, Spring DB, Munderloh SH: Spinal computed tomography scanning in the evaluation of metastatic disease. Cancer 54:253–258, 1984.
16. Coffre C, Vanel D, Contesso G, et al: Problems and pitfalls in the use of computed tomography for the local evaluation of long bone osteosarcoma: report on 30 cases. Skeletal Radiol 13:147–153, 1985.
17. Porter BA, Shields AF, Olson DO: Magnetic resonance imaging of bone marrow disorders. Radiol Clin North Am 24(2):269–289, 1986.
18. Porter BA: MR may become routine for imaging bone marrow. Diagn Imaging 9:104–108, 1987.
19. Shields AF, Porter BA, Churchley S, et al: The detection of bone marrow involvement by lymphoma using magnetic resonance imaging. J Clin Oncol 5:225–230, 1987.
20. Olson DO, Shields AF, Scheurich CJ, et al: Magnetic resonance imaging of the bone marrow in patients with leukemia, aplastic anemia, and lymphoma. Invest Radiol 21:540–546, 1986.
21. Colman LK, Porter BA, Redmond J, et al: Early diagnosis of spinal metastases by CT and MR studies. J Comput Assist Tomogr 12(3):423–426, 1988.
22. Moon KL, Genant JH, Helms CA, et al: Musculoskeletal applications of nuclear magnetic resonance. Radiology 147:161–171, 1983.
23. Ehman RL, Berquist TH, McLeod RA: MR imaging of the musculoskeletal system: a 5-year appraisal. Radiology 166:313–320, 1988.
24. Sartoris DJ, Resnick D: MR imaging of the musculoskeletal system: current and future status. AJR 149:457–467, 1987.
25. Cristy M: Active bone marrow distribution as a function of age in humans. Phys Med Biol 26:389–400, 1981.
26. Bydder GM, Young IR: MR imaging: clinical use of inversion recovery sequence. J Comput Assist Tomogr 9(4):659–675, 1985.
27. Bydder GM, Pennock M, Steiner RE, et al: The short TI inversion recovery sequence—an approach to MR imaging of the abdomen. Magn Reson Imaging 3:251–254, 1985.
28. Bydder GM, Steiner RE, Blumgart LH, et al: MR imaging of the liver using short TI inversion recovery sequences. J Comput Assist Tomogr 9:1084, 1985.
29. Steiner RE: Magnetic resonance imaging: its impact on diagnostic radiology. AJR 145:883–893, 1985.
30. Droege RT, Wiener SN, Rzeszotarski MS, et al: Nuclear magnetic resonance: a gray scale model for head images. Radiology 148:763–771, 1983.
31. Droege RT, Wiener SN, Rzeszotarski MS, et al: A strategy for magnetic resonance imaging of the head: results of a semi-empirical model. Part 1. Radiology 153:419, 1984.
32. Droege RT, Wiener SN, Rzeszotarski MS, et al: A strategy for magnetic resonance imaging of the head: results of a semi-empirical model. Part 2. Radiology 153:424, 1984.
33. Rapoport S, Sostman HD, Pope C, et al: Venous clots, evaluation with MR imaging. Radiology 162:527–530, 1987.
34. Moran PR, Kumar NG, Karstaedt N, et al: Tissue contrast enhancement: image reconstruction algorithm and selection of TI in inversion recovery MRI. Magn Reson Imaging 4:229–235, 1986.
35. Stimac GK, Porter BA, Olson DO, et al: Gadolinium-DTPA-enhanced MR imaging of spinal neoplasms: preliminary investigation and comparison with unenhanced spin-echo and STIR sequences. AJNR 9:839–846, 1988.
36. Nyberg DA, Porter BA, Olds MO, et al: MR imaging of hemorrhagic adnexal masses. J Comput Assist Tomogr 11(4):664–669, 1987.
37. Bertino RE, Porter BA, Stimac GK, et al: Imaging spinal osteomyelitis and epidural abscess with short TI inversion recovery (STIR). AJNR 9:563–564, 1988.
38. Porter BA: Low field, STIR advance MRI in clinical oncology. Diagn Imaging 10(11):222–230, 1988.
39. Porter BA, Schwartz A, Olson DO: Low-field STIR imaging of avascular necrosis, marrow edema, and infarction. Radiology 165(P):83, 1987.
40. Porter BA, Olson DO, Stimac G, et al: Low-field STIR imaging of marrow malignancies. Radiology 165(P):275, 1987.
41. Dubinsky T, Porter BA, Olson DO: Short TI inversion recovery MR imaging of chest wall malignancies. Radiology 165(P):197, 1987.
42. Porter BA, Redmond J, Dunning DM, et al: Low-field STIR imaging of spinal malignancies. Radiology 169(P):65, 1988.
43. Porter BA, Borrow JW: Low-field STIR imaging of lymphoma: clinical experience with 92 cases. Radiology 169(P):175, 1988.

44. Zimmer WD, Berquist TH, McLeod RA, et al: Bone tumors: magnetic resonance imaging versus computed tomography. Radiology 155:709–718, 1985.

45. Pettersson H, Gillespy T, Hamlin DJ, et al: Primary musculoskeletal tumors: examination with MR imaging compared with conventional modalities. Radiology 164:237–241, 1987.

46. Kricun ME: Red-yellow marrow conversion: its effect on the location of some solitary bone lesions. Skeletal Radiol 14:10–19, 1985.

47. Dooms GC, Fisher MR, Hricak H, et al: Bone marrow imaging: magnetic resonance studies related to age and sex. Radiology 155:429–432, 1985.

48. Sugimura K, Yamasaki K, Kitagaki H, et al: Bone marrow diseases of the spine: differentiation with T1 and T2 relaxation times in MR imaging. Radiology 165:541–544, 1987.

49. Hyman RA, Gorey MT: Imaging strategies for MR of the spine. Radiol Clin North Am 26:505–533, 1988.

50. Richardson ML: Optimizing pulse sequences for magnetic resonance imaging of the musculoskeletal system. Radiol Clin North Am 24:137–144, 1986.

51. Hendrick RE, Nelson TR, Hendee WR: Optimizing tissue contrast in magnetic resonance imaging. Magn Reson Imaging 2:193–204, 1984.

52. Porter BA, Hastrup W, Richardson ML, et al: Classification and investigation of artifacts in magnetic resonance imaging. RadioGraphics 7(2):271–287, 1987.

53. Wood ML, Runge VM, Henkelman RM: Overcoming motion in abdominal MR imaging. AJR 150:513–522, 1988.

54. Enzmann DR, Rubin JB: Cervical spine: MR imaging with a partial flip angle, gradient-refocused pulse sequence. Radiology 166:467–472, 1988.

55. Winkler ML, Ortendahl DA, Mills TC, et al: Characteristics of partial flip-angle and gradient reversal MR imaging. Radiology 166:17–26, 1988.

56. Mills TC, Ortendahl DA, Hylton NM, et al: Partial flip-angle MR imaging. Radiology 162:531–539, 1987.

57. Dixon WT: Simple proton spectroscopic imaging. Radiology 153:189–194, 1984.

58. Sepponen RE, Sipponen JT, Tanttu JI: A method for chemical shift imaging: demonstration of bone marrow involvement with proton chemical shift imaging. J Comput Assist Tomogr 8:585–587, 1984.

59. Wismer GL, Rosen BR, Buxton R, et al: Chemical shift imaging of bone marrow: preliminary experience. AJR 145:1031–1037, 1985.

60. McKinstry CS, Steiner RE, Young AT, et al: Bone marrow in leukemia and aplastic anemia: MR imaging before, during and after treatment. Radiology 162:701–707, 1987.

61. Rosen BR, Fleming DM, Kushner DC, et al: Hematologic bone marrow disorders: quantitative chemical shift MR imaging. Radiology 169:799–804, 1988.

62. Helms CA, Cann CE, Brunelle FO, et al: Detection of bone marrow metastases using quantitative computed tomography. Radiology 140:745–750, 1981.

63. Mink JH: Percutaneous bone biopsy in the patient with known or suspected osseous metastases. Radiology 161:191–194, 1986.

64. Mink JH, Weitz I, Kagan AR, et al: Bone scan-positive and radiograph- and CT-negative vertebral lesion in a woman with locally advanced breast cancer. AJR 148:341–343, 1987.

65. Rosenthal DI, Mayo-Smith W, Goodsitt MM, et al: Bone and bone marrow changes in Gaucher disease: evaluation with quantitative CT. Radiology 170:143–146, 1989.

66. Pagani JJ, Libshitz HI: Imaging bone metastases. Radiol Clin North Am 20(3):545–560, 1982.

67. Deutsch AL, Mink JH, Rosenfelt FP, et al: Incidental detection of hematopoietic hyperplasia on routine knee MR imaging. AJR 152:333–336, 1989.

68. Rao VM, Fishman M, Mitchell DG, et al: Painful sickle cell crisis: bone marrow patterns observed with MR imaging. Radiology 161:211–215, 1986.

69. Moore SG, Gooding CA, Brasch RC, et al: Bone marrow in children with acute lymphocytic leukemia: MR relaxation times. Radiology 160:237–240, 1986.

70. Cohen MD, Klatte EC, Baehner R, et al: Magnetic resonance imaging of bone marrow disease in children. Radiology 151:715–718, 1984.

71. Nidecker AC, Muller S, Aue WP, et al: Extremity bone tumors: evaluation by P-31 MR spectroscopy. Radiology 157:167–174, 1985.

72. Thompson JA, Shields AF, Porter BA, et al: Magnetic resonance imaging of bone marrow in hairy cell leukemia: correlation with clinical response to alpha-interferon. Leukemia 1:315–316, 1987.

73. Lanir A, Hadar H, Cohen I, et al: Gaucher disease: assessment with MR imaging. Radiology 161:239–244, 1986.

74. Rossleigh MA, Lovegrove FTA, Reynolds PM, et al: Serial bone scans in the assessment of response to therapy in advanced breast cancer. Clin Nucl Med 7:397–402, 1982.

75. Smith J, Bragg DG: Tumors of the skeletal system. In Bragg DC, et al, ed: Oncologic Imaging. Elmsford, NY, Pergamon Press, 1985, pp 501–529.

76. Sarpel S, Sarpel G, Yu E, et al: Early diagnosis of spinal-epidural metastasis by magnetic resonance imaging. Cancer 59:1112–1116, 1987.

77. Orzel JA, Sawaf NW, Richardson ML: Lymphoma of the skeleton: scintigraphic evaluation. AJR 150:1095–1099, 1988.

78. Dubinsky TJ, Porter BA, Olson DO: Short TI inversion-recovery MR imaging of chest wall malignancies. Radiology 165(P):197, 1987.

79. Mikhael MA, Paige NL: Hodgkin's disease of spine: computed tomography and magnetic resonance imaging. J Comput Tomogr 11:174–177, 1987.

79a. Mould JJ, Adam NM: The problem of avascular necrosis of bone in patients treated for Hodgkin's disease. Clin Radiol 34:231–236, 1983.

80. Pieters R, van Brenk AI, Veerman AJP, et al: Bone marrow magnetic resonance studies in childhood leukemia: evaluation of osteonecrosis. Cancer 60:2994–3000, 1987.

81. Kamby C, Vejborg I, Daugaard S, et al: Clinical and radiologic characteristics of bone metastases in breast cancer. Cancer 60:2524–2531, 1987.

82. Aoki J, Yamamoto I, Hino M, et al: Sclerotic bone metastasis: radiologic-pathologic correlation. Radiology 159:127–132, 1986.

83. Sartoris DJ, Clopton P, Nemcek A, et al: Vertebral-body collapse in focal and diffuse disease: patterns of pathologic processes. Radiology 160:479–483, 1986.

84. Brasch RC, Wesbey GE, Gooding CA, et al: Magnetic resonance imaging of transfusional hemosiderosis complicating thalassemia major. Radiology 150:767–771, 1984.

85. Ramsey RG, Zacharias CE: MRI imaging of the spine after radiation therapy: easily recognizable effects. AJR 144:1131–1135, 1985.

86. Porter BA, Olson DO, Stimac G, et al: STIR imaging of spinal malignancies. Radiology 169(P):65, 1988.

87. Dooms G, Maldague B, Malghem J, et al: MR differential diagnosis between benign and malignant vertebral collapses. Radiology 169(P):65, 1988.

88. Sze G, Abramson A, Krol G, et al: Gadolinium-DTPA in the evaluation of intradural extramedullary spinal disease. AJR 150:911–921, 1988.

89. de Santos LA, Goldstein HM, Murray JA, et al: Computed tomography in the evaluation of musculoskeletal neoplasms. Radiology 128:89–94, 1978.

90. Levine E, Lee KR, Neff JR, et al: Comparison of computed tomography and other imaging modalities in the evaluation of musculoskeletal tumors. Radiology 131:431–437, 1979.

91. Genant HK, Wilson JS, Bovill EG, et al: Computed tomography of the musculoskeletal system. J Bone Joint Surg 62A:1088–1101, 1980.

92. Boyko OB, Cory DA, Cohen MD, et al: MR imaging of osteogenic and Ewing's sarcoma. AJR 148:317–322, 1987.

93. Vanel D, Couanet D, Leclere J, et al: Early detection of bone metastases of Ewing's sarcoma by magnetic resonance imaging. Diagn Imaging Clin Med 55:381–383, 1986.

94. Bloem JL, Taminiau AHM, Eulderink F, et al: Radiologic staging of primary bone sarcoma: MR imaging, scintigraphy, angiography, and CT correlation with pathologic examination. Radiology 169:805–810, 1988.

95. Bloem JL, Falke THM, Taminiau AHM, et al: Magnetic resonance imaging of primary malignant bone tumors. RadioGraphics 5(6):853–886, 1985.

96. Bloem JL, Bluemm RG, Taminiau AHM, et al: Magnetic resonance imaging of primary malignant bone tumors. RadioGraphics 7(3):425–445, 1987.

97. Levin DN, Herrmann A, Spraggins T, et al: Musculoskeletal tumors: improved depiction with linear combinations of MR images. Radiology 163:545–549, 1980.

98. Zimmer WD, Berquist TH, McLeod RA, et al: Magnetic resonance imaging of osteosarcomas: comparison with computed tomography. Clin Orthop 208:289–299, 1986.

99. Beltran J, Simon DC, Katz W, et al: Increased MR signal intensity in skeletal muscle adjacent to malignant tumors: pathologic correlation and clinical significance. Radiology 162:251–255, 1987.

100. Hermann G, Wagner LD, Gendal ES, et al: Spinal cord compression in type I Gaucher disease. Radiology 170:147–148, 1989.

101. Rosenthal DI, Scott JA, Barranger J, et al: Evaluation of Gaucher disease using magnetic resonance imaging. J Bone Joint Surg 68A:802–808, 1986.

102. Mitchell DG, Kressel HY: MR imaging of early avascular necrosis. Radiology 169:281–282, 1988.

103. Mitchell DG, Rao VM, Dalinka M, et al: Hematopoietic and fatty bone marrow distribution in the normal and ischemic hip: new observations with 1.5T MR imaging. Radiology 161:199–202, 1986.

104. Glickstein MF, Burk DL, Scheibler ML, et al: Avascular necrosis versus other diseases of the hip: sensitivity of MR imaging. Radiology 169:213–215, 1988.

105. Thickman D, Axel L, Kressel HY, et al: Magnetic resonance imaging of avascular necrosis of the femoral head. Skeletal Radiol 15:133–140, 1986.

106. Totty WG, Murphy WA, Ganz WI, et al: Magnetic resonance imaging of the normal and ischemic femoral head. AJR 143:1273–1280, 1984.

107. Mitchell DG, Joseph PM, Fallon M, et al: Chemical-shift MR imaging of the femoral head: an in vitro study of normal hips and hips with avascular necrosis. AJR 148:1159–1164, 1987.

108. Lang P, Jergesen HE, Moseley ME, et al: Avascular necrosis of the femoral head: high-field-strength MR imaging with histologic correlation. Radiology 169:517–524, 1988.

109. Mitchell MD, Kundel HL, Steinberg ME, et al: Avascular necrosis of the hip: comparison of MR, CT, and scintigraphy. AJR 147:67–71, 1986.

110. Markisz JA, Knowles JR, Altchek DW, et al: Segmental patterns of avascular necrosis of the femoral heads: early detection with MR imaging. Radiology 162:717–720, 1987.

111. Wilson AJ, Murphy WA, Hardy DC, et al: Transient osteoporosis: transient bone marrow edema? Radiology 167:757–760, 1988.

112. Bloem JL: Transient osteoporosis of the hip: MR imaging. Radiology 167:753–755, 1988.

113. Kaplan PA, Asleson RJ, Klassen LW, et al: Bone marrow patterns in aplastic anemia: observations with 1.5T MR imaging. Radiology 164:441–444, 1987.

114. Stafford SA, Rosenthal DI, Gebhardt MC, et al: MRI in stress fracture. AJR 147:553–556, 1986.

115. Lee JK, Yao L: Stress fractures: MR imaging. Radiology 169:217–220, 1988.

116. Stoller DW, Genant HK, Helms CA, et al: Magnetic Resonance Imaging in Orthopaedics and Rheumatology. Philadelphia, JB Lippincott, 1989, pp 167–172.

117. Modic MT, Feiglin DH, Piraino DW, et al: Vertebral osteomyelitis: assessment using MR. Radiology 157:157–166, 1985.

118. Unger E, Moldofsky P, Gatenby R, et al: Diagnosis of osteomyelitis by MR imaging. AJR 150:605–610, 1988.

119. Beltran J, Noto AM, McGhee RB, et al: Infections of the musculoskeletal system: high-field-strength MR imaging. Radiology 164:449–454, 1987.

120. Van Lom KJ, Kellerhouse LE, Pathria MN, et al: Infection versus tumor in the spine: criteria for distinction with CT. Radiology 166:851–855, 1988.

121. Laredo JD, Reizine D, Bard M, et al: Vertebral hemangiomas: radiologic evaluation. Radiology 161:183–189, 1986.

122. Ross JS, Masaryk TJ, Modic MT, et al: Vertebral hemangiomas: MR imaging. Radiology 165:165–169, 1987.

123. Hajek PC, Baker LL, Goobar JE, et al: Focal fat deposition in axial bone marrow: MR characteristics. Radiology 162:245–249, 1987.

124. LeBlanc AD, Schonfeld E, Schneider VS, et al: The spine: changes in T2 relaxation times from disuse. Radiology 169:105–107, 1988.

125. Rao VM, Dalinka MK, Mitchell DG, et al: Osteopetrosis: MR characteristics at 1.5T. Radiology 161:217–220, 1986.

126. Lee JK, Yao L, Wirth CR: MR imaging of solitary osteochondromas: report of eight cases. AJR 149:557–560, 1987.

126a. Beltran J, Simon DC, Levy M, et al: Aneurysmal bone cysts: MR imaging at 1.5T. Radiology 158:689–690, 1986.

127. Dahlin DC, McLeod RA: Aneurysmal bone cyst and other non-neoplastic conditions. Skeletal Radiol 8:243–250, 1982.

128. Sundaram M, Awwad EE: Magnetic resonance imaging of arachnoid cysts destroying the sacrum. AJR 146:359–360, 1986.

129. Porter BA, Olson DO, Shields AF, et al: Differential diagnosis of marrow lesions on MR imaging. Proceedings: Society of Magnetic Resonance in Medicine, 5th Annual Meeting, August 1986, pp 1180–1181.

130. Porter BA, Olson DO, Shields AF, et al: Differential diagnosis of marrow lesions on MR imaging. Radiology 161(P):24, 1986.

131. Bohndorf K, Reiser M, Lochner B, et al: Magnetic resonance imaging of primary tumours and tumour-like lesions of bone. Skeletal Radiol 15:511–517, 1986.

132. Brown KT, Kattapuram SV, Rosenthal DL: Computed tomography analysis of bone tumors: patterns of cortical destruction and soft tissue extension. Skeletal Radiol 15:448–451, 1986.

133. Coleman RE, Rubens RD, Fogelman I: Reappraisal of the baseline bone scan in breast cancer. J Nucl Med 29:1045–1049, 1988.

134. Coleman RE, Mashiter G, Whitaker KB, et al: Bone scan flare predicts successful systemic therapy for bone metastases. J Nucl Med 29:1354–1359, 1988.

135. de Roos A, Kressel H, Spritzer C, et al: MR imaging of marrow changes adjacent to end-plates in degenerative lumbar disk disease. AJR 149:531–534, 1987.

136. Drace J, Baker LL, Chang P, et al: Preliminary results of MR imaging of lymphoma: distinguishing active tumor from benign residue. Radiology 165(P):201, 1987.

137. Engel IA, Straus DJ, Lacher M, et al: Osteonecrosis in patients with malignant lymphoma. Cancer 48:1245–1250, 1981.

138. Frager DH, Goldman MJ, Seimon LP, et al: Computed tomography guidance for skeletal biopsy. Skeletal Radiol 16:644–646, 1987.

139. Genez BM, Wilson MR, Houk RW, et al: Early osteonecrosis of the femoral head: detection in high-risk patients with MR imaging. Radiology 168:521–524, 1988.

140. Gillespy T, Genant KH, Helms CA: Magnetic resonance imaging of osteonecrosis. Radiol Clin North Am 24:193–208, 1986.

141. Glass RBJ, Poznanski AK, Fisher MR, et al: MR imaging of osteoid osteoma. J Comput Assist Tomogr 10:1065–1067, 1986.

142. Ginsberg HN, Swayne LC: Three-phase bone scanning in chronic myelogeneous leukemia. Clin Nucl Med 12:823–824, 1987.

143. Jensen KE, Grube T, Thomsen C, et al: Prolonged bone marrow T1 relaxation in patients with polycythemia vera. Magn Reson Imaging 6:291–295, 1988.

144. Mahboubi S: CT appearance of nidus in osteoid osteoma. J Comput Assist Tomogr 10:457–459, 1986.

145. Modic MT, Masaryk T, Paushter D: Magnetic resonance imaging of the spine. Radiol Clin North Am 24(2):229–245, 1986.

146. Modic MT, Pflanze W, Feiglin DHI, et al: Magnetic resonance imaging of musculoskeletal infections. Radiol Clin North Am 24(2):247–258, 1986.

147. Modic MT, Steinberg PM, Ross JS, et al: Degenerative disc disease: assessment of changes in vertebral body marrow with MR imaging. Radiology 166:193–199, 1988.
148. Quinn SF, Murray W, Clark RA, et al: MR imaging of chronic osteomyelitis. J Comput Assist Tomogr 12:113–117, 1988.
149. Rafii M, Firooznia H, Golimbu C, et al: Radiation induced fractures of sacrum: CT diagnosis. J Comput Assist Tomogr 12:231–235, 1988.
150. Vasquez TE, Frey C, Walker LN, et al: False-negative bone image with radiographically evident osteoblastic lesions in prostatic carcinoma. Clin Nucl Med 11:817–818, 1986.
151. Vanel D, Lacombe M, Couanet D, et al: Musculoskeletal tumors: follow-up with MR imaging after treatment with surgery and radiation therapy. Radiology 164:243–245, 1987.
152. Hudson TM, Hamlin DJ, Fitzsimmons JR: Magnetic resonance imaging of fluid levels in an aneurysmal bone cyst and in anticoagulated human blood. Skeletal Radiol 13:267–270, 1985.

INDEX

Note: Page numbers in *italics* indicate figures; those followed by *t* indicate tables.